Respiratory Care Calculations

FOURTH EDITION

David W. Chang, EdD, RRT-NPS

Professor
Department of Cardiorespiratory Care
University of South Alabama
Mobile, Alabama, U.S.A.

In loving memory of my mother Tsung-yuin Chang
(1916–2016)

Contents

Section 3

Ventilator Waveform **277**

Section 4

Basic Statistics and Educational Calculations **299**

Section 5

Answer Key to Self-Assessment Questions **321**

Section 6

Symbols and Abbreviations **331**

Section 7

Appendices **337**

Listing by Subject Areas

REVIEW

TEMPERATURE CONVERSIONS

VENTILATION

Introduction

The purpose of this book is to provide respiratory therapists, nurses, and other healthcare professionals a concise source of information for respiratory care calculations. It is suitable for use in the classroom, laboratory, and clinical settings.

Respiratory care equations are some of the most useful tools available. Not only do the equations provide answers to clinical questions, they help practitioners learn the variables in an equation and how the variables may be altered to achieve better clinical outcomes. When an equation is calculated correctly, the data can be interpreted in a meaningful way. The patients benefit from the accurate answer and appropriate application of data.

Why I wrote this text

Over 24 years ago, Dr. Donald F. Egan wrote in the 1st edition Foreword about the pioneering days of inhalation therapy, "In that early phase of development, most therapists had a fearful opinion of mathematics, but fortunately arithmetic skills had little relevance to the work of most therapists — a far cry from today's needs." Dr. Egan's comment written in 1994 remains accurate today. It is my sincere trust that healthcare professionals will continue to excel in the calculation and application of clinical data.

New to the fourth edition

- Full color design for the entire book.
- Hard copy and eBook formats.
- Step-by-step method for easy calculation and accurate answer.
- Over 800 self-assessment questions to reinforce correct calculation and retainment of knowledge.
- Self-assessment questions follow the examination format of the National Board for Respiratory Care (NBRC).
- New chapters on intravenous fluid infusion rate by drips, IV flow, or body weight.
- Notes and discussions for each topic provide relevant information for clinical practice.

Organization

The organization of this book makes its contents easy-to-navigate. **Section 1:** Review of Basic Math Function. This refresher of mathematical skills ensures correct manipulation of numbers and variables in an equation.

Respiratory care calculations are presented alphabetically in **Section 2**, which allows the reader to locate specific calculations easily. The same search function is available in the index.

Section 3: Ventilator Waveform has 26 different illustrations covering waveforms from volume-time to flow-volume waveforms. **Section 4:** Basic Statistics and Educational Calculations should be useful for educators. **Section 5** lists the answers to self-assessment questions. **Section 6** provides the Symbols and Abbreviations commonly used in respiratory care. Concluding this book are appendices in **Section 7** that covers clinical topics ranging from Barometric Pressures at Selected Altitudes to Pressure Conversions.

Features

Each calculation is presented with the equation followed by normal values, examples, and exercises. Bibliography is provided at the end of this book for further study. Supplemental information and clinical notes appear in the margin to provide additional explanation or clarification of the equation. Self-Assessment Questions, in NBRC format, can be found at the end of each calculation to enhance and reinforce learning and retention. Answers for these questions are listed in Section 5 of the book. With its comprehensive coverage of respiratory care calculations and extensive additional learning resources readers will find this book useful in preparing for their clinical practice and credentialing examinations.

About the author

David W. Chang, EdD, RRT-NPS, is professor of cardiorespiratory care at the University of South Alabama in Mobile, Alabama. Over the years, he has served in different capacities in the American Association for Respiratory Care, Commission on Accreditation for Respiratory Care, and National Board for Respiratory Care. Dr. Chang has also authored Clinical Application of Mechanical Ventilation. He may be reached at **dchang@southalabama.edu**.

Acknowledgments

I would like to recognize my colleagues for their time and efforts in reviewing the manuscript during different stages of its development. They provided factual corrections and thoughtful comments and suggestions. This 4th edition would not be in its current form without their expert assistance. My deepest appreciation goes to:

Lisa A. Conry, MA, RRT
Director of Clinical Education
Spartanburg Community College
Spartanburg, South Carolina

Tammy A. Miller, MEd, RRT
Program Chair
Southern Regional Technical College
Thomasville, Georgia

William V. Wojciechowski, MS, RRT
Professor Emeritus
University of South Alabama
Mobile, Alabama

Publishing a textbook involves many tedious steps, from conception of the contents to copyediting and typesetting of the book. I am extremely grateful for the superb job of layout, typesetting, and cover design created by:

Zoltán Sárkány
Tîrgu Mureș, Romania

Review of Basic Math Functions

Review of Basic Math Functions

1. Add numbers with decimals.
   Note: Line up the decimals properly.

   EXAMPLE 43.45 + 10.311 + 0.25 = 54.011

   $$\begin{array}{r} 43.45 \\ 10.311 \\ +0.25 \\ \hline 54.011 \end{array}$$

2. Subtract numbers with decimals.
   Note: Line up the decimals properly.

   EXAMPLE 198.24 − 40.015 = 158.225

   $$\begin{array}{r} 198.24 \\ -40.015 \\ \hline 158.225 \end{array}$$

3. Multiply numbers with decimals.
   Note: Count the total number of digits after the decimals in the numbers and place the decimal in the answer accordingly.

   EXAMPLE 50.6 × 0.002 = 0.1012 can be treated as

   $$\begin{array}{r} 506 \\ \times \quad 2 \\ \hline 1,012 \end{array}$$

   There are a total of 4 digits (1 in 50.6 and 3 in 0.002) after the decimals in the numbers. The decimal in the product 1,012 comes after the 2 (1,012.0); moving it 4 places to the left gives an answer of 0.1012.

4. Divide numbers with decimals.

   Terminology: $\dfrac{\text{Dividend}}{\text{Divisor}} = \text{Answer}$

   Step 1. Count and compare the number of digits after the decimal in the dividend and after the decimal in the divisor.

   Step 2. Move the decimal points for both dividend and divisor to the right so that they become whole numbers. Remember to move decimals the same number of places to the right in both the dividend and divisor.

   EXAMPLE $\dfrac{0.68}{3.4}$ can be changed to $\dfrac{68}{340} = 0.2$

   Move the decimal points two places to the right for both the dividend and the divisor (0.68 is changed to 68 and 3.4 is changed to 340).

EXAMPLE $\dfrac{2.4}{0.006}$ can be changed to $\dfrac{2,400}{6} = 400$

Move the decimal points three places to the right for the dividend and the divisor (2.4 is changed to 2,400 and 0.006 is changed to 6).

5. Add/subtract and multiply/divide
   Note: Perform multiplication/division **before** addition/subtraction.

EXAMPLE 1
$$12 \times 6 - 2 = (12 \times 6) - 2$$
$$= 72 - 2$$
$$= 70$$

EXAMPLE 2
$$116 - \frac{455}{5} = 116 - \left(\frac{455}{5}\right)$$
$$= 116 - 91$$
$$= 25$$

6. Parantheses
   Note: Perform calculation within parentheses in the order ( ), [ ], and { }.

EXAMPLE 1
$$12 \times (6 - 2) = 12 \times 4$$
$$= 48$$

EXAMPLE 2
$$194 - \{[20 \times (9 - 5)] + 14\} = 194 - \{[20 \times 4] + 14\}$$
$$= 194 - \{80 + 14\}$$
$$= 194 - 94$$
$$= 100$$

7. Ratio
   Note: A ratio compares two related quantities or measurements. It is usually expressed in the form 1:2, as in *I:E* ratio.

EXAMPLE 1 *I:E* ratio of 1:2 means that the expiratory phase (*E*) is two times as long as the inspiratory phase (*I*). A ratio is dimensionless: it does not include units such as seconds or inches. An *I:E* ratio of 1:2 may mean that the inspiratory time (*I* time) is 1 second and expiratory time (*E* time) is 2 seconds *or* the *I* time is 2 seconds and the *E* time is 4 seconds.

EXAMPLE 2 Inverse *I:E* ratio of 2:1 means that the inspiratory phase is two times as long as the expiratory phase.

EXAMPLE 3 Oxygen: air entrainment ratio of 1:4 means that 1 part of oxygen is combined with 4 parts of air.

8. Percentage
   Note: Percentage expresses a value in parts of 100. It is written in the form 65% or 0.65, as in F_IO_2.

   EXAMPLE 1   An intrapulmonary shunt of 15% means that 15 of 100 units of perfusion do not take part in gas exchange.

   EXAMPLE 2   An arterial oxygen content of 21 vol% means that 21 of 100 units of arterial blood are saturated with oxygen.

9. Relationships of X and Y in equation $A = \dfrac{X^*}{Y}$

   [When A is constant, X and Y are directly related]

   EXAMPLE 1 $\text{Resistance} = \dfrac{\text{Pressure change } (\Delta P)}{\text{Flow}}$

   When airway resistance is constant, an **increase** in driving pressure generates a **higher** flow. Likewise, a **decrease** in driving pressure yields a **lower** flow.

   EXAMPLE 2 $\text{Compliance} = \dfrac{\text{Volume change } (\Delta V)}{\text{Pressure change } (\Delta P)}$

   When compliance is constant, an **increase** in pressure generates a **higher** lung volume. By the same token, a **decrease** in pressure **lowers** the lung volume.

10. Relationships of A and X in equation $A = \dfrac{X}{Y}$

    [When Y is constant, A and X are directly related]

    EXAMPLE 1 $\text{Resistance} = \dfrac{\text{Pressure change } (\Delta P)}{\text{Flow}}$

    In order to maintain a constant flow, an **increase** in driving pressure is needed to overcome a **higher** resistance. If the resistance is **low**, **less** pressure is needed to maintain a constant flow.

    EXAMPLE 2 $\text{Compliance} = \dfrac{\text{Volume change } (\Delta V)}{\text{Pressure change } (\Delta P)}$

    When a constant peak inspiratory pressure is used on a pressure-controlled ventilator, the volume delivered is **increased** in the presence of **high** compliance. On the other hand, the volume delivered by a pressure-controlled ventilator is **decreased** with **low** compliance.

---

* $A = \dfrac{X}{Y}$ *can be rewritten as* $X = AY$ *or* $Y = \dfrac{X}{A}$. *When any two of three values are known, the third can be calculated.*

11. Relationships of A and Y in equation $A = \dfrac{X}{Y}$

[When X is constant, A and Y are inversely related]

EXAMPLE 1

$$\text{Resistance} = \frac{\text{Pressure change } (\Delta P)}{\text{Flow}}$$

In the presence of **increasing** airway resistance, air flow to the lungs is **decreased** if the pressure (work of breathing or ventilator work) remains constant. On the other hand, with **decreasing** airway resistance, air flow to the lungs is **increased** at constant pressure (work of breathing or ventilator work).

EXAMPLE 2

$$\text{Compliance} = \frac{\text{Volume change } (\Delta V)}{\text{Pressure change } (\Delta P)}$$

During volume-controlled ventilation, the peak inspiratory pressure of the ventilator **increases** in the presence of **decreasing** compliance. As the compliance **improves (increases)**, the inspiratory pressure **decreases**.

12. Relationships of A, B and X, Y in equation $\dfrac{A}{B} = \dfrac{X}{Y}$ [same as $AY = BX$]

[A or Y is directly related to B or X. A and Y are inversely related to each other]
[B or X is directly related to A or Y. B and X are inversely related to each other]

Respiratory Care Calculations

1

Airway Resistance: Estimated (R_{aw})

EQUATION

$$R_{aw} = \frac{(PIP - P_{PLAT})^*}{Flow}$$

R_{aw} : Airway resistance in cm H_2O/L/sec
PIP : Peak inspiratory pressure in cm H_2O
P_{PLAT} : Plateau pressure in cm H_2O (static pressure)
Flow : Flow rate in L/sec

NORMAL VALUE

0.6 to 2.4 cm H_2O/L/sec at flow rate of 0.5 L/sec (30 L/min). If the patient is intubated, use serial measurements to establish trend.

EXAMPLE

Calculate the estimated airway resistance of a patient where peak inspiratory pressure is 25 cm H_2O and plateau pressure is 10 cm H_2O. The ventilator flow rate is set at 60 L/min (1 L/sec).

$$R_{aw} = \frac{(PIP - P_{PLAT})}{Flow}$$

$$= \frac{25 - 10}{1}$$

$$= 25 - 10$$

$$= 15 \text{ cm } H_2O/L/sec$$

EXERCISE

Given: Peak inspiratory pressure = 45 cm H_2O
Plateau pressure = 35 cm H_2O
Inspiratory flow = 50 L/min (0.83 L/sec)

Calculate the estimated airway resistance.

[Answer: R_{aw} = 12 cm H_2O/L/sec]

NOTES

This equation estimates the airflow resistance in the airway. ($PIP - P_{PLAT}$) represents the pressure gradient in the presence of flow. In ventilators with constant flow patterns, the inspiratory flow rate can be used in this equation. Otherwise, a pneumotachometer may be needed to measure the inspiratory flow rate at PIP. Flow rates in L/min should first be changed to L/sec by dividing L/min by 60. For example:

$$40 \text{ L/min} = \frac{40 \text{ (L/min)}}{60}$$

$$= 0.67 \text{ L/sec}$$

Some conditions leading to an increase in airway resistance include bronchospasm, retained secretions, and use of a small endotracheal or tracheostomy tube. These increases in airway resistance can be minimized by using bronchodilators for bronchospasm, frequent suctioning for retained secretions, and the largest appropriate endotracheal or tracheostomy tube.

In nonintubated subjects, a body plethysmography must be used to measure and calculate the airway resistance by $R_{aw} = \frac{(P_{ao} - P_{alv})}{Flow}$, where P_{ao} is the pressure at the airway opening and P_{alv} is the alveolar pressure.

SELF-ASSESSMENT QUESTIONS

1a. During volume-controlled ventilation, the (PIP – P_{PLAT}) gradient is directly related to the:

A. airflow resistance
B. frequency
C. F_IO_2
D. lung compliance

1b. Calculate the estimated airway resistance (R_{aw} est) of a patient whose peak inspiratory pressure is 60 cm H_2O and plateau pressure is 40 cm H_2O. The ventilator constant flow rate is set at 60 L/min (1 L/sec).

A. 10 cm H_2O/L/sec
B. 20 cm H_2O/L/sec
C. 50 cm H_2O/L/sec
D. 100 cm H_2O/L/sec

1c. Given: PIP = 60 cm H_2O, P_{PLAT} = 40 cm H_2O, PEEP = 10 cm H_2O. Calculate the estimated R_{aw} if the constant flow rate is 50 L/min (0.83 L/sec).

A. 20 cm H_2O/L/sec
B. 24 cm H_2O/L/sec
C. 28 cm H_2O/L/sec
D. 32 cm H_2O/L/sec

1d. A patient's airway pressures are as follows: peak inspiratory pressure = 45 cm H_2O, plateau pressure = 15 cm H_2O. The ventilator constant flow rate is set at 60 L/min (1 L/sec). Calculate the estimated airway resistance.

A. 15 cm H_2O/L/sec
B. 20 cm H_2O/L/sec
C. 30 cm H_2O/L/sec
D. 60 cm H_2O/L/sec

1e. Given: PIP = 60 cm H_2O, P_{PLAT} = 30 cm H_2O, PEEP = 5 cm H_2O. Calculate the estimated R_{aw} if the constant flow rate is 50 L/min (0.83 L/sec).

A. 10 cm H_2O/L/sec
B. 20 cm H_2O/L/sec
C. 30 cm H_2O/L/sec
D. 36 cm H_2O/L/sec

>> Go to **rtexam.com** for more learning resources

Alveolar-Arterial O$_2$ Tension Gradient: $P(A-a)O_2$

EQUATION

$$P(A-a)O_2 = P_AO_2 - P_aO_2$$

$P(A-a)O_2$: Alveolar-arterial oxygen tension gradient in mm Hg

P_AO_2 : Alveolar-arterial oxygen tension in mm Hg

P_aO_2 : Arterial oxygen tension in mm Hg

NORMAL VALUE

(1) On *room air*, the $P(A-a)O_2$ should be less than 4 mm Hg for every 10 years in age. For example, the $P(A-a)O_2$ should be less than 24 mm Hg for a 60-year-old patient.

(2) On *100% oxygen*, every 50 mm Hg difference in $P(A-a)O_2$ approximates 2% shunt.

EXAMPLE 1

Given: P_AO_2 = 100 mm Hg
$\quad\quad\quad\quad P_aO_2$ = 85 mm Hg
$\quad\quad\quad\quad F_IO_2$ = 21%
$\quad\quad$ Patient age = 40 years

Calculate $P(A-a)O_2$. Is it abnormal for this patient?

$$
\begin{aligned}
P(A-a)O_2 &= P_AO_2 - P_aO_2 \\
&= (100 - 85)\ \text{mm Hg} \\
&= 15\ \text{mm Hg}
\end{aligned}
$$

$P(A-a)O_2$ of 15 mm Hg is normal for a 40-year-old patient.

EXAMPLE 2

Given: P_AO_2 = 660 mm Hg
$\quad\quad\quad\quad P_aO_2$ = 360 mm Hg
$\quad\quad\quad\quad F_IO_2$ = 100%

Calculate $P(A-a)O_2$. What is the estimated physiologic shunt in percent?

$$
\begin{aligned}
P(A-a)O_2 &= P_AO_2 - P_aO_2 \\
&= (660 - 360)\ \text{mm Hg} \\
&= 300\ \text{mm Hg}
\end{aligned}
$$

NOTES

The value of $P(A-a)O_2$ (also known as $A-a$ gradient) can be used to estimate (1) the degree of hypoxemia and (2) the degree of physiologic shunt. It is derived from a rarely used shunt equation:

$$\frac{Q_S}{Q_T} = \frac{(P_AO_2 - P_aO_2 \times 0.003)}{(C_aO_2 - C_{\bar{v}}O_2) + (P_AO_2 - P_aO_2) \times 0.003}$$

The $P(A-a)O_2$ is increased when hypoxemia results from V/Q mismatch, diffusion defect, or shunt. In the absence of cardiopulmonary disease, it increases with aging.

Since every 50 mm Hg difference in $P(A-a)O_2$ approximates 2% shunt, 300 mm Hg $P(A-a)O_2$ difference is estimated to be 12% shunt:

$$50 \text{ mm Hg} = 2\%$$

$$\frac{50 \text{ mm Hg}}{300 \text{ mm Hg}} = \frac{2\%}{x\%}$$

$$x = \frac{2 \times 300}{50}\%$$

$$x = \frac{600}{50}\%$$

$$= 12\%$$

EXERCISE 1 Given: $P_AO_2 = 93$ mm Hg
$P_aO_2 = 60$ mm Hg
$F_IO_2 = 21\%$
Patient age $= 65$ years

Calculate $P(A-a)O_2$. Is the $P(A-a)O_2$ normal or abnormal based on the patient's age?

[Answer: $P(A-a)O_2$ 33 mm Hg. It is abnormal because 33 mm Hg is more than 26 mm Hg, the allowable difference for patient's age.]

EXERCISE 2 Given: $P_AO_2 = 646$ mm Hg
$P_aO_2 = 397$ mm Hg
$F_IO_2 = 100\%$

Calculate $P(A-a)O_2$ and estimate the percent physiologic shunt.

[Answer: $P(A-a)O_2$ 249 mm Hg. The estimated shunt is 10% because every 50 mm Hg $P(A-a)O_2$ difference represents about 2% shunt:

$$50 \text{ mm Hg} = 2\%$$

$$\frac{50 \text{ mm Hg}}{249 \text{ mm Hg}} = \frac{2\%}{x\%}$$

$$x = \frac{2 \times 249}{50}\%$$

$$x = \frac{498}{50}\%$$

$$= 9.96\% \text{ or } 10\%]$$

SELF-ASSESSMENT QUESTIONS

2a. Given the following values obtained from breathing room air: $P_AO_2 = 105$ mm Hg, $P_aO_2 = 70$ mm Hg. What is the $P(A - a)O_2$? Is it normal for a 70-year-old patient?

    A. 70 mm Hg; normal
    B. 70 mm Hg; abnormal
    C. 35 mm Hg; normal
    D. 35 mm Hg; abnormal

2b. If a patient's P_aO_2 is 70 mm Hg and $P(A - a)O_2$ is 30 mm Hg, what is the calculated P_AO_2?

    A. 30 mm Hg
    B. 40 mm Hg
    C. 70 mm Hg
    D. 100 mm Hg

2c. If a patient's $P(A - a)O_2$ is 50 mm Hg and the calculated P_AO_2 is 240 mm Hg, what is the patient's P_aO_2?

    A. 100 mm Hg
    B. 140 mm Hg
    C. 190 mm Hg
    D. 290 mm Hg

2d. While breathing 100% oxygen, for each 50 mm Hg difference in $P(A - a)O_2$ approximates:

    A. 2% shunt
    B. 4% shunt
    C. 5% shunt
    D. 10% shunt

2e. Given: $P_AO_2 = 638$ mm Hg, $P_aO_2 = 240$ mm Hg, $F_IO_2 = 100\%$. What is the calculated $P(A - a)O_2$ and the estimated physiologic shunt?

    A. 240 mm Hg; 12%
    B. 240 mm Hg; 16%
    C. 398 mm Hg; 16%
    D. 398 mm Hg; 22%

» Go to **rtexam.com** for more learning resources

Alveolar Oxygen Tension (P_AO_2)

NOTES

The P_AO_2 is mainly determined by the F_IO_2 and P_B. Low inspired F_IO_2 and high altitude ($\downarrow P_B$) reduce the calculated P_AO_2. High inspired F_IO_2 and low altitude ($\uparrow P_B$ as in diving below sea level) increase the P_AO_2. P_AO_2 is primarily used for other calculations such as alveolar-arterial oxygen tension gradient ($A - a$ gradient) and arterial/alveolar oxygen tension (a/A) ratio.

The respiratory exchange ratio (1/0.8 or 1.25) is not used when the F_IO_2 is ≥60%.

EQUATION

$$P_AO_2 = (P_B - P_{H_2O}) \times F_IO_2 - (P_aCO_2 \times 1.25)^*$$

P_AO_2 : Alveolar oxygen tension in mm Hg
P_B : Barometric pressure in mm Hg
P_{H_2O} : Water vapor pressure, 47 mm Hg saturated at 37 °C
F_IO_2 : Inspired oxygen concentration in percent
P_aCO_2 : Arterial carbon dioxide tension in mm Hg
1.25 : $\dfrac{1}{0.8}\left(\dfrac{1}{\text{Normal respiratory exchange ratio}}\right)$

*This ratio is omitted when F_IO_2 is ≥60%.

*Modified from

$$P_AO_2 = (P_B - P_{H_2O}) \times F_IO_2 - P_aCO_2 \times \left[F_IO_2 + \frac{1 - F_IO_2}{R} \right],$$

where R is the respiratory exchange ratio, normally 0.8.

NORMAL VALUES

The normal values vary according to the F_IO_2 and P_B.

EXAMPLE

Given:
P_B = 760 mm Hg
P_{H_2O} = 47 mm Hg
F_IO_2 = 40% or 0.4
P_aCO_2 = 30 mm Hg
P_AO_2 = $(P_B - P_{H_2O}) \times F_IO_2 - (P_aCO_2 \times 1.25)^*$
= $(760 - 47) \times 0.4 - (30 \times 1.25)$
= $713 \times 0.4 - 31.5$
= $285.2 - 31.5$
= 247.7 or 248 mm Hg

EXERCISE

Given:
P_B = 750 mm Hg
P_{H_2O} = 47 mm Hg
F_IO_2 = 50% or 0.5
P_aCO_2 = 40 mm Hg

Calculate the P_AO_2.

[Answer: P_AO_2 = 301.5 or 302 mm Hg]

SELF-ASSESSMENT QUESTIONS

3a. Which of the following is the clinical equation to calculate the partial pressure of oxygen in the alveoli?

A. $P_AO_2 = (P_B - P_{H_2O}) \times F_IO_2 - (P_aCO_2 \times 1.25)$
B. $P_AO_2 = (P_B - P_{H_2O}) \times F_IO_2$
C. $P_AO_2 = (P_B \times F_IO_2) - (P_aCO_2 - P_{H_2O})$
D. $P_AO_2 = (P_B \times F_IO_2) - P_{H_2O}$

3b. In the alveolar oxygen tension (P_AO_2) equation, the respiratory exchange ratio is omitted when the F_IO_2 is greater than:

A. 50%
B. 60%
C. 70%
D. 80%

3c. Given: P_B = 760 mm Hg, P_{H_2O} = 47 mm Hg, F_IO_2 = 0.7, P_aCO_2 = 50 mm Hg. The P_AO_2 is about: (Do not use respiratory exchange ratio in equation because F_IO_2 is greater than 60%.)

A. 403 mm Hg
B. 417 mm Hg
C. 428 mm Hg
D. 449 mm Hg

3d. Calculate the alveolar oxygen tension (P_AO_2), given the following values: P_B = 750 mm Hg, P_{H_2O} = 47 mm Hg, F_IO_2 = 30% or 0.3, and P_aCO_2 = 40 mm Hg.

A. 30 mm Hg
B. 100 mm Hg
C. 161 mm Hg
D. 170 mm Hg

3e. Given: P_B = 520 mm Hg (at 10,000 ft altitude), P_{H_2O} = 47 mm Hg, F_IO_2 = 21%, and P_aCO_2 = 40 mm Hg. What is the calculated alveolar oxygen tension (P_AO_2)? What is the P_AO_2 if the person hyperventilates to a P_aCO_2 of 30 mm Hg?

A. 69 mm Hg; 81 mm Hg
B. 100 mm Hg; 110 mm Hg
C. 82 mm Hg; 88 mm Hg
D. 49 mm Hg; 62 mm Hg

>> Go to **rtexam.com** for more learning resources

4

Anion Gap

Anion gap helps to evaluate the overall electrolyte balance between the cations and anions in the extracellular fluid. Potassium is not included in the calculation because it contributes little to the extracellular cation concentration. If potassium is included in the equation, the normal value range would be 15 to 20 mEq/L.

Metabolic acidosis in the presence of a normal anion gap is usually caused by a loss of base. It is known as hyperchloremia metabolic acidosis because this condition is usually related to loss of HCO_3^- and accumulation of chloride ions.

Metabolic acidosis in the presence of an increased anion gap is usually the result of increased fixed acids. These fixed acids may be produced (e.g., renal failure, diabetic ketoacidosis, lactic acidosis), or they may be added to the body (e.g., poisoning by salicylates, methanol, and ethylene glycol).

Fluid and electrolyte therapy is indicated when there is a significant anion gap (>16 mEq/L).

EQUATION

$$\text{Anion gap} = Na^+ - (Cl^- + HCO_3^-)$$

Na^+	:	Serum sodium concentration in mEq/L
Cl^-	:	Serum chloride concentration in mEq/L
HCO_3^-	:	Serum bicarbonate concentration in mEq/L

NORMAL VALUES

10 to 14 mEq/L

15 to 20 mEq/L if potassium (K^+) is included in the equation

EXAMPLE

Given: Na^+ = 140 mEq/L
Cl^- = 105 mEq/L
HCO_3^- = 22 mEq/L

Calculate the anion gap.

$$\begin{aligned}
\text{Anion gap} &= Na^+ - (Cl^- + HCO_3^-) \\
&= 140 - (105 + 22) \\
&= 140 - 127 \\
&= 13 \text{ mEq/L}
\end{aligned}$$

EXERCISE 1

Given: Na^+ = 130 mEq/L
Cl^- = 92 mEq/L
HCO_3^- = 20 mEq/L

What is the calculated anion gap?

[Answer: Anion gap = 18 mEq/L]

EXERCISE 2

A patient with metabolic acidosis has these electrolyte data: Na^+ = 138 mEq/L, Cl^- = 107 mEq/L, HCO_3^- = 18 mEq/L. Is the metabolic acidosis due to loss of base or increase of fixed acid?

What is the calculated anion gap?

[Answer: Anion gap = 13 mEq/L; metabolic acidosis due to loss of base]

SELF-ASSESSMENT QUESTIONS

4a. A physician asks the therapist to evaluate a patient's overall status of electrolyte balance. The therapist should use the following set of electrolyes to calculate the anion gap:

A. Na^+, H^+, Cl^-, HCO_3^-
B. Na^+, K^+, HCO_3^-
C. Na^+, Cl^-, HCO_3^-
D. Na^+, Ca^{++}, Cl^-, HCO_3^-

4b. Given: $Na^+ = 138$ mEq/L, $Cl^- = 102$ mEq/L, $HCO_3^- = 25$ mEq/L. Calculate the anion gap.

A. 36 mEq/L
B. 25 mEq/L
C. 12 mEq/L
D. 11 mEq/L

4c. Given: $Na^+ = 135$ mEq/L, $Cl^- = 96$ mEq/L, $HCO_3^- = 22$ mEq/L. What is the calculated anion gap?

A. 15 mEq/L
B. 17 mEq/L
C. 20 mEq/L
D. 22 mEq/L

4d. Metabolic acidosis with a normal anion gap is typically caused by a:

A. gain of acid
B. gain of base
C. loss of acid
D. loss of base

4e. Metabolic acidosis with an increased anion gap is usually the result of:

A. increased fixed acid
B. increased fixed base
C. decreased fixed acid
D. decreased fixed base

» Go to **rtexam.com** for more learning resources

5

Arterial/Alveolar Oxygen Tension (a/A) Ratio

NOTES

The a/A ratio is an indicator of the efficiency of oxygen transport. A low a/A ratio reflects ventilation/perfusion (V/Q) mismatch, diffusion defect, or shunt.

This ratio is often used to calculate the approximate F_IO_2 needed to obtain a desired P_aO_2.

EQUATION

$$a/A \text{ ratio} = \frac{P_aO_2}{P_AO_2}$$

a/A ratio : Arterial/alveolar oxygen tension ratio in percent
P_aO_2 : Arterial oxygen tension in mm Hg
P_AO_2 : Alveolar oxygen tension in mm Hg

NORMAL VALUE   >60%

EXAMPLE   Calculate the a/A ratio if the $P_aO_2 = 100$ mm Hg and $P_AO_2 = 248$ mm Hg.

$$a/A \text{ ratio} = \frac{P_aO_2}{P_AO_2}$$

$$= \frac{100}{248}$$

$$= 0.403 \text{ or } 40\%$$

EXERCISE 1   Given: $P_AO_2 = 320$ mm Hg
                     $P_aO_2 = 112$ mm Hg

Calculate the a/A ratio.

[Answer: a/A ratio = 0.35 or 35%]

EXERCISE 2   Given: $P_AO_2 = 109$ mm Hg
                     $P_aO_2 = 76$ mm Hg

Calculate the a/A ratio.

[Answer: a/A ratio = 0.70 or 70%]

EXERCISE 3   Given: $P_AO_2 = 540$ mm Hg
                     $P_aO_2 = 105$ mm Hg

Calculate the a/A ratio.

[Answer: a/A ratio = 0.19 or 19%]

SELF-ASSESSMENT QUESTIONS

5a. Calculate the a/A ratio if the $P_aO_2 = 80$ mm Hg and $P_AO_2 = 170$ mm Hg.

    A. 80%
    B. 47%
    C. 34%
    D. 66%

5b. What is the a/A ratio if the $P_aO_2 = 150$ mm Hg and $P_AO_2 = 500$ mm Hg.

    A. 30%
    B. 40%
    C. 50%
    D. 60%

5c. Given: $P_AO_2 = 210$ mm Hg, $P_aO_2 = 45$ mm Hg. Calculate the a/A ratio. Is it normal?

    A. 12%; abnormal
    B. 21%; abnormal
    C. 60%; normal
    D. 74%; normal

5d. The calculated P_AO_2 is 300 mm Hg and the arterial PO_2 is 180 mm Hg. What is the a/A ratio?

    A. 54%; normal
    B. 54%; abnormal
    C. 60%; normal
    D. 60; abnormal

5e. V/Q mismatch and intrapulmonary shunting typically lead to a(n):

    A. increased P_aO_2
    B. increased P_AO_2
    C. increased a/A ratio
    D. decreased a/A ratio

» Go to **rtexam.com** for more learning resources

6

Arterial–Mixed Venous Oxygen Content Difference $[C(a-\bar{v})O_2]$

NOTES

Measurements of arterial mixed venous oxygen content difference $[C(a-\bar{v})O_2]$ are useful in assessing changes in oxygen consumption and cardiac output. Under conditions of normal oxygen consumption and cardiac output, about 25% of the available oxygen is used for tissue metabolism.

Therefore, a $C(a-\bar{v})O_2$ of 5 vol% (CaO_2 20 vol% – $C_{\bar{v}}O_2$ 15 vol%) reflects a balanced relationship between oxygen consumption and cardiac output (**Figure 2-1**).

According to the cardiac output equation (Fick's estimated method)

$$Q_T = \frac{VO_2}{[C(a-\bar{v})O_2]}$$

the arterial-mixed venous oxygen content difference $C(a-\bar{v})O_2$ is directly related to the oxygen consumption (VO_2) and inversely related to the cardiac output (Q_T).

Relationship of $C(a-\bar{v})O_2$ and oxygen consumption

If the cardiac output stays unchanged or is unable to compensate for hypoxia, an increase of oxygen consumption (e.g., increased metabolic rate) will cause an increase in $C(a-\bar{v})O_2$. A decrease of oxygen consumption will cause a decrease in $C(a-\bar{v})O_2$.

EQUATION

$$C(a-\bar{v})O_2 = C_aO_2 - C_{\bar{v}}O_2$$

$C(a-\bar{v})O_2$: Arterial – mixed venous oxygen content difference in vol%

C_aO_2 : Arterial oxygen content in vol%

$C_{\bar{v}}O_2$: Mixed venous oxygen content in vol%

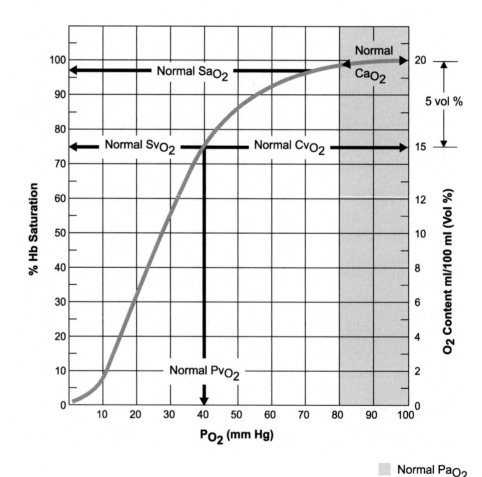

FIGURE 2-1. Oxygen dissociation curve. The normal oxygen content difference between arterial and venous blood is about 5 vol%. Note that both the right side and the left side of the graph illustrate that approximately 25% of the available oxygen is used for tissue metabolism, and the hemoglobin returning to the lungs is normally about 75% saturated with oxygen.

TABLE 2-1. Factors that increase the $C(a-\bar{v})O_2$

Decreased cardiac output
Periods of increased oxygen consumption
    Exercise
    Seizures
    Shivering
    Hyperthermia

TABLE 2-2. Factors that decrease the $C(a-\bar{v})O_2$

Increased cardiac output
Skeletal muscle relaxation (e.g., induced by drugs)
Peripheral shunting (e.g., sepsis, trauma)
Certain poisons (e.g., cyanide prevents cellular metabolism)
Hypothermia

NORMAL VALUES   4 to 5 vol% for healthy or critically ill patients with cardiopulmonary compensation.

EXAMPLE

Given: C_aO_2 = 18.3 vol%
          $C_{\bar{v}}O_2$ = 14.1 vol%
          $C(a-\bar{v})O_2$ = $C_aO_2 - C_{\bar{v}}O_2$
                   = (18.3 – 14.1) vol%
                   = 4.2 vol%

EXERCISE 1

Given: C_aO_2 = 16.2 vol%
          $C_{\bar{v}}O_2$ = 13.1 vol%

Calculate the $C(a-\bar{v})O_2$. What is the interpretation for a critically ill patient?

[Answer: $C(a-\bar{v})O_2$ = 3.1 vol%. The patient has adequate cardiopulmonary compensation.]

EXERCISE 2

Given: C_aO_2 = 16.8 vol%
          $C_{\bar{v}}O_2$ = 10.6 vol%

Calculate the $C(a-\bar{v})O_2$. What is the interpretation for a critically ill patient?

[Answer: $C(a-\bar{v})O_2$ = 6.2 vol%. The patient does not have adequate cardiopulmonary compensation.]

NOTES *(continued)*

Relationship of $C(a-\bar{v})O_2$ and cardiac output

When oxygen consumption remains constant, the $C(a-\bar{v})O_2$ becomes an indicator of the cardiac output. A decrease of $C(a-\bar{v})O_2$ is indicative of an increase of cardiac output, and an increase of $C(a-\bar{v})O_2$ reflects a decrease of cardiac output.

For a summary of factors that change the $C(a-\bar{v})O_2$ values, see **Tables 2-1** and **2-2**.

SELF-ASSESSMENT QUESTIONS

6a. In critically ill patients with adequate cardiopulmonary compensation, the normal range for $C(a-\bar{v})O_2$ is:

A. 5 to 6 vol%
B. 4 to 5 vol%
C. 6 to 7 vol%
D. 5 to 7 vol%

6b. A patient's oxygen content measurements are: $C_aO_2 = 20$ vol%, $C_{\bar{v}}O_2 = 14$ vol%. Calculated the $C(a-\bar{v})O_2$. Is it normal?

A. 5 vol%; yes
B. 6 vol%; no
C. 7 vol%; no
D. 8 vol%; no

6c. Given the following measurements obtained from a critically ill patient: $C_aO_2 = 20.5$ vol%, $C_{\bar{v}}O_2 = 16$ vol%. What is the $C(a-\bar{v})O_2$? What is the interpretation?

A. 3.5 vol%; with adequate cardiopulmonary compensation
B. 3.5 vol%; without adequate cardiopulmonary compensation
C. 4.5 vol%; with adequate cardiopulmonary compensation
D. 4.5 vol%; without adequate cardiopulmonary compensation

6d. A critically ill patient has the following oxygen content measurements: $C_aO_2 = 20$ vol%, $C_{\bar{v}}O_2 = 14$ vol%. What is the arterial-mixed venous oxygen content difference $C(a-\bar{v})O_2$? What is the interpretation?

A. 4 vol%; with adequate cardiopulmonary compensation
B. 4 vol%; without adequate cardiopulmonary compensation
C. 6 vol%; with adequate cardiopulmonary compensation
D. 6 vol%; without adequate cardiopulmonary compensation

6e. The following oxygen content measurements are obtained from a critically ill patient: $C_cO_2 = 21.0$ vol%, $C_aO_2 = 19.3$ vol%, $C_{\bar{v}}O_2 = 14.8$ vol%. What is the calculated arterial-mixed venous oxygen content difference $C(a-\bar{v})O_2$? What is the interpretation?

A. 4 vol%; with adequate cardiopulmonary compensation
B. 4 vol%; without adequate cardiopulmonary compensation
C. 4.5 vol%; with adequate cardiopulmonary compensation
D. 4.5 vol%; without adequate cardiopulmonary compensation

» Go to **rtexam.com** for more learning resources

7

ATPS to BTPS

EQUATION

$Volume_{BTPS} = Volume_{BTPS} \times Factor$

$Volume_{BTPS}$: Gas volume saturated with water at body temperature (37°C) and ambient pressure

$Volume_{ATPS}$: Gas volume saturated with water at ambient (room) temperature and pressure

Factor : Factors for converting gas volumes from ATPS to BTPS (**Table 7-1**)

EXAMPLE

A tidal volume measured under the ATPS condition is 600 mL. What is the corrected tidal volume if the room temperature is 25°C? (See **Table 7-1** for conversion factor)

$$
\begin{aligned}
Volume_{BTPS} &= Volume_{ATPS} \times Factor \\
&= Volume \times Factor \ at \ 25°C \\
&= 600 \times 1.075 \\
&= 645 \ mL
\end{aligned}
$$

EXERCISE 1

A tidal volume was recorded at 23°C. What should be the factor for converting this measurement from ATPS to BTPS at normal body temperature (37°C)? (See **Table 7-1**)

[Answer: Conversion factor = 1.085]

EXERCISE 2

A peak flow of 120 L/min was recorded at 27°C. What is the corrected flow rate at body temperature (37°C)? (See **Table 7-1**)

[Answer: Flow rate at 37°C = 120 L/min × 1.063 = 127.56 or 128 L/min]

NOTES

According to Charles' law, lung volumes and flow rates measured at room temperature should be corrected to values at body temperature. The conversion factors from ATPS to BTPS (**Table 7-1**) should be used if the pulmonary function device does not correct for temperature change.

TABLE 7-1. Conversion factors from ATPS to BTPS

Gas temperature (°C)	Factors to Convert to 37°C Saturated*	Water Vapor Pressure (mm Hg)
22	1.091	19.8
23	1.085	21.1
24	1.080	22.4
25	1.075	23.8
26	1.068	25.2
27	1.063	26.7
28	1.057	28.3
29	1.051	30.0
30	1.045	31.8
31	1.039	33.7
32	1.032	35.7
33	1.026	37.7
34	1.020	39.9
35	1.014	42.2
36	1.007	44.6
37	1.000	47.0
38	0.993	49.8
39	0.986	52.5
40	0.979	55.4

*Conversion factors are based on P_B = 760 mm Hg. For other barometric pressures and temperatures, use the following equation: $\dfrac{P_B - P_{H_2O}}{P_B - 47} \times \dfrac{310}{(273 + °C)}$

SELF-ASSESSMENT QUESTIONS

7a. A conversion is needed because gas volume measured at room temperature (e.g., 25°C) is:

   A. greater than the volume at body temperature
   B. greater than the volume at any temperature
   C. lower than the volume at body temperature
   D. lower than the volume at any temperature

7b. What is the conversion factor from ATPS to BTPS at 26°C?

   A. 1.068
   B. 1.063
   C. 1.075
   D. 1.000

7c. The forced vital capacity (FVC) measured at 27°C is 2,000 mL. What is the corrected FVC at BTPS?

   A. 2,053 mL
   B. 2,126 mL
   C. 2,287 mL
   D. 2,320 mL

7d. The vital capacity (VC) measured under ATPS conditions is 4,800 mL at 26°C. What is the corrected VC at BTPS?

   A. 4,860 mL
   B. 4,977 mL
   C. 5,048 mL
   D. 5,126 mL

7e. The FEV_1 measured at 25°C is 1.0 L/sec. What is the corrected FVC at BTPS?

   A. 1.075 L/sec
   B. 1.750 L/sec
   C. 2.024 L/sec
   D. 2.320 L/sec

» Go to **rtexam.com** for more learning resources

8

Bicarbonate Corrections of Base Deficit

NOTES

This equation calculates the amount of sodium bicarbonate needed to correct severe metabolic acidosis. The value 1/4 in the equation represents the amount of extracellular water in the body.

During cardiopulmonary resuscitation or when the patient's perfusion is unsatisfactory, the entire calculated amount is given. Bicarbonate should not be given to correct respiratory acidosis because this condition is best managed by establishing a patent airway and providing adequate ventilation. If bicarbonate is indicated, half of the calculated amount is given initially to prevent overcompensation (i.e., from acidosis to alkalosis). Bicarbonate may not be needed when the arterial pH is greater than 7.20 or the base deficit is less than 10 mEq/L. For patients with diabetic ketoacidosis, bicarbonate may best be withheld until the pH is less than 7.10. According to the *Textbook of Advanced Cardiac Life Support by AHA*, use of bicarbonate in cardiopulmonary resuscitation is not recommended. However, in severe pre-existing metabolic acidosis, 1 mEq/kg of sodium bicarbonate may be used. Subsequent doses should not exceed 33% to 50% of the calculated bicarbonate requirement. Refer to the current ACLS guidelines for specific indications.

EQUATION

$$HCO_3^- = \frac{(BD \times kg)}{4}$$

HCO_3^- : Sodium bicarbonate needed to correct severe base deficit, in mEq/L

BD : Base deficit in mEq/L, or negative base excess (−BE) as determined by arterial blood gases

kg : Body weight in kilograms

EXAMPLE

How many mEq/L of bicarbonate are needed to correct a base deficit of 12 mEq/L if the patient's body weight is 60 kg? If the initial dose is 1/2 of the calculated amount, what is the initial dose?

$$HCO_3^- = \frac{(BD \times kg)}{4}$$

$$= \frac{(12 \times 60)}{4}$$

$$= \frac{(720)}{4}$$

$$= 180 \text{ mEq/L}$$

Initial dose $= \frac{1}{2} \times 180$ or 90 mEq/L

EXERCISE 1

Calculate the amount of bicarbonate needed for a 70-kg patient whose BE is −18 mEq/L.

What is the initial dose?

[Answer: HCO_3^- = 315 mEq/L; initial dose = 158 mEq/L]

EXERCISE 2

The BE for a 100-kg patient is −16 mEq/L. What is the initial dose?

[Answer: Initial dose = 200 mEq/L]

SELF-ASSESSMENT QUESTIONS

8a. Calculating the amount of bicarbonate needed to correct severe metabolic acidosis requires the patient's:

A. base deficit
B. base deficit and weight
C. base deficit and height
D. height and weight

8b. In respiratory care, the base deficit (– base excess) is determined by performing a(n):

A. arterial blood gases
B. shunt study
C. pulmonary function study
D. blood chemistry

8c. The blood gas results of a 70-kg patient show a base deficit (BD) of 20 mEq/L. What is the bicarbonate needed to correct the BD?

A. 90 mEq/L
B. 140 mEq/L
C. 200 mEq/L
D. 350 mEq/L

8d. A 60-kg patient has a base deficit of 30 mEq/L. Calculate the base deficit (BD). What should be the initial dose?

A. BD = 45 mEq/L; 22.5 mEq/L
B. BD = 90 mEq/L; 45 mEq/L
C. BD = 450 mEq/L; 225 mEq/L
D. BD = 900 mEq/L; 450 mEq/L

8e. Calculate the amount of bicarbonate needed to correct a base deficit of 20 mEq/L for a patient weighing 80 kg. If the initial dose is 1/2 of the calculated amount, what should be the initial dose?

A. 800 mEq/L; initial dose = 400 mEq/L
B. 400 mEq/L; initial dose = 200 mEq/L
C. 200 mEq/L; initial dose = 100 mEq/L
D. 80 mEq/L; initial dose = 40 mEq/L

» Go to **rtexam.com** for more learning resources

Body Surface Area

The body surface area (BSA) is used to calculate the cardiac index, the stroke volume index, or the drug dosages for adults and children. One way to find the body surface area is to use the DuBois Body Surface Chart (**Figure 9-1**). If the chart is not available, this BSA equation can be used.

To use the equation, the patient's body weight in kilograms must be known. Divide the body weight in pounds by 2.2 to get kilograms.

EQUATION

$$BSA = \frac{(4 \times kg) + 7}{kg + 90}$$

BSA : Body surface area in m^2
kg : Body weight in kilograms

EQUATION 2

$$BSA = 0.04950 \times kg^{0.6046}$$

(This formula requires a calculator with power function.)

NORMAL VALUE   Adult average BSA = 1.7 m^2

EXAMPLE

What is the calculated BSA of a child weighing 44 pounds?

$$44 \text{ pounds} = \frac{44}{2.2} \text{ kg}$$

$$= 20 \text{ kg}$$

$$BSA = \frac{(4 \times kg) + 7}{kg + 90}$$

$$= \frac{(4 \times 20) + 7}{20 + 90}$$

$$= \frac{80 + 7}{110}$$

$$= \frac{87}{110}$$

$$= 0.79 \text{ m}^2$$

EXERCISE 1

Calculate the body surface area of a 132-lb patient.

[Answer: BSA = 1.65 m^2]

EXERCISE 2

Use the DuBois Body Surface Chart (**Figure 9-1**) to find the body surface area of a person who is 5'6" and 140 lb. Using the equation and weight provided, calculate the body surface area.

[Answer: BSA (**Figure 9-1**) = 1.72 m^2; BSA (calculated) = 1.70 m^2]

DIRECTIONS

To find body surface of a patient, locate the height in inches (or centimeters) on Scale I and the weight in pounds (or kilograms) on Scale II and place a straight edge (ruler) between these two points, which will intersect Scale III at the patient's surface area.

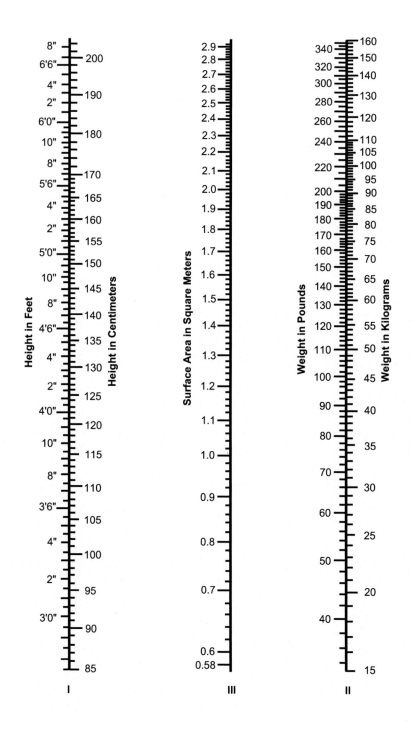

FIGURE 9-1. DuBois Body Surface Chart

Adapted from DuBois, Eugene F. Basal Metabolism in Health and Disease. Philadelphia: Lea and Febiger, 1924.
Source: Des Jardin, T.R. Cardiopulmonary Anatomy and Physiology: Essentials for Respiratory Care, 5th ed. Clifton Park, NY: Delmar Cengage Learning, 2008.

SELF-ASSESSMENT QUESTIONS

9a. Calculate the body surface area (BSA) of a person weighing 80 kg.

A. 1.92 m
B. 1.92 m²
C. 3.14 m
D. 3.14 m²

9b. The calculated body surface area (BSA) of a 200-kg person is:

A. 1.88 m
B. 2.78 m
C. 1.88 m²
D. 2.78 m²

9c. To use the DuBois Body Surface Chart, the following must be known:

A. age and height
B. gender and weight
C. height
D. height and weight

9d. For a 70-kg and 5'6" tall person, what is the approximate body surface area using the DuBois Body Surface Chart?

A. 1.4 m²
B. 1.6 m²
C. 1.8 m²
D. 1.9 m²

9e. What is the calculated body surface area (BSA) of a person weighing 120 lb? (2.2 lb = 1 kg.) If the same person is 5'5" tall, what is the body surface area using the DuBois Body Surface Chart?

A. 1.56 m²; 1.60 m²
B. 1.76 m²; 1.60 m²
C. 1.89 m²; 1.70 m²
D. 1.93 m²; 1.70 m²

» Go to **rtexam.com** for more learning resources

10

Cardiac Index (CI)

EQUATION

$$CI = \frac{CO}{BSA}$$

CI :   Cardiac index in L/min/m²
CO :   Cardiac output in L/min (Q_T)
BSA :   Body surface area in m²

NORMAL VALUE   2.5 to 3.5 L/min/m²

EXAMPLE

Given: Cardiac output   = 4 L/min
         Body surface area = 1.4 m²

Calculate the cardiac index.

$$CI = \frac{CO}{BSA}$$

$$= \frac{4}{1.4}$$

$$= 2.86 \ \text{L/min/m}^2$$

EXERCISE 1

Given: Cardiac output   = 4 L/min
         Body surface area = 2.5 m²

Find the cardiac index (CI).

[Answer: CI = 1.6 L/min/m²]

EXERCISE 2

Given: Cardiac output   = 5 L/min
         Body surface area = 1.8 m²

Calculate the cardiac index (CI).

[Answer: CI = 2.8 L/min/m²]

EXERCISE 3

What is the CI of a patient who has a cardiac output of 4.5 L/min and a BSA of 1.5 m²?

[Answer: CI = 3 L/min/m²]

NOTES

Normal cardiac output for a resting adult ranges from 4 to 8 L/min.

Cardiac index (CI) is used to normalize cardiac output measurements among patients of varying body sizes. For instance, a cardiac output of 4 L/min may be normal for an average-sized person but low for a large-sized person. The cardiac index will be able to distinguish this difference based on body size.

CI values between 1.8 and 2.5 L/min/m² indicate hypoperfusion. Values less than 1.8 may indicate cardiogenic shock.

SELF-ASSESSMENT QUESTIONS

10a. What is the normal range of cardiac index?

A. 2.5 to 3.5 L/min/m^2
B. 4 to 5 L/min/m^2
C. 4 to 8 L/min/m^2
D. 6 to 10 L/min/m^2

10b. Given the following measurements from a patient in the coronary intensive care unit: cardiac output = 5 L/min, body surface area = 1.7 m^2. What is the patient's cardiac index? Is it normal for this patient?

A. 2.9 L/min/m^2; abnormal
B. 2.9 L/min/m^2; normal
C. 3.3 L/min/m^2; abnormal
D. 3.3 L/min/m^2; normal

10c. An 85-kg patient has the following measurements: cardiac output = 5 L/min, body surface area = 2.9 m^2. What is the calculated cardiac index? Is it normal for this patient?

A. 1.7 L/min/m^2; abnormal
A. 1.7 L/min/m^2; normal
B. 14.5 L/min/m^2; normal
C. 14.5 L/min/m^2; abnormal

10d. The following measurements are obtained from a patient whose admitting diagnosis is obstructive sleep apnea: cardiac output (CO) = 6 L/min, body surface area = 3.3 m^2. Is the patient's cardiac output within the normal range? Is the cardiac index (CI) normal?

A. CO and CI abnormal
B. CO and CI within normal range
C. CO abnormal; CI within normal range
D. CO within normal range; CI abnormal

10e. The following values are obtained from a 50-year-old patient with congestive heart failure: cardiac output = 3.0 L/min, body surface area = 1.0 m^2. Is the patient's cardiac output (CO) normal? Cardiac index (CI)?

A. CO within normal range; CI abnormal
B. CO and CI within normal range
C. CO abnormal; CI within normal range
D. CO and CI abnormal

» Go to **rtexam.com** for more learning resources

11

Cardiac Output (CO): Fick's Estimated Method

EQUATION 1

$$CO = \frac{O_2 \text{ consumption}}{C_aO_2 - C_{\bar{v}}O_2}$$

EQUATION 2

$$CO = \frac{130 \times BSA}{C_aO_2 - C_{\bar{v}}O_2}$$

CO	: Cardiac output in L/min; same as total perfusion (Q_T)
O_2 consumption	: Estimated to be 130 × BSA, in mL/min (VO_2)
C_aO_2	: Arterial oxygen content in vol%
$C_{\bar{v}}O_2$	: Mixed venous oxygen content in vol%
130	: Estimated O_2 consumption rate of an adult, in mL/min/m²
BSA	: Body surface area in m²

NORMAL VALUE CO = 4 to 8 L/min

EXAMPLE

Given: Body surface area = 1.6 m²
        Arterial O_2 content = 20 vol%
        Mixed venous O_2 content = 15 vol%

Calculate the cardiac output (CO) using Fick's estimated method.

$$CO = \frac{O_2 \text{ consumption}}{C_aO_2 - C_{\bar{v}}O_2}$$

$$= \frac{130 \times BSA}{C_aO_2 - C_{\bar{v}}O_2}$$

$$= \frac{130 \times 1.6}{20\% - 15\%}$$

$$= \frac{208}{5\%}$$

$$= \frac{208}{0.05}$$

$$= 4,160 \text{ mL/min or } 4.16 \text{ L/min}$$

The CO equation is used to calculate the cardiac output per minute.

The O_2 consumption (130 × BSA) used in the equation is an estimate of the oxygen consumption rate of an adult. This estimate is easier and faster to use than an actual measurement, but it may give inaccurate cardiac output determinations, particularly in patients with unusually high or low metabolic (O_2 consumption) rates.

Under normal conditions, the cardiac output is directly related to oxygen consumption (i.e., the cardiac output would increase in cases of increased oxygen consumption). If the cardiac output fails to keep up with the oxygen consumption needs, the $C(a-\bar{v})O_2$ increases.

EXERCISE   Given: BSA $= 1.2\ m^2$
$C_aO_2 = 19\ vol\%$
$C_{\bar{v}}O_2 = 14\ vol\%$

Calculate the cardiac output using Fick's estimated method.

[Answer: CO = 3,120 mL/min or 3.12 L/min]

SELF-ASSESSMENT QUESTIONS

11a. The normal cardiac output for adults ranges from:

A. 4 to 6 L/min
B. 4 to 8 L/min
C. 5 to 6 L/min
D. 5 to 8 L/min

11b. Since oxygen consumption in mL/min can be estimated by using the formula 130 mL/min/m² × BSA m², what is the estimated O_2 consumption for a patient whose body surface area (BSA) is 1.5 m²?

A. 100 mL/min
A. 130 mL/min
B. 150 mL/min
C. 195 mL/min

11c. Given: oxygen consumption = 156 mL/min, arterial O_2 content (C_aO_2) = 19 vol%, mixed venous O_2 content ($C_{\bar{v}}O_2$) = 15 vol%. Calculate the cardiac output using Fick's estimated method.

A. 156 mL/min
B. 892 mL/min
C. 2.3 L/min
D. 3.9 L/min

11d. The following hemodynamic values are obtained from a patient in the intensive care unit: estimated oxygen consumption = 180 mL, arterial O_2 content (C_aO_2) = 18.4 vol%, mixed venous O_2 content = 14.4 vol%. Calculate the cardiac output using Fick's estimated method. Is it normal?

A. 4.5 L/min; normal
B. 5.5 L/min; normal
C. 6 L/min; abnormal
D. 6.5 L/min; abnormal

11e. A patient whose body surface area is about 1.4 m² has the following oxygen content values: C_aO_2 = 19.5 vol%, $C_{\bar{v}}O_2$ = 14.5 vol%. What is the cardiac output based on Fick's estimated method?

    A. 2.73 L/min
    B. 2.98 L/min
    C. 3.64 L/min
    D. 4.52 L/min

11f. Using Fick's estimated method, calculate the cardiac output with these data: O_2 consumption = 200 mL/min, C_cO_2 = 20 vol%, C_aO_2 = 19.5 vol%, C_vO_2 = 14.5 vol%.

    A. 3 L/min
    B. 4 L/min
    C. 5 L/min
    D. 6 L/min

11g. The oxygen consumption may be estimated by using the following formula: (BSA = Body Surface Area)

    A. 100 / BSA
    B. 130 / BSA
    C. 100 × BSA
    D. 130 × BSA

11h. Given: BSA = 2 m², C_cO_2 = 20.1 vol%, C_aO_2 = 20 vol%, C_vO_2 = 16 vol%. Calculate the CO using Fick's estimated method.

    A. 5.5 L/min
    B. 6.0 L/min
    C. 6.5 L/min
    D. 7.0 L/min

11i. Assuming a steady cardiac output, an increase of oxygen consumption would cause:

    A. an increase of $C_aO_2 - C_vO_2$ gradient
    B. an increase of $C_cO_2 - C_vO_2$ gradient
    C. a decrease of $C_cO_2 - C_aO_2$ gradient
    D. a decrease of $C_aO_2 - C_vO_2$ gradient

12

Cerebral Perfusion Pressure

To calculate the CPP, the MAP and ICP must have the same unit of measurement (mm Hg). The MAP may be obtained directly from the monitor of an indwelling arterial catheter. MAP may also be calculated from the indirect blood pressure measurements:

$$MAP = \frac{(systolic\ BP + 2 \times diastolic\ BP)}{3}$$

The ICP is obtained directly from the intra-cranial pressure monitor.

The CPP has a normal limit of 70 to 80 mm Hg. Low CPP indicates that the cerebral perfusion is inadequate and it is associated with a high mortality rate. There is no class I evidence for the optimum level of CPP, but the critical threshold is believed to be from 70 to 80 mm Hg. Mortality increased about 20% for each 10 mm Hg drop in CPP. In studies involving severe head injuries, 35% reduction in mortality was achieved when the CPP was maintained above 70 mm Hg.

Since CPP is the difference between MAP and ICP, changes in MAP or ICP will directly affect the CPP. A higher CPP can be achieved by raising the MAP or lowering the ICP. In the absence of hemorrhage, the MAP should be managed initially by fluid balance, followed by a vasopressor such as norepinephrine or dopamine. Systemic hypotension (SBP <90 mm Hg) should be avoided and controlled as soon as possible because early hypotension is associated with increased morbidity and mortality following severe brain injury.

The ICP for normal subjects is 8 to 12 mm Hg. In practice, the ICP clinical limit is up to 20 mm Hg.

EQUATION 1

$$CPP = MAP - ICP$$

CPP : Cerebral perfusion pressure
MAP : Mean arterial pressure
ICP : Intracranial pressure

NORMAL VALUE

70 to 80 mm Hg

EXAMPLE 1

Calculate the CPP given the following data:

MAP = 90 mm Hg, ICP = 14 mm Hg. Is the calculated CCP within normal limits?

$$
\begin{aligned}
CPP &= MAP - ICP \\
&= 90\ mm\ Hg - 14\ mm\ Hg \\
&= 76\ mm\ Hg
\end{aligned}
$$

CPP is within normal limit of 70 to 80 mm Hg.

EXAMPLE 2

The arterial blood pressure of a patient is 110/60 mm Hg. The ICP measured at the same time is 18 mm Hg. Is the calculated CCP normal?

$$
\begin{aligned}
MAP &= \frac{(systolic\ BP + 2 \times diastolic\ BP)}{3} \\
&= \frac{(110 + 2 \times 60)}{3} \\
&= \frac{(110 + 120)}{3} \\
&= \frac{230}{3} \\
&= 76.66\ or\ 77\ mm\ Hg
\end{aligned}
$$

$$
\begin{aligned}
CPP &= MAP - ICP \\
&= 77\ mm\ Hg - 18\ mm\ Hg \\
&= 59\ mm\ Hg
\end{aligned}
$$

EXERCISE 1

Given: MAP = 86 mm Hg, ICP = 14 mm Hg. Calculate the CCP. Is it within the normal limit?

[Answer: CPP = 72 mm Hg; within normal limit of 70 to 80 mm Hg]

EXERCISE 2 A patient has blood pressure of 80/40 mm Hg and intracranial pressure of 8 mm Hg. Calculate the cerebral perfusion pressure (CPP). Is it within normal limits?

[Answer: CPP = 45 mm Hg; below normal limit of 70 to 80 mm Hg]

SELF-ASSESSMENT QUESTIONS

12a. Which of the following conditions is indicative of poor patient outcome resulting from lack of perfusion to the brain?

A. high arterial blood pressure
B. low cerebral perfusion pressure
C. high mean arterial pressure
D. low intracranial pressure

12b. Calculate the cerebral perfusion pressure given the following data: mean arterial pressure = 70 mm Hg, intracranial pressure = 18 mm Hg. Is the calculated CCP within normal limits?

A. 52 mm Hg; lower than normal limit
B. 52 mm Hg; higher than normal limit
C. 98 mm Hg; within normal limit
D. 98 mm Hg; higher than normal limit

12c. The mean arterial pressure of a patient is 100 mm Hg. The intracranial pressure is 22 mm Hg. What is the calculated cerebral perfusion pressure? Is it normal?

A. 78 mm Hg; abnormal
B. 78 mm Hg; normal
C. 122 mm Hg; abnormal
D. 122 mm Hg; normal

12d. The arterial blood pressure of a patient is 90/50 mm Hg. The ICP on the monitor shows 20 mm Hg. What is the calculated CPP? Is it normal?

A. 76 mm Hg; normal
B. 66 mm Hg; normal
C. 43 mm Hg; abnormal
D. 53 mm Hg; abnormal

12e. A patient has an arterial blood pressure of 120/70 mm Hg and an intracranial pressure of 28 mm Hg. What is the calculated CPP? Is the CPP within the normal limit?

A. 64 mm Hg; within normal limit of 60 to 70 mm Hg
B. 64 mm Hg; lower than normal limit of 70 to 80 mm Hg
C. 59 mm Hg; within normal limit of 50 to 60 mm Hg
D. 59 mm Hg; lower than normal limit of 70 to 80 mm Hg

12f. The normal cerebral perfusion pressure (CPP) ranges from:

A. 30 to 40 mm Hg
B. 40 to 50 mm Hg
C. 50 to 60 mm Hg
D. 70 to 80 mm Hg

12g. The cerebral perfusion pressure (CPP) equals to:

A. MAP + ICP
B. MAP × ICP
C. MAP – ICP
D. MAP / ICP

12h. When an arterial catheter is not available, the mean arterial pressure (MAP) may be estimated by:

A. MAP = (systolic pressure + 2 × diastolic pressure) / 3
B. MAP = (systolic pressure + diastolic pressure) / 3
C. MAP = (2 x systolic pressure – diastolic pressure) / 3
D. MAP = (systolic pressure – diastolic pressure) / 3

12i. Vital signs of a patient show irregular heart rate of 140/min, arterial blood pressure of 100/45 mm Hg, intracranial pressure of 13 mm Hg. What is the calculated cerebral perfusion pressure? Is it higher or lower than the normal range?

A. 40 mm Hg; higher than the normal range
B. 50 mm Hg; higher than the normal range
C. 40 mm Hg; lower than the normal range
D. 50 mm Hg; lower than the normal range

13

Compliance: Dynamic $\left(C_{\text{dyn}}\right)$

EQUATION

$$C_{\text{dyn}} = \frac{\Delta V}{\Delta P}$$

C_{dyn} : Dynamic compliance in mL/cm H_2O
ΔV : Corrected tidal volume in mL
ΔP : Pressure change (Peak inspiratory pressure − PEEP) in cm H_2O

NORMAL VALUE

30 to 40 mL/cm H_2O

If the patient is intubated, use serial measurements to establish trend.

EXAMPLE

Given: ΔV = 500 mL
Peak inspiratory pressure = 30 cm H_2O
PEEP = 10 cm H_2O

Calculate the dynamic compliance.

$$\begin{aligned}
C_{\text{dyn}} &= \frac{\Delta V}{\Delta P} \\
&= \frac{500}{30-10} \\
&= \frac{500}{20} \\
&= 25 \text{ mL/cm } H_2O
\end{aligned}$$

NOTES

Dynamic compliance is used to assess changes in the nonelastic (airway) resistance to air flow. When the air flow resistance is increases, the peak inspiratory pressure rises while the dynamic compliance remains unchanged. Therefore the dynamic compliance is reduced (due to ↑PIP) while the static compliance remains unchanged (due to unchanged plateau pressure).

The dynamic compliance can change *independently* without corresponding change in static compliance. This is indicative of airway resistance changes. If the dynamic compliance decreases with minimal or no decrease in static compliance, it is likely caused by an increase in nonelastic (airway) resistance. Examples include bronchospasm, main-stem intubation, mucus plug, kinked ventilator tubing or endotracheal tube.

Instead of the set tidal volume, the corrected tidal volume is used in the equation to account for the volume loss due to ventilator circuit expansion during inspiration.

Elastance (E) is the reciprocal of compliance (C) where $E = \Delta P/\Delta V$ and $C = \Delta V/\Delta P$. In clinical settings, compliance is used to describe the elastic characteristics of the lungs or chest wall.

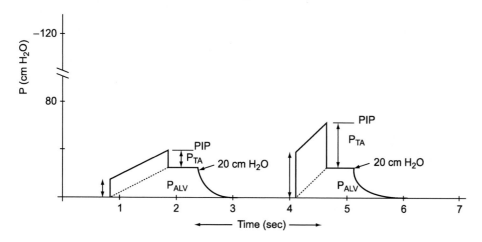

FIGURE 13-1. (from left to right) Shows an increase of transairway pressure (P_{TA}). Airway resistance is increased because the PIP is increased while the P_{ALV} (lung compliance) remains unchanged.

EXERCISE

Given: Corrected tidal volume   = 600 mL
            Peak inspiratory pressure = 40 cm H_2O
            PEEP   = 5 cm H_2O

Calculate the dynamic compliance.

[Answer: C_{dyn} = 17.1 or 17 mL/cm H_2O]

SELF-ASSESSMENT QUESTIONS

13a. **The normal range for dynamic compliance is:**

A. 30 to 40 mL/cm H_2O
B. 20 to 40 mL/cm H_2O
C. 10 to 20 mL/cm H_2O
D. 10 to 30 mL/cm H_2O

13b. **Given: corrected tidal volume = 650 mL, peak inspiratory pressure = 32 cm H_2O. Calculate the dynamic compliance.**

A. 10 mL/cm H_2O
B. 14 mL/cm H_2O
C. 18 mL/cm H_2O
D. 20 mL/cm H_2O

13c. **What is the patient's dynamic compliance if the corrected tidal volume = 600 mL, peak inspiratory pressure = 45 cm H_2O, and PEEP = 15 cm H_2O?**

A. 14 mL/cm H_2O
B. 20 mL/cm H_2O
C. 26 mL/cm H_2O
D. 40 mL/cm H_2O

13d. **A mechanically ventilated patient has these measurements: corrected tidal volume = 600 mL, peak inspiratory pressure = 35 cm H_2O, plateau (alveolar) pressure = 25 cm H_2O, and PEEP = 5 cm H_2O. What is the dynamic compliance?**

A. 30 mL/cm H_2O
B. 24 mL/cm H_2O
C. 20 mL/cm H_2O
D. 15 mL/cm H_2O

13e. If a patient's corrected tidal volume is 500 mL and the corresponding peak inspiratory pressure is 20 cm H_2O, what is the calculated dynamic compliance?

    A. 16 mL/cm H_2O
    B. 20 mL/cm H_2O
    C. 25 mL/cm H_2O
    D. 40 mL/cm H_2O

13f. The dynamic compliance is calculated by:

    A. corrected tidal volume / plateau pressure
    B. corrected tidal volume / peak inspiratory pressure
    C. corrected tidal volume × plateau pressure
    D. corrected tidal volume × peak inspiratory pressure

13g. Given: corrected tidal volume 600 mL, peak inspiratory pressure 30 cm H_2O, plateau pressure 20 cm H_2O, mean airway pressure 26 cm H_2O. What is the dynamic compliance?

    A. 20 mL/cm H_2O
    B. 23 mL/cm H_2O
    C. 27 mL/cm H_2O
    D. 30 mL/cm H_2O

13h. Mr. West has the following data from the ventilator flow sheet: corrected tidal volume 500 mL, peak inspiratory pressure 65 cm H_2O, plateau pressure 35 cm H_2O, positive end-expiratory pressure (PEEP) 15 cm H_2O. Calculate the dynamic compliance.

    A. 4 mL/cm H_2O
    B. 6 mL/cm H_2O
    C. 8 mL/cm H_2O
    D. 10 mL/cm H_2O

13i. A mechanically ventilated patient has the following data: corrected tidal volume = 600 mL, peak inspiratory pressure = 40 cm H_2O, plateau pressure = 20 cm H_2O, and PEEP = 10 cm H_2O. What is the dynamic compliance?

    A. 10 mL/cm H_2O
    B. 20 mL/cm H_2O
    C. 30 mL/cm H_2O
    D. 60 mL/cm H_2O

» Go to **rtexam.com** for more learning resources

Compliance: Static (C_{st})

Static compliance reflects changes of the elastic (lung parenchymal) resistance to air flow in the lungs. The static and dynamic compliance measurements are directly related because changes in the plateau pressure will invoke similar and proportional changes in the peak inspiratory pressure. Lung parenchymal diseases (e.g., pneumonia) reduce the static compliance *and* dynamic compliance. Improvement of lung parenchymal disease will increase the static *and* dynamic compliance.

Plateau pressure is same as alveolar pressure. It is measured by applying a brief inspiratory pause immediately following end-inspiration of a mechanical tidal volume.

Instead of the set tidal volume, the corrected tidal volume is used in the equation to account for the volume loss due to ventilator circuit expansion during inspiration.

Elastance (E) is the reciprocal of compliance (C) where $E = \Delta P / \Delta V$ and $C = \Delta V / \Delta P$. In clinical settings, compliance is used to describe the elastic characteristics of the lungs or chest wall.

EQUATION

$$C_{st} = \frac{\Delta V}{\Delta P}$$

C_{st} : Static compliance in mL/cm H_2O
ΔV : Corrected tidal volume in mL
ΔP : Pressure change (Plateau pressure – PEEP) in cm H_2O

NORMAL VALUE

40 to 60 mL/cm H_2O

If the patient is intubated, use serial measurements to establish trend.

EXAMPLE

Given: ΔV = 500 mL
Plateau pressure = 20 cm H_2O
PEEP = 5 cm H_2O

Calculate the static compliance.

$$
\begin{aligned}
C_{st} &= \frac{\Delta V}{\Delta P} \\
&= \frac{500}{20-5} \\
&= \frac{500}{15} \\
&= 33.3 \text{ or } 33 \text{ mL/cm } H_2O
\end{aligned}
$$

EXERCISE

Given: Corrected tidal volume = 600 mL
Plateau pressure = 25 cm H_2O
PEEP = 5 cm H_2O

Calculate the static compliance.

[Answer: C_{st} = 30 mL/cm H_2O]

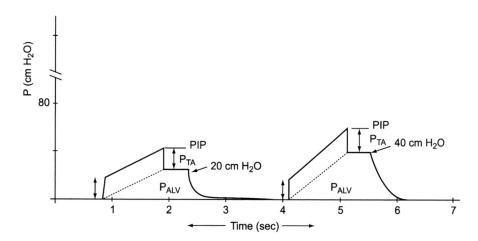

FIGURE 14-1. (from left to right) Shows an increase of P_{ALV} and PIP. The increase in P_{ALV} is due to a decrease in lung compliance. The increase in PIP is due to an increase of the P_{ALV} (plateau pressure). Airway resistance is unchanged because the P_{TA} measurements remain unchanged.

SELF-ASSESSMENT QUESTIONS

14a. The normal static compliance ranges from:

    A. 20 to 30 L/cm H_2O
    B. 20 to 40 L/cm H_2O
    C. 40 to 50 L/cm H_2O
    D. 40 to 60 L/cm H_2O

14b. Static compliance is calculated by dividing the corrected tidal volume by:

    A. plateau pressure
    B. positive end-expiratory pressure
    C. peak inspiratory pressure
    D. transpulmonary pressure

14c. Given the following ventilation parameters, corrected tidal volume = 600 mL, plateau pressure = 30 cm H_2O, calculate the static compliance.

    A. 14 mL/cm H_2O
    B. 16 mL/cm H_2O
    C. 18 mL/cm H_2O
    D. 20 mL/cm H_2O

14d. Calculate the static compliance with these data: corrected tidal volume = 650 mL, plateau pressure = 30 cm H_2O, and PEEP = 10 cm H_2O.

    A. 65 mL/cm H_2O
    B. 33 mL/cm H_2O
    C. 22 mL/cm H_2O
    D. 18 mL/cm H_2O

14e. The following measurements are obtained from a mechanically ventilated patient: corrected tidal volume = 600 mL, peak inspiratory pressure = 55 cm H_2O, plateau pressure = 35 cm H_2O, and PEEP = 10 cm H_2O. What is the static compliance?

A. 13 mL/cm H_2O
B. 24 mL/cm H_2O
C. 26 mL/cm H_2O
D. 28 mL/cm H_2O

14f. Of the 4 sets of data below, which has the highest static compliance?

	Corrected tidal volume	Plateau pressure	PEEP
A.	650 mL	20 cm H_2O	0 cm H_2O
B.	650 mL	22 cm H_2O	0 cm H_2O
C.	650 mL	24 cm H_2O	0 cm H_2O
D.	650 mL	26 cm H_2O	0 cm H_2O

14g. Given: 4 sets of data from a PEEP titration trial. Which of the following yields the best (highest) static compliance?

	Corrected tidal volume	Plateau pressure	PEEP
A.	700 mL	32 cm H_2O	8 cm H_2O
B.	700 mL	31 cm H_2O	10 cm H_2O
C.	700 mL	32 cm H_2O	12 cm H_2O
D.	700 mL	36 cm H_2O	14 cm H_2O

14h. Four sets of data are obtained during PEEP titration. Which of the following yields the best (highest) static compliance?

	Corrected tidal volume	Plateau pressure	PEEP
A.	600 mL	26 cm H_2O	6 cm H_2O
B.	600 mL	28 cm H_2O	8 cm H_2O
C.	600 mL	28 cm H_2O	10 cm H_2O
D.	600 mL	32 cm H_2O	12 cm H_2O

» Go to **rtexam.com** for more learning resources

15

Compliance: Total (C_T)

EQUATION

$$\frac{1}{C_T} = \frac{1}{C_L} + \frac{1}{C_{cw}}$$

$\dfrac{1}{C_T}$: Reciprocal of total compliance (lung and chest wall)

$\dfrac{1}{C_L}$: Reciprocal of lung compliance

$\dfrac{1}{C_{cw}}$: Reciprocal of chest-wall compliance

NOTES

This equation describes the relationship among total compliance, lung compliance, and chest-wall compliance. It is essential to note that the reciprocals of these values are related.

With an intact lung-thorax system, the lung compliance equals the chest-wall compliance. When this condition exists, the total compliance is half of the lung compliance or chest-wall compliance.

EXAMPLE

If the lung and chest-wall compliance values are both 0.2 L/cm H_2O, find the total compliance.

$$\frac{1}{0.2} + \frac{1}{0.2} = \frac{(1+1)}{0.2} \text{ (reciprocal of total compliance)}$$

$$= \frac{2}{0.2}$$

$$= \frac{1}{0.1}$$

[Answer: Total compliance = 0.1 L/cm H_2O]

EXERCISE

Calculate the total compliance if the lung and chest-wall compliance values are both 0.18 L/cm H_2O.

[Answer: Total compliance = 0.09 L/cm H_2O]

SELF-ASSESSMENT QUESTIONS

15a. Which of the following groups of compliance values equal one another in an intact lung-thorax system?

A. lung compliance and chest-wall compliance
B. total compliance and chest-wall compliance
C. total compliance and lung compliance
D. total compliance, lung compliance, and chest-wall compliance

15b. Total compliance is about ___ L/cm H_2O, ___ the normal lung compliance value.

A. 0.1; twice
B. 0.1; half of
C. 0.2; twice
D. 0.2; half of

15c. The normal chest-wall compliance is about ___ L/cm H_2O, ___ the normal lung compliance value.

A. 0.1; twice
B. 0.1; same as
C. 0.2; half of
D. 0.2; same as

15d. Under normal conditions, all of the following statements are true *except*:

A. Chest-wall compliance is similar to lung compliance.
B. Chest-wall compliance is greater than total compliance.
C. Lung compliance is greater than total compliance.
D. The sum of lung and chest wall compliance is greater than total compliance.

15e. Under normal conditions, the sum of the *reciprocals* of chest wall compliance and lung compliance equals to the:

A. total compliance
B. lung compliance
C. reciprocals of total compliance
D. chest wall compliance

» Go to **rtexam.com** for more learning resources

16

Corrected Tidal Volume (V_T)

EQUATION

Corrected V_T = Expired V_T – Tubing volume

Expired V_T : Expired tidal volume in mL
Circuit volume : Volume "lost" in ventilator circuit during inspiratory phase (Pressure change × 3 mL/cm H_2O)*

EXAMPLE

Expired V_T = 650 mL
Peak inspiratory pressure = 25 cm H_2O
Positive end-expiratory pressure (PEEP) = 5 cm H_2O
Circuit compression factor = 3 mL/cm H_2O*

Calculate the corrected tidal volume.

Circuit volume = Pressure change × 3 mL/cm H_2O
= (25 – 5) cm H_2O × 3 mL/cm H_2O
= 20 cm H_2O × 3 mL/cm H_2O
= 60 mL

Corrected V_T = Expired V_T – Circuit volume
= 650 mL – 60 mL
= 590 mL

EXERCISE

Expired V_T = 600 mL
Peak inspiratory pressure = 45 cm H_2O
PEEP = 10 cm H_2O
Circuit compression factor = 2 mL/cm H_2O

Calculate the corrected tidal volume.

[Answer: Corrected V_T = 530 mL]

NOTES

During mechanical ventilation (volume-controlled or pressure-controlled), a majority of the tidal volume goes to the lungs. A small portion of this tidal volume expands the ventilator circuit during inspiration. On exhalation, volumes from the lungs and circuit are shown as expired tidal volume. The volume "lost" in the circuit is calculated by multiplying the peak inspiratory (minus PEEP, if used) and the circuit compliance factor.

The circuit compression factor can be determined by: (1) Set the frequency at 10 to 16/min and the tidal volume between 100 and 200 mL with minimum flow rate and maximum pressure limit; (2) completely occlude the patient Y-connection of the ventilator circuit; (3) record the expired volume (mL) and the peak inspiratory pressure (cm H_2O); and (4) divide the expired volume by the peak inspiratory pressure. The answer is the circuit compression factor in mL/cm H_2O.

The circuit compression factor varies depending on the (1) ventilator, (2) characteristics of circuit (e.g., elastic material) and humidifier (e.g., water level).

SELF-ASSESSMENT QUESTIONS

16a. The ventilator circuit compression factor is dependent on the:

A. characteristics of circuit
B. type of ventilator
C. characteristics of humidifier
D. All of the above

16b. What is the circuit compression volume if the circuit compression factor is 2 mL/cm H_2O and the pressure change is 30 cm H_2O?

A. 30 mL
B. 33 mL
C. 60 mL
D. 90 mL

16c. Given the following data, calculate the corrected tidal volume: expired V_T = 700 mL; peak inspiratory pressure = 40 cm H_2O; PEEP = 0 cm H_2O; circuit compression factor = 3 mL/cm H_2O.

A. 540 mL
B. 580 mL
C. 600 mL
D. 620 mL

16d. Calculate the corrected tidal volume with the following data: expired V_T = 780 mL; peak inspiratory pressure = 45 cm H_2O; PEEP = 5 cm H_2O; circuit compression factor = 2 mL/cm H_2O.

A. 700 mL
B. 690 mL
C. 680 mL
D. 670 mL

16e. Calculate the corrected tidal volume with the following measurements: expired V_T = 650 mL; peak inspiratory pressure = 35 cm H_2O; plateau pressure = 25 cm H_2O; PEEP = 5 cm H_2O; circuit compression factor = 3 mL/cm H_2O.

A. 510 mL/cm H_2O
B. 540 mL/cm H_2O
C. 560 mL/cm H_2O
D. 590 mL/cm H_2O

Go to **rtexam.com** for more learning resources

17

Correction Factor

NOTES

A correction factor should be used when the measured values are *consistently* different from the expected value. The correction factor is greater than 1 if the expected value is greater than the measured value. A correction factor is not needed if the expected and measured values are the same. The correction factor is less than 1 if the expected value is less than the measured value.

EQUATION

$$\text{Correction Factor} = \frac{\text{Expected}}{\text{Measured}}$$

Expected : Expected (input) measurements such as barometric pressure, volume in calibration syringe

Measured : Actual (output) measurements such as pressure in ventilator circuit, volume recorded by spirometry

NORMAL VALUE

The correction factor is dependent on the expected and measured values.

EXAMPLE 1

The volume (expected) of a pulmonary function calibration syringe is 3 L. During calibration on three separate trials, the measured volumes are consistently 2.98 L. The correction factor is therefore 3.00/2.98 or 1.007. When the same device is used to measure lung volumes and capacities, the measurements should be "corrected" using this correction factor.

If the measured vital capacity is 4.2 L, the corrected vital capacity becomes 4.2 L × 1.007 or 4.23 L.

EXAMPLE 2

In Example 1, the measured volume is smaller than the expected volume during calibration and the calculated correction factor is greater than 1. In this example, the measured volume is 3.02 L, which is larger than the expected volume of 3 L in the calibration syringe. The correction factor is therefore 3.00/3.02 or 0.993.

If the measured vital capacity is 4.2 L, the corrected vital capacity becomes 4.2 L × 0.993 or 4.17 L.

EXERCISE 1

A pressure manometer has a calibrated pressure of 50 cm H_2O. If the actual pressure measurements of a known 50 cm H_2O source are consistently 52 cm H_2O, what should be the correction factor?

[Answer: Correction factor = 0.961]

EXERCISE 2   A 3-L calibration syringe is used to calibrate the pulmonary function spirometer. If the spirometer records a volume of 2.88 L, what should be the correction factor for subsequent volume measurements?

[Answer: Correction factor = 1.042]

What should be the correction factor if the spirometer records a volume of 3.07 L?

[Answer: Correction factor = 0.977]

SELF-ASSESSMENT QUESTIONS

17a. The correction factor used in calibration of a pulmonary function spirometer or other similar device can be calculated by using the following solution:

A. expected value + actual value
B. expected value – actual value
C. expected value × actual value
D. expected value / actual value

17b. 3.0 L of air from a calibration syringe is used to calibrate the pulmonary function spirometer. The recorded volumes are consistently 2.89 L. Calculate the correction factor for subsequent volumes measured by this spirometer.

A. 0.926
B. 0.963
C. 1.038
D. 1.045

17c. A known flow rate at precisely 4 L/sec is introduced into the spirometer, and the spirometer consistently records flow rates of 4.07 L/sec. What should be the correction factor for subsequent flow rate measurements?

A. 0.983
B. 0.973
C. 1.025
D. 1.018

17d. If the correction factor for a spirometer is 0.993 and the spirometer measures a vital capacity of 3.8 L, what should be the corrected vital capacity?

A. 3.61 L
B. 3.77 L
C. 3.84 L
D. 3.89 L

17e. An infrared temperature sensing device is calibrated at 37 °C. In 3 separate measurements at a known temperature of 37 °C, the actual readings were consistently 37.6 °C. What should be the correction factor?

A. 1.016
B. 0.921
C. 0.984
D. 0.952

17f. The calibrated standard pressure of a manometer is 2,000 psig. If the actual pressure measurements of a known 2,000 psig source are consistently 2,080 psig, what should be the correction factor for the manometer?

A. 0.962
B. 1.021
C. 1.040
D. 1.064

17g. A 3-L calibration syringe is used for volume calibration in the pulmonary function lab. If the spirometer consistently measures a volume of 3.04 L, what should be the correction factor?

A. 0.991
B. 0.987
C. 1.013
D. 1.022

17h. If the correction factor for a weight scale is 1.04 and the weight measurement records 200 lbs, what is the corrected weight?

A. 188 lbs
B. 192 lbs
C. 200 lbs
D. 208 lbs

» Go to **rtexam.com** for more learning resources

18

Dalton's Law of Partial Pressure

NOTES

Dalton's law, named for the English chemist John Dalton (1766–1844), states that the total pressure exerted by a gas mixture is equal to the sum of the partial pressures of all gases in the mixture. Water vapor is a gas and it exerts water vapor pressure. **Table 18-1** shows the gases that compose the barometric pressure in the absence of water vapor.

In unusual atmospheric environments, individual gas pressures increase in hyperbaric conditions (e.g., hyperbaric chamber, under water below sea level) and decrease in hypobaric conditions (e.g., high altitude).

EQUATION

Total pressure	=	P1 + P2 + P3 + ...
Total pressure	:	Pressure of all gases in mixture
P1	:	Pressure of gas 1 in gas mixture
P2	:	Pressure of gas 2 in gas mixture
P3	:	Pressure of gas 3 in gas mixture
...	:	Pressure of other gases

TABLE 18-1. Gases That Compose the Barometric Pressure

Gas	% of Atmosphere	Partial Pressure of Dry Gas (mm Hg)
Nitrogen (N_2)	78.08	593
Oxygen (O_2)	20.95	159
Argon (Ar)	0.93	7
Carbon Dioxide (CO_2)	0.03	0.2

EXAMPLE

Calculate the P_IO_2 of a gas sample at a barometric pressure (P_B) of 300 mm Hg. ($F_IO_2 = 21\%$)

$$P_IO_2 = F_IO_2 \times P_B$$
$$= 21\% \times 300 \text{ mm Hg}$$
$$= 63 \text{ mm Hg}$$

EXERCISE

What is the calculated P_IO_2 at 3 barometric pressure (2,280 mm Hg)?

[Answer: $P_IO_2 = 479$ mm Hg]

SELF-ASSESSMENT QUESTIONS

18a. The sum of partial pressures exerted by all gases in the atmosphere equals to the barometric pressure. This is a statement of:

A. Dalton's law
B. Henry's law
C. Charles' law
D. Graham's law

18b. On an F_IO_2 of 20.95%, the inspired PO_2 (P_IO_2) is 159 mm Hg at one barometric pressure (760 mm Hg). What is the P_IO_2 if the barometric pressure is doubled to 1,520 mm Hg as in a hyperbaric chamber?

A. 322 mm Hg
B. 318 mm Hg
C. 259 mm Hg
D. 179 mm Hg

18c. The P_IO_2 at 10,000 ft above sea level should be _____ the P_IO_2 at sea level because of the _____ condition at high altitude.

A. higher than; hyperbaric
B. higher than; hypobaric
C. lower than; hyperbaric
D. lower than; hypobaric

18d. The F_IO_2 and P_IO_2 in dry ambient air at sea level are about:

A. 21% and 159 mm Hg
B. 21% and 100 mm Hg
C. 40% and 159 mm Hg
D. 40% and 100 mm Hg

18e. The altitude in Denver Colorado is about 6,000 ft, and the corresponding barometric pressure is 609 mm Hg. What is the P_IO_2? Is it higher or lower than the P_IO_2 at sea level (159 mm Hg)? (Note: F_IO_2 remains 21% and does not change at high altitude.)

A. 164 mm Hg; higher
B. 172 mm Hg; higher
C. 128 mm Hg; lower
D. 140 mm Hg; lower

Go to **rtexam.com** for more learning resources

19

Deadspace to Tidal Volume Ratio (V_D/V_T)

NOTES

V_D/V_T ratio reflects the portion of tidal volume not taking part in gas exchange (i.e., wasted ventilation). A large V_D/V_T ratio indicates ventilation is in excess of perfusion. Emphysema, positive-pressure ventilation, pulmonary embolism, and hypotension are some causes of increased deadspace ventilation.

For patients receiving mechanical ventilation, V_D/V_T ratio of up to 60% is considered acceptable. This value is consistent with a normal V_D/V_T after the patient is weaned off mechanical ventilation and extubated.

EQUATION

$$\frac{V_D}{V_T} = \frac{(P_aCO_2 - P_{\bar{E}}CO_2)}{P_aCO_2}$$

$\dfrac{V_D}{V_T}$: Deadspace to tidal volume ratio in %

P_aCO_2 : Arterial carbon dioxide tension in mm Hg

$P_{\bar{E}}CO_2$: Mixed expired carbon dioxide tension in mm Hg*

NORMAL VALUE

20 to 40% in patients breathing spontaneously

40 to 60% in intubated patients receiving mechanical ventilation

EXAMPLE

Given: P_aCO_2 = 40 mm Hg

$P_{\bar{E}}CO_2$ = 30 mm Hg

Calculate the V_D/V_T ratio.

$$\frac{V_D}{V_T} = \frac{(P_aCO_2 - P_{\bar{E}}CO_2)}{P_aCO_2}$$

$$= \frac{40 - 30}{40}$$

$$= \frac{10}{40}$$

$$= 0.25 \text{ or } 25\%$$

EXERCISE

Given: P_aCO_2 = 30 mm Hg

$P_{\bar{E}}CO_2$ = 15 mm Hg

Calculate the V_D/V_T ratio.

[Answer: V_D/V_T = 0.50 or 50%]

* $P_{\bar{E}}CO_2$ is measured by analyzing the PCO_2 of a sample of expired gas collected on the exhalation port of the ventilator circuit or via a one-way valve for spontaneously breathing patients. A 5-L bag can be used for sample collection. To prevent contamination of the gas sample, sigh breaths should not be included in this sample and exhaled gas should be completely isolated from the patient circuit. The P_aCO_2 is measured by analyzing an arterial blood gas sample obtained while collecting the exhaled gas sample.

SELF-ASSESSMENT QUESTIONS

19a. A mixed, expired gas sample is required for calculation of:

A. $I:E$ ratio
B. air entrainment ratio
C. V_D/V_T ratio
D. cardiac index

19b. The deadspace to tidal volume ratio (V_D/V_T) requires measurements of:

A. arterial and mixed expired PO_2
B. arterial and mixed expired PCO_2
C. arterial and mixed venous PO_2
D. arterial and mixed venous PCO_2

19c. For intubated patients on mechanical ventilation, it is acceptable to have a V_D/V_T ratio of up to:

A. 30%
B. 40%
C. 50%
D. 60%

19d. Given: $P_aCO_2 = 35$ mm Hg, $P_{\bar{E}}CO_2 = 20$ mm Hg, $P_aO_2 = 80$ mm Hg, pH = 7.45. What is the V_D/V_T ratio?

A. 43%
B. 41%
C. 38%
D. 33%

19e. A mechanically ventilated patient has the following measurements: $P_aCO_2 = 45$ mm Hg, $P_{\bar{E}}CO_2 = 25$ mm Hg. What is the patient's deadspace to tidal volume ratio? Is it normal?

A. 44%; normal
B. 44%; abnormal
C. 55%; normal
D. 55%; abnormal

Density (D) of Gases

EQUATION

$$D = \frac{gmw \text{ (g)}}{22.4 \text{ (L)}}$$

D : Density of gas in g/L
gmw : Gram molecular weight in g*

EXAMPLE 1

Calculate the density of carbon dioxide (CO_2).

$$D = \frac{gmw \text{ (g)}}{22.4 \text{ (L)}}$$

$$= \frac{\text{atomic weight of C} + (\text{atomic weight of O} \times 2)}{22.4}$$

$$= \frac{12 + (16 \times 2)}{22.4}$$

$$= \frac{12 + 32}{22.4}$$

$$= \frac{44}{22.4}$$

$$= 1.96 \text{ g/L}$$

EXAMPLE 2

Calculate the density of air (21% O_2, 78% N_2, 1% Ar).

$$D = \frac{gmw \text{ (g)}}{22.4 \text{ (L)}}$$

$$= \frac{0.21 \times (\text{wt. of O} \times 2) + 0.78 \times (\text{wt. of N} \times 2) + 0.01 \times (\text{wt. of Ar})}{22.4}$$

$$= \frac{0.21 \times (16 \times 2) + 0.78 \times (14 \times 2) + 0.01 \times (40)}{22.4}$$

$$= \frac{0.21 \times 32 + 0.78 \times 28 + 0.01 \times 40}{22.4}$$

$$= \frac{6.72 + 21.84 + 0.4}{22.4}$$

$$= \frac{28.96}{22.4}$$

$$= 1.29 \text{ g/L}$$

gmw = Atomic weight × Number of atoms per molecule

EXERCISE 1

Use **Figure 20-1** Periodic Table of Common Elements and find the atomic weight and gram molecular weight (*gmw*) of oxygen (O_2).

[Answer: Atomic weight of O = 16 g; *gmw* of O_2 = 32 g]

EXERCISE 2

What is the density (D) of oxygen (O_2)?

[Answer: D = 1.429 g/L]

EXERCISE 3

Calculate the density of a gas mixture of 70% helium (He) and 30% oxygen (O_2).

[Answer: D = 0.554 g/L]

SELF-ASSESSMENT QUESTIONS

20a. Calculate the density of nitrogen (N_2) given the atomic weight for nitrogen (N) is 14.

A. 0.31 g/L
B. 0.63 g/L
C. 1.25 g/L
D. 2.5 g/L

20b. Given: atomic weight of helium (He) = 4 g. What is its gas density?

A. 0.18 g/L
B. 1.8 g/L
C. 18 g/L
D. 4 g/L

20c. Calculate the density of carbon dioxide (CO_2) given that the atomic weights for carbon and oxygen are 12 and 16, respectively.

A. 1.48 g/L
B. 1.61 g/L
C. 1.75 g/L
D. 1.96 g/L

20d. Calculate the density of a helium/oxygen mixture (80% He, 20% O_2). The atomic weights for helium and oxygen are 4 and 16, respectively.

A. 0.43 g/L
B. 0.55 g/L
C. 0.68 g/L
D. 0.79 g/L

20e. Which of the following gas element/molecules is the most dense? N_2, CO, O_2, or CO_2? Calculate and report their densities. The molecular weights for N_2, CO, O_2, and CO_2 are 28, 28, 32, and 44, respectively.

A. N_2: 1.25 g/L
B. CO: 1.25 g/L
C. O_2: 1.43 g/L
D. CO_2: 1.96 g/L

20f. Refer to Figure 20-1; the atomic mass (weight) of oxygen (O) is:

A. 8 g/mol
B. 16 g/mol
C. 24 g/mol
D. Insufficient information to obtain answer

20g. Refer to Figure 20-1; what is the molecular mass (weight) of an oxygen (O_2) molecule?

A. 8 g/mol
B. 16 g/mol
C. 32 g/mol
D. Insufficient information to obtain answer

20h. Refer to Figure 20-1; what is the density of oxygen (O_2) molecule?

A. 1.256 g/L
B. 1.429 g/L
C. 1.503 g/L
D. 1.772 g/L

Go to **rtexam.com** for more learning resources

Periodic Table of Common Elements

1 IA 1A																		18 VIIIA 8A
1 H hydrogen 1.008	2 IIA 2A											13 IIIA 3A	14 IVA 4A	15 VA 5A	16 VIA 6A	17 VIIA 7A	**2 He** helium 4.003
3 Li lithium 6.941	**4 Be** beryllium 9.012												**5 B** boron 10.811	**6 C** carbon 12.011	**7 N** nitrogen 14.007	**8 O** oxygen 15.999	**9 F** fluorine 18.998	**10 Ne** neon 20.180
11 Na sodium 22.990	**12 Mg** magnesium 24.305	3 IIIB 3B	4 IVB 4B	5 VB 5B	6 VIB 6B	7 VIIB 7B	8 VIII 8	9 VIII 8	10	11 IB 1B	12 IIB 2B		**13 Al** aluminum 26.982	**14 Si** silicon 28.086	**15 P** phosphorus 30.974	**16 S** sulfur 32.066	**17 Cl** chlorine 35.453	**18 Ar** argon 39.948
19 K kalium 39.098	**20 Ca** calcium 40.078	**21 Sc** scandium 44.956	**22 Ti** titanium 47.88	**23 V** vanadium 50.942	**24 Cr** chromium 52.996	**25 Mn** manganese 54.938	**26 Fe** iron 55.933	**27 Co** cobalt 58.933	**28 Ni** nickel 58.693	**29 Cu** copper 63.546	**30 Zn** zinc 65.39	**31 Ga** gallium 69.732	**32 Ge** germanium 72.61	**33 As** arsenic 74.922	**34 Se** selenium 78.972	**35 Br** bromine 79.904	**36 Kr** krypton 84.80
37 Rb rubidium 84.468	**38 Sr** strontium 87.62	**39 Y** yttrium 88.906	**40 Zr** zirconium 91.224	**41 Nb** niobium 92.906	**42 Mo** molybdenum 95.95	**43 Tc** technetium 98.907	**44 Ru** ruthenium 101.07	**45 Rh** rhodium 102.906	**46 Pd** palladium 106.42	**47 Ag** silver 107.868	**48 Cd** cadmium 112.411	**49 In** indium 114.818	**50 Sn** tin 118.71	**51 Sb** antimony 121.760	**52 Te** tellurium 127.6	**53 I** iodine 126.901	**54 Xe** xenon 131.29
55 Cs caesium 132.905	**56 Ba** barium 137.327	57–71	**72 Hf** hafnium 178.49	**73 Ta** tantalum 180.948	**74 W** tungsten 183.85	**75 Re** rhenium 186.207	**76 Os** osmium 190.23	**77 Ir** iridium 192.22	**78 Pt** platinum 195.08	**79 Au** gold 196.967	**80 Hg** mercury 200.59	**81 Tl** thallium 204.383	**82 Pb** lead 207.2	**83 Bi** bismuth 208.980	**84 Po** polonium [208.982]	**85 At** astatine 209.987	**86 Rn** radon 222.018
87 Fr francium 223.020	**88 Ra** radium 226.025	89–103	**104 Rf** rutherfordium [261]	**105 Db** dubnium [262]	**106 Sg** seaborgium [266]	**107 Bh** bohrium [264]	**108 Hs** hassium [269]	**109 Mt** meitnerium [268]	**110 Ds** darmstadtium [269]	**111 Rg** roentgenium [272]	**112 Cn** copernicium [277]	**113 Nh** nihonium [286]	**114 Fl** flerovium [289]	**115 Mc** moscovium [290]	**116 Lv** livermorium [293]	**117 Ts** tennessine [294]	**118 Og** oganesson [294]

57 La lanthanum 138.91	**58 Ce** cerium 140.12	**59 Pr** praseodymium 140.91	**60 Nd** neodymium 144.24	**61 Pm** promethium [145]	**62 Sm** samarium 150.36	**63 Eu** europium 151.96	**64 Gd** gadolinium 157.25	**65 Tb** terbium 158.93	**66 Dy** dysprosium 162.50	**67 Ho** holmium 164.93	**68 Er** erbium 167.26	**69 Tm** thulium 168.93	**70 Yb** ytterbium 173.05	**71 Lu** lutetium 174.97
89 Ac actinium [227]	**90 Th** thorium 232.04	**91 Pa** protactinium 231.04	**92 U** uranium 238.03	**93 Np** neptunium [237]	**94 Pu** plutonium [244]	**95 Am** americium [243]	**96 Cm** curium [247]	**97 Bk** berkelium [247]	**98 Cf** californium [251]	**99 Es** einsteinium [252]	**100 Fm** fermium [257]	**101 Md** mendelevium [258]	**102 No** nobelium [259]	**103 Lr** lawrencium [262]

FIGURE 20-1. The Periodic Table of Common Elements

21

Dosage – IV Infusion Dosage Based on Infusion Rate (mcg/kg/min)

EQUATION

Infusion dosage = Dosage desired × Body weight

Infusion dosage : Amount of drug infused in mcg/min or mcg/hr
Dosage desired : Amount of drug ordered in mcg
Body weight : Body weight in kg

NORMAL VALUE Not applicable

EXAMPLE

An order reads continuous IV infusion of dopamine at 2 mcg/kg/min to keep systolic blood pressure ≥ 100 mm Hg. The patient's body weight is 150 lbs. Calculate the infusion dosage in mcg/min and mcg/hr.

(Step 1) Change body weight to kg

$$150 \text{ lbs} = (150/2.2) \text{ kg}$$
$$= 68 \text{ kg}$$

(Step 2) Infusion dosage = Dosage desired × Body weight
$$= 2 \text{ mcg/kg/min} \times 68 \text{ kg}$$
$$= 136 \text{ mcg/min}$$

(Step 3) 136 mcg/min = 136 × 60 mcg/60 min (multiply numerator and denominator by 60)
$$= 8,160 \text{ mcg/hr or } 8.16 \text{ mg/hr}$$

EXERCISE

A 200 mL IV solution contains 160 mg of dopamine. The desired infusion rate for a 200-lb patient is 5 mcg/kg/min. Calculate the infusion dosage in mcg/min and mcg/hr.

[Answer: 455 mcg/min or 27,300 mcg/hr]

SELF-ASSESSMENT QUESTIONS

21a. Given: body weight 83 kg, infusion rate 16 mcg/kg/min. Calculate the infusion dosage in mcg/min.

    A. 99 mcg/min
    B. 1,328 mcg/min
    C. 2,008 mcg/min
    D. 2,518 mcg/min

21b. The infusion rate of dopamine for a 130-lb (59-kg) patient is 5 mcg/kg/min. Calculate the infusion dosage in mcg/min and mcg/hr.

    A. 295 mcg/min or 17,700 mcg/hr (17.7 mg/hr)
    B. 310 mcg/min or 18,600 mcg/hr (18.6 mg/hr)
    C. 322 mcg/min or 19,320 mcg/hr (19.32 mg/hr)
    D. 337 mcg/min or 20,200 mcg/hr (20.2 mg/hr)

21c. A 160-lb (73-kg) patient is to receive an IV infusion of dobutamine at a rate of 5 mcg/kg/min. What is the infusion dosage in mcg/min and mcg/hr?

    A. 185 mcg/min or 11,100 mcg/hr (11.1 mg/hr)
    B. 220 mcg/min or 13,200 mcg/hr (13.2 mg/hr)
    C. 365 mcg/min or 21,900 mcg/hr (21.9 mg/hr)
    D. 800 mcg/min or 48,000 mcg/hr (48 mg/hr)

21d. A patient is receiving an infusion dose of nesiritide (Netrecor) for heart failure at a rate of 0.01 mcg/kg/min. Since the patient's body weight is 140 lbs, what is the infusion dosage in mcg/min?

    A. 0.014 mcg/min
    B. 1.4 mcg/min
    C. 0.064 mcg/min
    D. 0.64 mcg/min

21e. Ms. Worth, a 130-lb patient, is receiving a continuous infusion of fentanyl for pain management. The infusion rate is 1 mcg/kg/hr. What is the infusion dosage of fentanyl per hour?

    A. 59 mcg/hr
    B. 65 mcg/hr
    C. 82 mcg/hr
    D. 130 mcg/hr

21f. The infusion rate of dopamine ranges from 2 to 10 mcg/kg/min. For a 150-lb patient, what is the *range* of infusion dosage?

A. 108 mcg/min to 540 mcg/min
B. 114 mcg/min to 570 mcg/min
C. 122 mcg/min to 610 mcg/min
D. 136 mcg/min to 680 mcg/min

21g. The maintenance infusion rate of propofol is 0.1 to 0.2 mg/kg/min. What is the *range* of infusion dosage for a 110-lb patient?

A. 1 mg/min to 2 mg/min
B. 5 mg/min to 10 mg/min
C. 10 mg/min to 20 mg/min
D. 50 mg/min to 100 mg/min

Go to **rtexam.com** for more learning resources

22

Dosage – IV Infusion Dosage Based on Infusion Rate (mL/hr or mL/min)

EQUATION

Infusion dosage = IV drug concentration × Infusion rate

Infusion dosage	: Amount of drug infused in mcg/min or mcg/hr
IV drug concentration	: Available concentration of drug solution in mcg/mL or mg/mL
Infusion rate	: Desired infusion rate in mL/hr or mL/min

NORMAL VALUE Not applicable.

EXAMPLE 1 (mg/hr)

A dopamine IV solution has a concentration of 400 mg in 500 mL of D5W. The desired infusion rate is 30 mL/hr. At this infusion rate, what is the infusion dosage of dopamine per *hour*?

Infusion dosage = IV drug concentration × Infusion rate

$$= \frac{400 \text{ mg}}{500 \text{ mL}} \times \frac{30 \text{ mL}}{\text{hr}}$$

$$= \frac{12,000}{500}$$

$$= 24 \text{ mg/hr or } 24,000 \text{ mcg/hr}$$

At an infusion rate of 30 mL/hr, the infusion dosage of dopamine is 24 mg/hr.

EXAMPLE 2 (mg/min)

A dopamine IV solution has a concentration of 400 mg in 500 mL of D5W. The desired infusion rate is 30 mL/hr. At this infusion rate, what is the infusion dosage of dopamine per *minute*?

Refer to Example 1, 24 mg of dopamine are infusion at an infusion rate of 30 mL/hr. To change the infused dosage per *minute*, divide the answer by 60 (i.e., one hr = 60 minutes)

Infusion dosage/min = 24 mg/60

$$= 0.4 \text{ mg/min or } 400 \text{ mcg/min}$$

NOTES

To change mg to mcg, multiple mg by 1,000.

To change infusion dosage per hr to per min, divide infusion dosage by 60.

Example 1 shows the answer in mg/hr. See below for the conversion of units from equation to answer.

$$\frac{400 \text{ mg}}{500 \text{ mL}} \times \frac{30 \text{ mL}}{\text{hr}} = 24 \text{ mg/hr}$$

EXERCISE

A dopamine IV solution has a concentration of 800 mg in 500 mL of D5W. The infusion rate is set at 20 mL/hr. At this infusion rate, calculate the infusion dosage of dopamine (A) per hour and (B) per minute.

[Answer: (A) 32 mg/hr or 32,000 mcg/hr; (B) 0.533 mg/min or 533 mcg/min]

SELF-ASSESSMENT QUESTIONS

22a. An IV solution contains 5 mg of drug in 200 mL of D5W. It is being infused at a rate of 60 mL/hr, calculate the infusion dosage of this drug in mcg per hour and mcg per minute. (Hint: change 5 mg to 5,000 mcg)

A. 800 mcg/hr or 13.3 mcg/min
B. 1,000 mcg/hr or 16.7 mcg/min
C. 1,200 mcg/hr or 20 mcg/min
D. 1,500 mcg/hr or 25 mcg/min

22b. The concentration of an epinephrine solution is 1 mg in 1,000 mL. This intravenous solution is infused at a rate of 120 mL/hr. At this infusion rate, calculate the infusion dosage of epinephrine in mcg per hour and mcg per minute.

A. 120 mcg/hr or 2 mcg/min
B. 180 mcg/hr or 3 mcg/min
C. 240 mcg/hr or 4 mcg/min
D. 300 mcg/hr or 5 mcg/min

22c. A 1,000 mL IV solution contains 1 mg of epinephrine. This solution is being infused at a rate of 240 mL/hr. What is the infusion dosage of epinephrine in mcg per hour and per minute?

A. 120 mcg/hr or 2 mcg/min
B. 180 mcg/hr or 3 mcg/min
C. 240 mcg/hr or 4 mcg/min
D. 300 mcg/hr or 5 mcg/min

22d. A 100-mL IV solution contains 50 mcg of fentanyl. When this solution is infused at a rate of 50 mL per hour, what is the infusion dosage in mcg per hour and per minute?

A. 15 mcg/hr or 0.25 mcg/min
B. 25 mcg/hr or 0.42 mcg/min
C. 50 mcg/hr or 0.83 mcg/min
D. 100 mcg/hr or 1.67 mcg/min

22e. A 200-mL IV solution is mixed with 50 mcg of fentanyl. The infusion rate is set at 60 mL/hr. Calculate the infusion dosage in mcg per hour and mcg per minute.

    A. 15 mcg/hr or 0.25 mcg/min
    B. 25 mcg/hr or 0.42 mcg/min
    C. 50 mcg/hr or 0.83 mcg/min
    D. 100 mcg/hr or 1.67 mcg/min

22f. A nitroglycerin IV solution has a concentration of 25 mg in 500 mL of 0.9% saline. At an infusion rate of 60 mL/hr, calculate the infusion dosage in mcg/hr and mcg/min.

    A. 1,800 mcg/hr or 30 mcg/min
    B. 2,400 mcg/hr or 40 mcg/min
    C. 3,000 mcg/hr or 50 mcg/min
    D. 3,600 mcg/hr or 60 mcg/min

22g. An IV solution contains 50 mg of nitroglycerin in 500 mL of D5W. The infusion rate is set at 120 mL/hr. What is the infusion dose of nitroglycerin in mcg/hr and mcg/min?

    A. 9,000 mcg/hr or 150 mcg/min
    B. 12,000 mcg/hr or 200 mcg/min
    C. 15,000 mcg/hr or 250 mcg/min
    D. 18,000 mcg/hr or 300 mcg/min

Dosage — IV Infusion Rate Based on Drips

23

NOTES

An electronic infusion pump is required to deliver a precise volume of intravenous solution (with or without drugs). If infusion pumps are not available in situations such as mass casualty incidents, power failure or away from hospitals, the IV fluid may be administered by gravity using a tubing drip system. A regular drip system is 10, 12 or 15 drops per mL. A micro drip system is 60 drops per mL.

EQUATION

Drip rate = Infusion rate × Drop factor × Time conversion

Drip rate	: Drops of IV solution in drops/min (gtt/min)
Infusion rate	: Infusion flow rate in mL/hr
Drop factor	: Conversion factor in drops per mL (e.g., 15 gtt/mL; micro drip 60 gtt/mL)
Time conversion	: Conversion between 1 hr and 60 min

NORMAL VALUE Not applicable

EXAMPLE 1 **Regular drip 15 gtt/mL**

An order reads "Administer intravenous (IV) infusion with 1,000 mL of D5W solution over 8 hours." The IV tubing has a drop factor of 15 gtt/mL. Calculate the drip rate.

Drip rate = Infusion rate × Drop factor × Time factor

$$= \frac{1{,}000 \text{ mL}}{8 \text{ hrs}} \times \frac{15 \text{ gtt}}{1 \text{ mL}} \times \frac{1 \text{ hr}}{60 \text{ min}}$$

$$= \frac{15{,}000 \text{ drops}}{480 \text{ min}}$$

$$= 31.25 \text{ or } 31 \text{ drops/min}$$

EXAMPLE 2 **Micro drip 60 gtt/mL**

Using Example 1 with a microdrip system at 60 drops/min. An order reads "Administer intravenous (IV) infusion with 1,000 mL of D5W solution over 8 hours." The IV tubing has a drop factor of 60 gtt/mL. Calculate the drip rate.

Drip rate = Infusion rate × Drop factor × Time factor

$$= \frac{1{,}000 \text{ mL}}{8 \text{ hrs}} \times \frac{60 \text{ gtt}}{1 \text{ mL}} \times \frac{1 \text{ hr}}{60 \text{ min}}$$

$$= \frac{60{,}000 \text{ drops}}{480 \text{ min}}$$

$$= 125 \text{ drops/min}$$

EXERCISE 1   **Regular drip 15 drops/mL**

A patient is to receive 900 mL of D5W over 4 hours. The drip system delivers 15 drops per mL. Calculate the drip rate in drops per min.

Drip rate = Infusion rate × Drop factor × Time factor

$$= \frac{900 \text{ mL}}{4 \text{ hrs}} \times \frac{15 \text{ gtt}}{1 \text{ mL}} \times \frac{1 \text{ hr}}{60 \text{ min}}$$

$$= \frac{13{,}500 \text{ drops}}{240 \text{ min}}$$

$$= 56.25 \text{ or } 56 \text{ drops/min}$$

EXERCISE 2   **Micro drip 60 drops/mL**

A patient is to receive 500 mL of D5W over 8 hours. The drip system delivers 60 drops per mL. Calculate the drip rate in drops per min.

Drip rate = Infusion rate × Drop factor × Time factor

$$= \frac{500 \text{ mL}}{8 \text{ hrs}} \times \frac{60 \text{ gtt}}{1 \text{ mL}} \times \frac{1 \text{ hr}}{60 \text{ min}}$$

$$= \frac{30{,}000 \text{ drops}}{480 \text{ min}}$$

$$= 62.5 \text{ or } 63 \text{ drops/min}$$

SELF-ASSESSMENT QUESTIONS

23a. Using the drip method to deliver intravenous solutions and drugs, the micro drip system delivers:

A. 10 drops/mL
B. 12 drops/mL
C. 15 drops/mL
D. 60 drops/mL

23b. The physician order reads "IV 300 mL of D5W over 2 hours". The drip system delivers 15 drops per mL. Calculate the drip rate in drops per min.

A. 26 drops/min
B. 38 drops/min
C. 42 drops/min
D. 44 drops/min

23c. A patient is to receive 500 mL of D5W over 4 hours. The micro drip system delivers 60 drops per mL. What should be the drip rate in drops per min?

A. 100 drops/min
B. 116 drops/min
C. 125 drops/min
D. 132 drops/min

23d. A 400 mL of 0.9% NaCl solution with KCl added is to be given intravenously over 6 hrs. What is the drip rate if the drip system delivers 20 drops per mL?

A. 22 drops/min
B. 24 drops/min
C. 26 drops/min
D. 28 drops/min

23e. An insulin solution of 40 units in 500 mL is to be given to the patient over 4 hours. What is the drip rate if the drip system delivers 15 drops per mL?

A. 22 drops/min
B. 25 drops/min
C. 28 drops/min
D. 31 drops/min

23f. An order reads "IV 300 mL of D5W over 4 hours". The micro drip system delivers 60 drops per mL. Calculate the drip rate in drops per min for this 300 mL solution.

A. 65 drops/min
B. 70 drops/min
C. 75 drops/min
D. 80 drops/min

23g. The physician has ordered an IV solution with 400 mL of D5W over 2 hours. What is the drip rate if the drip system delivers 12 drops per mL?

A. 40 drops/min
B. 60 drops/min
C. 80 drops/min
D. 100 drops/min

24

Dosage – IV Infusion Rate Based on Infusion Dosage (mcg/min)

EQUATION

$$\text{Infusion rate} = \frac{\text{Infusion dosage}}{\text{IV drug concentration}}$$

Infusion rate : Desired infusion rate in mL/min or mL/hr

Infusion dosage : Amount of drug infused in mcg/min or mcg/hr

IV drug concentration : Available concentration of drug solution in mg/mL or mcg/mL

NORMAL VALUE Not applicable

EXAMPLE An order reads continuous IV infusion of norepinephrine (Levophed) at 4 mcg/min to maintain systolic blood pressure ≥100 mm Hg. The available Levophed concentration is 2 mg of Levophed in 250 mL of D5W solution. Calculate the infusion rate in mL/min and mL/hr.

$$\text{Infusion rate} = \frac{\text{Infusion dosage}}{\text{IV drug concentration}}$$

$$= \frac{4\,\text{mcg/min}}{2\,\text{mg/250 mL}}$$

$$= \frac{4\,\text{mcg/min}}{2{,}000\,\text{mcg/250 mL}} \quad (1\,\text{mg} = 1{,}000\,\text{mcg})$$

$$= \frac{4\,\text{mcg} \times 250\,\text{mL}}{2{,}000\,\text{mcg} \times \text{min}} \quad (\text{cancel out both mcg})$$

$$= \frac{1{,}000\,\text{mL}}{2{,}000\,\text{min}}$$

$$= 0.5\,\text{mL/min or } 30\,\text{mL/hr}$$

(Note: To change mL/min to mL/hr, multiply numerator *and* denominator by 60. 60 min = 1 hr)

NOTES

A fraction consists of two integers (numbers). The number on top of a fraction is the numerator. The number on bottom of a fraction is the denominator.

When dividing a fraction (A) by another fraction (B), there are 2 steps.

Step 1 – Multiply the numerator of fraction A and the denominator of fraction B. This becomes the numerator of the new fraction.

Step 2 – Multiply the denominator of fraction A and the numerator of fraction B. This becomes the denominator of the new fraction.

Example: fraction A is $\frac{3}{4}$ and fraction B is $\frac{1}{2}$.

$$\frac{\frac{3}{4}}{\frac{1}{2}} = \frac{3 \times 2}{4 \times 1} = \frac{6}{4} = 1.5$$

EXERCISE   The physician order reads continuous IV infusion of isoproterenol (Isuprel) at 6 mcg/min. The prepared drug concentration is 2 mg of Isuprel in 250 mL of D5W solution. Calculate the infusion rate in mL/min and mL/hr.

[Answer: 0.75 mL/min or 45 mL/hr]

SELF-ASSESSMENT QUESTIONS

24a.   The available concentration of a fentanyl solution is 50 mcg in 200 mL of D5W. The desired fentanyl infusion dosage is 0.25 mcg/min. What should be the infusion rate in mL/min and mL/hr?

A. 0.1 mL/min or 6 mL/hr
B. 0.5 mL/min or 30 mL/hr
C. 1 mL/min or 60 mL/hr
D. 2 mL/min or 120 mL/hr

24b.   A nitroglycerin IV solution has a concentration of 25 mg in 500 mL of 0.9% saline. For an infusion dosage of 50 mcg/min, calculate the infusion rate in mL/min and mL/hr.

A. 0.5 mL/min or 30 mL/hr
B. 1 mL/min or 60 mL/hr
C. 1.5 mL/min or 90 mL/hr
D. 2 mL/min or 120 mL/hr

24c.   An IV solution contains 50 mg of nitroglycerin in 500 mL of D5W. The desired infusion dosage is 200 mcg/min. Calculate the infusion rate of nitroglycerin in mL/min and mL/hr.

A. 0.5 mL/min or 30 mL/hr
B. 1 mL/min or 60 mL/hr
C. 1.5 mL/min or 90 mL/hr
D. 2 mL/min or 120 mL/hr

24d.   An IV solution contains 5 mg of drug in 500 mL of D5W. The physician order reads continuous infusion at a dosage of 25 mcg/min. What should be the infusion rate in mL/min and mL/hr?

A. 2.5 mL/min or 150 mL/hr
B. 3 mL/min or 180 mL/hr
C. 3.5 mL/min or 210 mL/hr
D. 4 mL/min or 240 mL/hr

24e. The concentration of an epinephrine IV solution is 1 mg in 1,000 mL. This intravenous solution is infused at a dosage of 1 mcg/min. At this infusion dosage, calculate the infusion rate of epinephrine in mL/min and mL/hr.

A. 1 mL/min or 60 mL/hr
B. 1.5 mL/min or 90 mL/hr
C. 2 mL/min or 120 mL/hr
D. 2.5 mL/min or 150 mL/hr

24f. A 1,000 mL IV solution contains 1 mg of epinephrine. The infusion dosage is 4 mcg/min. What is the infusion rate in mL/min and mL/hr?

A. 1 mL/min or 60 mL/hr
B. 2 mL/min or 120 mL/hr
C. 3 mL/min or 180 mL/hr
D. 4 mL/min or 240 mL/hr

24g. A 100-mL IV solution contains 50 mcg of fentanyl. The desired infusion dosage is 0.5 mcg/min. What is the infusion rate in mL/min and mL/hr?

A. 0.5 mL/min or 30 mL/hr
B. 1 mL/min or 60 mL/hr
C. 1.5 mL/min or 90 mL/hr
D. 2 mL/min or 120 mL/hr

25

Dosage – IV Infusion Rate Based on Infusion Dosage by Weight (mcg/kg/min)

A fraction consists of two integers (numbers). The number on top of a fraction is the numerator. The number on bottom of a fraction is the denominator.

When dividing a fraction (A) by another fraction (B), there are 2 steps.

Step 1 – Multiply the numerator of fraction A and the denominator of fraction B. This becomes the numerator of the new fraction.

Step 2 – Multiply the denominator of fraction A and the numerator of fraction B. This becomes the denominator of the new fraction.

Example: fraction A is $\frac{3}{4}$ and fraction B is $\frac{1}{2}$.

$$\frac{\frac{3}{4}}{\frac{1}{2}} = \frac{3 \times 2}{4 \times 1} = \frac{6}{4} = 1.5$$

EQUATION

$$\text{Infusion rate} = \frac{(\text{Infusion dosage} \times \text{Kg})}{\text{IV drug concentration}}$$

Infusion rate	: Desired infusion rate in mL/min or mL/hr
Infusion dosage	: Amount of drug infused in mcg/kg/min
kg	: Body weight in kg
IV drug concentration	: Available concentration of drug solution in mg/mL or mcg/mL

NORMAL VALUE   Not applicable

EXAMPLE

The physician order reads "continuous IV infusion of nitroprusside (Nipride) at 3 mcg/kg/min to keep systolic blood pressure below 140 mm Hg." The available Nipride concentration is 50 mg of Nipride in 250 mL of D5W solution. The patient's weight is 50 kg. Calculate the infusion rate in mL/min and mL/hr.

$$\text{Infusion rate} = \frac{(\text{Infusion dosage} \times \text{Kg})}{\text{IV drug concentration}}$$

$$= \frac{3 \text{ mcg/Kg/min} \times 50 \text{ Kg}}{50 \text{ mg/250 mL}}$$

$$= \frac{150 \text{ mcg/min}}{50,000 \text{ mcg/250 mL}} \quad (1 \text{ mg} = 1,000 \text{ mcg})$$

$$= \frac{150 \text{ mcg} \times 250 \text{ mL}}{50,000 \text{ mcg} \times \text{min}} \quad (\text{cancel out both mcg})$$

$$= \frac{37,500 \text{ mL}}{50,000 \text{ min}}$$

$$= 0.75 \text{ mL/min or } 45 \text{ mL/hr}$$

(Note: To change mL/min to mL/hr, multiply numerator and denominator by 60. 60 min = 1 hr)

EXERCISE The physician order reads "Infuse Nipride at 4 mcg/kg/min to keep systolic blood pressure below 140 mm Hg." The prepared Nipride concentration is 50 mg in 250 mL of D5W. The patient's weight is 70 kg. Calculate the infusion rate in mL/min and mL/hr.

[Answer: 1.4 mL/min or 84 mL/hr]

SELF-ASSESSMENT QUESTIONS

25a. An IV solution contains 20 mg of drug in 100 mL of D5W. The physician order reads continuous infusion at a dosage of 1 mcg/kg/min for the 80-kg patient. What should be the infusion rate in mL/min and mL/hr?

A. 0.1 mL/min or 6 mL/hr
B. 0.2 mL/min or 12 mL/hr
C. 0.3 mL/min or 18 mL/hr
D. 0.4 mL/min or 24 mL/hr

25b. An IV solution has 10 mg of propofol (Diprivan) in 50 mL of saline. It is to be infused at a rate of 0.005 mg/kg/min for a 70-kg patient. Calculate the infusion rate in mL/min and mL/hr.

A. 0.5 mL/min or 30 mL/hr
B. 1 mL/min or 60 mL/hr
C. 1.75 mL/min or 105 mL/hr
D. 2.25 mL/min or 135 mL/hr

25c. The concentration of dobutamine (Dobutrex) is 500 mg in 250 mL of D5W. An 80-kg patient is to receive the infusion at 5 mcg/kg/min. What should be the infusion rate in mL/min and mL/hr?

A. 0.2 mL/min or 12 mL/hr
B. 0.5 mL/min or 30 mL/hr
C. 1 mL/min or 60 mL/hr
D. 1.5 mL/min or 90 mL/hr

25d. A milrinone (Primacor) IV solution has a concentration of 200 mcg in 200 mL of solution. The infusion dosage for a 50-kg patient is 0.25 mcg/kg/min. Calculate the infusion rate in mL/min and mL/hr.

A. 6 mL/min or 360 mL/hr
B. 8.5 mL/min or 510 mL/hr
C. 10 mL/min or 600 mL/hr
D. 12.5 mL/min or 750 mL/hr

25e. An IV solution contains 1.5 mg nesiritide (Natrecor) in 250 mL of D5W. The desired infusion dosage is 0.01 mcg/kg/min. Calculate the infusion rate for a 60-kg patient in mL/min and mL/hr.

 A. 0.1 mL/min or 6 mL/hr
 B. 0.5 mL/min or 30 mL/hr
 C. 1 mL/min or 60 mL/hr
 D. 1.5 mL/min or 90 mL/hr

25f. The concentration of a dopamine IV solution is 400 mg in 250 mL. An 80-kg patient is to receive an infusion dose of 10 mcg/kg/min. At this infusion dosage, calculate the infusion rate of dopamine in mL/min and mL/hr.

 A. 0.25 mL/min or 15 mL/hr
 B. 0.5 mL/min or 30 mL/hr
 C. 1 mL/min or 60 mL/hr
 D. 1.5 mL/min or 90 mL/hr

25g. The physician order for a 60-kg patient reads "Nipride at 2 mcg/kg/min to keep systolic blood pressure below 140 mm Hg." The Nipride concentration is 50 mg in 250 mL of D5W. Calculate the infusion rate in mL/min and mL/hr.

 A. 0.3 mL/min or 18 mL/hr
 B. 0.6 mL/min or 36 mL/hr
 C. 1 mL/min or 60 mL/hr
 D. 2 mL/min or 120 mL/hr

26

[Handwritten at top: $1\% = \dfrac{1\,gram}{100\,ml} \rightarrow \dfrac{1,000\,mg}{100\,ml}$ $10\,mg/ml$]

Dosage for Aerosol Therapy: Percent (%) Solutions

EQUATION 1	Dosage = Volume used × Concentration of original solution

EQUATION 2

$$\text{Volume} = \frac{\text{Dosage desired}}{\text{Concentration of original solution}}$$

EXAMPLE 1

How many mg of isoproterenol are in 0.5 mL of a 1:100 (1%) drug solution?

SOLUTION A. [This calculation gives the answer in g. It may be converted to mg.]

Dosage = Volume used × Concentration of original solution
   = 0.5 × 1%
   = 0.5 × 0.01
   = 0.005 g (or 5 mg)

SOLUTION B. [This calculation gives the answer in mg.]

The 1:100 or 1% solution is same as 10 mg/mL as shown below:

$$1\% = \frac{1\,g}{100\,mL}$$

[Handwritten: $\cdot 10$ $10g = 1,000\,mL$]

$$= \frac{1,000\,mg}{100\,mL}$$

$$= 10\,mg/mL$$

Dosage = Volume used × Concentration of original solution
   = 0.5 mL × 1%
   = 0.5 mL × 10 mg/mL
   = 5 mg

EXAMPLE 2

An isoproterenol solution has a concentration of 1:200. How much volume is needed to obtain 2.5 mg of active ingredient?

$$\text{Volume} = \frac{\text{Dosage desired}}{\text{Concentration of original solution}}$$

$$= \frac{2.5\,mg}{1:200}$$

$$= \frac{2.5 \text{ mg}}{(1\text{g}/200 \text{ mL})}$$

$$= \frac{2.5 \text{ mg}}{(1{,}000 \text{ mg}/200 \text{ mL})}$$

$$= \frac{2.5 \text{ mg}}{5 \text{ mg/mL}}$$

$$= 0.5 \text{ mL}$$

EXERCISE 1	How many mg of active ingredient are in 0.5 mL of a 0.5% albuterol sulfate solution?
	[Answer: Dosage = 2.5 mg]

EXERCISE 2	How much of a 0.5% drug solution is needed to obtain 5 mg of active ingredient?
	[Answer: Volume = 1 mL]

SELF-ASSESSMENT QUESTIONS

26a. A 1:1,000 (0.1%) drug solution is same as:

A. 0.1 mg/mL
B. 1 mg/mL
C. 10 mg/mL
D. 100 mg/mL

26b. How many mg of active ingredient are present in 0.5 mL of a 1:100 (1%) drug solution?

A. 5 mg
B. 10 mg
C. 15 mg
D. 20 mg

26c. How many mg of active ingredient are in 1 mL of a 1:200 drug solution?

A. 1 mg
B. 2 mg
C. 5 mg
D. 10 mg

26d. A 30-mL stock bottle of racemic epinephrine has a concentration of 2.25%. How much volume should be drawn from the bottle if 10 mg of the active ingredient are needed?

A. 0.12 mL

B. 0.25 mL

C. 0.36 mL

D. 0.44 mL

26e. How many mg of active ingredient are present in 0.25 mL of a 2.25% racemic epinephrine solution?

A. 5.6 mg

B. 6.4 mg

C. 7.2 mg

D. 8.8 mg

26f. How much of a 0.5% drug solution is needed for 5 mg of active ingredient?

A. 0.25 mL

B. 0.5 mL

C. 1 mL

D. 1.5 mL

26g. A stock bottle of acetylcysteine (Mucomyst) has a concentration of 10%. How many mg of active ingredient are present if 2 mL of this drug are used?

A. 5 mg

B. 10 mg

C. 20 mg

D. 200 mg

26h. How much of a 20% solution of acetylcysteine (Mucomyst) is needed for 400 mg of active ingredient?

A. 0.2 mL

B. 2 mL

C. 20 mL

D. 200 mL

Dosage for Aerosol Therapy: Unit Dose

NOTES

In dosage calculation, 1% means 1 g of drug (active ingredient) in 100 mL of solution. A 1% solution is same as 10 mg/mL. See below:

1% = 1 g in 100 mL = 1,000 mg in 100 mL = 10 mg in 1 mL

[Shortcut: multiple the number of % by 10 to get _____ mg/mL.
For example, 5% = 5x10 mg/mL = 50 mg/mL]

EQUATION 1

Dosage = Volume used × Concentration of unit dose

EQUATION 2

$$\text{Volume} = \frac{\text{Dosage desired}}{\text{Concentration of unit dose}}$$

EXAMPLE 1

A 2.5 mL unit dose of drug has a concentration of 0.2%. How many mg of active ingredient are in this unit dose?

SOLUTION A. [This calculation gives an answer in g. It may be converted to mg.]

$$
\begin{aligned}
\text{Dosage} &= \text{Volume used} \times \text{Concentration of unit dose} \\
&= 2.5 \text{ mL} \times 0.2\% \\
&= 2.5 \text{ mL} \times 0.002 \text{ g/mL} \\
&= 0.005 \text{ g (or 5 mg)}
\end{aligned}
$$

SOLUTION B. [This calculation gives an answer in mg.]

The 0.2% solution can be rewritten as follows:

$$
\begin{aligned}
0.2\% &= \frac{0.2 \text{ g}}{100 \text{ mL}} \\
&= \frac{200 \text{ mg}}{100 \text{ mL}} \\
&= 2 \text{ mg/mL}
\end{aligned}
$$

$$
\begin{aligned}
\text{Dosage} &= \text{Volume used} \times \text{Concentration of unit dose} \\
&= 2.5 \text{ mL} \times 0.2\% \\
&= 2.5 \text{ mL} \times 2 \text{ mg/mL} \\
&= 5 \text{ mg}
\end{aligned}
$$

EXAMPLE 2

A unit dose of albuterol sulfate contains 3.0 mL in a 0.83 mg/mL concentration. How many mg of active ingredient are in this unit dose?

$$
\begin{aligned}
\text{Dosage} &= \text{Volume used} \times \text{Concentration of unit dose} \\
&= 3.0 \text{ mL} \times 0.83 \text{ mg/mL} \\
&= 2.49 \text{ or } 2.5 \text{ mg}
\end{aligned}
$$

EXAMPLE 3

A unit dose of albuterol sulfate contains 3.0 mL in a 0.83 mg/mL concentration. How much volume is needed for 1.5 mg of active ingredient?

$$\text{Volume} = \frac{\text{Dosage desired}}{\text{Concentration of unit dose}}$$

$$= \frac{1.5 \text{ mg}}{0.83 \text{ mg/mL}}$$

$$= 1.8 \text{ mL}$$

EXERCISE 1

A 2.5 mL unit dose of drug solution has a concentration of 0.6%. How many mg of active ingredient are in this unit dose? How much active ingredient is in half a unit dose?

[Answer: Dosage = 15 mg; $\frac{1}{2}$ unit dose = 7.5 mg]

EXERCISE 2

A 3.0 mL unit dose of albuterol sulfate has a concentration of 0.042%. What is the total amount of active ingredient in this unit dose?

[Answer: Dosage in 3.0 mL = 1.26 mg]

EXERCISE 3

A 3.0 mL unit dose of albuterol sulfate has a concentration of 0.83 mg/mL. How much of this unit dose should be used if 1.66 mg of active ingredient are needed?

[Answer: Volume of unit dose solution needed = 2 mL]

SELF-ASSESSMENT QUESTIONS

27a. A unit dose of bronchodilator contains 5.0 mL in a 0.5 mg/mL concentration. How much active ingredient is in this unit dose?

A. 0.5 mg
B. 1.0 mg
C. 2.5 mg
D. 5.0 mg

27b. A unit dose of drug contains 2.5 mL in a 0.2% concentration. How many mg of active ingredient are in this unit dose?

A. 0.5 mg
B. 1.25 mg
C. 2.5 mg
D. 5 mg

27c. A unit dose of levalbuterol (Xopenex) contains 3.0 mL in a 0.0417% concentration. How many mg of active ingredient are in this unit dose?

A. 0.125 mg
B. 1.25 mg
C. 12.5 mg
D. 125 mg

27d. A unit dose of levalbuterol (Xopenex) contains 3.0 mL in a 0.0417% concentration. How much *solution* is needed for 2.5 mg of active ingredient?

A. 2 mL
B. 4 mL
C. 6 mL
D. 8 mL

27e. A unit dose of levalbuterol (Xopenex) contains 3.0 mL in a 0.0417% concentration. How many unit doses are needed for 2.5 mg of active ingredient?

A. 2 unit doses
B. 3 unit doses
C. 4 unit doses
D. 5 unit doses

27f. A unit dose of albuterol sulfate contains 3.0 mL in a 0.083% concentration. If eight unit doses are used in a large-volume aerosol treatment, the total amount of active ingredient in the nebulizer is about:

A. 2.5 mg
B. 5 mg
C. 10 mg
D. 20 mg

27g. A 3-mL unit dose of levalbuterol HCl contains 0.63 mg of active ingredient. If 2 unit doses are used, how many mg of active ingredient are used?

A. 1.26 mg
B. 2.40 mg
C. 2.86 mg
D. 3.14 mg

27h. A 0.5 mL unit dose of Racepinephrine inhalation solution has a concentration of 2.25%. What is the dosage in *one* unit dose?

A. 5.63 mg
B. 11.25 mg
C. 22.5 mg
D. 45 mg

27i. A 0.5 mL unit dose of racemic epinephrine inhalation solution has a concentration of 2.25%. What is the dosage in *two* unit doses?

    A. 5.63 mg
    B. 11.25 mg
    C. 45 mg
    D. 22.5 mg

27j. An ipratropium bromide (Atrovent) unit dose contains 2.5 mL in a 0.02% concentration. How many mg of active ingredient are in one unit dose?

    A. 0.25 mg
    B. 0.5 mg
    C. 1 mg
    D. 2 mg

27k. The physician orders two unit doses of ipratropium bromide (Atrovent). If each unit dose contains 2.5 mL in a 0.02% concentration, how many mg of ipratropium bromide (Atrovent) are ordered?

    A. 1 mg
    B. 2 mg
    C. 3 mg
    D. 4 mg

27l. A unit dose of drug solution contains 3 mL in a 0.5% concentration. How many mg of active ingredient are in this unit dose?

    A. 10 mg
    B. 15 mg
    C. 20 mg
    D. 40 mg

27m. A 5-mL unit dose of drug solution has a concentration of 0.1%. How many mg of active ingredient are in this unit dose?

    A. 1 mg
    B. 0.5 mg
    C. 5 mg
    D. 10 mg

» Go to **rtexam.com** for more learning resources

28

Dosage for Children: Young's Rule

NOTES

Young's rule of dosage calculation requires the child's age. It should be used for children ranging from 1 to 12 years of age.

If the child's weight is not in proportion to age, Clark's rule for dosage calculation should be used. See *Dosage for Infants and Children: Clark's Rule*. Since an effective drug dosage varies greatly among individuals and conditions, the calculated dosage must be carefully evaluated before drug administration.

EQUATION

$$\text{Child's dose} = \left[\frac{\text{Age}}{(\text{Age}+12)} \right] \times \text{Adult dose}$$

Child's dose : Estimated child's drug dosage
Age : Age of child in years
Adult dose : Normal adult drug dosage

EXAMPLE

What should be the dosage for an 8-year-old if the adult dose is 50 mg?

$$\text{Child's dose} = \left[\frac{\text{Age}}{(\text{Age}+12)} \right] \times \text{Adult dose}$$

$$= \left[\frac{8}{(8+12)} \right] \times 50 \text{ mg}$$

$$= \left[\frac{8}{20} \right] \times 50 \text{ mg}$$

$$= 0.4 \times 50 \text{ mg}$$

$$= 20 \text{ mg}$$

EXERCISE

If the adult dose is 30 mg, what is the calculated pediatric dose for a 6-year-old patient?

[Answer: Dosage = 10 mg]

SELF-ASSESSMENT QUESTIONS

28a. If the child's age is known and is within the range of 1 to 12 years, the drug dosage for this child can be estimated by using:

A. Golden's rule
B. Fried's rule
C. Clark's rule
D. Young's rule

28b. If the drug dosage for an adult is 15 mg, what is the pediatric dosage for a 6-year-old patient using Young's rule for dosage calculation?

    A. 1 mg
    B. 2 mg
    C. 5 mg
    D. 10 mg

28c. Using Young's rule of dosage calculation for children, what should be the dosage for a 5-year-old child if the adult dose of a medication is 10 mg?

    A. 1.88 or 1.9 mg
    B. 2.12 or 2.1 mg
    C. 2.58 or 2.6 mg
    D. 2.94 or 2.9 mg

28d. If the adult dosage of a medication is 25 mg, what should be the dosage for a 10-year-old child based on Young's rule?

    A. 11.36 or 11 mg
    B. 12.41 or 12 mg
    C. 13.09 or 13 mg
    D. 14.44 or 14 mg

28e. An adult dose of a liquid decongestant is 3 mL. Using Young's Rule, what should be the dosage for a 6 year-old child?

    A. 0.5 mL
    B. 1 mL
    C. 1.5 mL
    D. 2 mL

28f. Young's rule for dosage calculation is based on a child's:

    A. age
    B. weight
    C. height
    D. height and weight

28g. Young's rule is suitable for children up to a(n):

    A. weight of 80 lbs
    B. height of 36 inches
    C. age of 12 years
    D. grade level of 8th grade

» Go to **rtexam.com** for more learning resources

29

Dosage for Infants and Children: Clark's Rule

NOTES

Clark's rule of dosage calculation requires the infant's or child's weight. Clark's rule can be used in infants or children. It provides a more reasonable estimate of drug dosage than Young's rule when the patient's body weight is not in proportion to age.

Because an effective drug dosage varies greatly among individuals and conditions, the calculated dosage must be carefully evaluated before drug administration.

EQUATION

$$\text{Infant or child's dose} = \left[\frac{\text{Weight in lb}}{150}\right] \times \text{Adult dose}$$

Infant's or child's dose	: Estimated infant's or child's dosage
Weight in lb	: Weight of infant or child in pounds
Adult dose	: Normal adult drug dosage
150	: A constant number

EXAMPLE

What should be the dosage for a 50-lb child if the adult dose is 30 mg?

$$\text{Infant or child's dose} = \left[\frac{\text{Weight in lb}}{150}\right] \times \text{Adult dose}$$

$$= \left[\frac{50}{150}\right] \times 30 \text{ mg}$$

$$= \frac{1}{3} \times 30 \text{ mg}$$

$$= 10 \text{ mg}$$

EXERCISE

If the adult dose is 50 mg, what is the calculated dosage for a 3-lb infant?

[Answer: Dosage = 1 mg]

SELF-ASSESSMENT QUESTIONS

29a. With Clark's rule of dosage calculation for infants and children, what should be the dosage for a 30-lb child if the adult dose is 30 mg?

A. 6 mg
B. 8 mg
C. 10 mg
D. 12 mg

29b. Use Clark's rule of dosage calculation for infants and children to calculate the dosage for a 50-lb child. The normal adult dose is 30 mg.

    A. 2 mg
    B. 5 mg
    C. 10 mg
    D. 20 mg

29c. If the weight of an infant or child is known, the drug dosage for this infant or child can be estimated by using:

    A. Young's rule
    B. Clark's rule
    C. Fried's rule
    D. Pickwick's rule

29d. The adult oral dose for a cough syrup is 10 mL. What should be the dosage for a 20-kg child? (1 kg = 2.2 lb)

    A. 2.9 or 3 mL
    B. 4.1 or 4 mL
    C. 4.9 or 5 mL
    D. 5.8 or 6 mL

29e. Clark's rule for dosage calculation is based on the infant's or child's:

    A. height in inches
    B. height in centimeters
    C. weight in kilogram
    D. weight in pounds

29f. With the Clark's rule for dosage calculation, the dosage would exceed the adult dose when the body weight of a child exceeds:

    A. 80 lbs
    B. 100 lbs
    C. 120 lbs
    D. 150 lbs

29g. The normal adult dose of an over-the-counter analgesic is two tablets. With the Clark's rule, the number of tablets for a 75-lb child should be:

    A. half of a tablet
    B. one tablet
    C. one and a half tablet
    D. two tablets

» Go to **rtexam.com** for more learning resources

30

Dosage for Infants and Children: Fried's Rule

NOTES

Fried's rule of dosage calculation requires the infant's or child's *age in months*.

Fried's rule can be used for infants and children up to two years of age.

If the body weight of the infant or child is not in proportion to age, Clark's rule for dosage calculation should be used.

Since an effective drug dosage varies greatly among individuals and conditions, the calculated dosage must be carefully evaluated before drug administration.

EQUATION

$$\text{Infant or child's dose} = \left(\frac{\text{Age in months}}{150} \right) \times \text{Adult dose}$$

Infant's or child's dose : Estimated infant's or child's dosage
Age in months : Age of infant or child in months, up to 24 months
Adult dose : Normal adult drug dosage
150 : A constant number

EXAMPLE

What should be the dosage for a 15-month-old child if the adult dose is 30 mg?

$$\text{Infant or child's dose} = \left(\frac{\text{Age in months}}{150} \right) \times \text{Adult dose}$$

$$= \left(\frac{15}{150} \right) \times 30 \text{ mg}$$

$$= \frac{1}{10} \times 30 \text{ mg}$$

$$= 3 \text{ mg}$$

EXERCISE

If the adult dose is 50 mg, what is the calculated dosage for a 2-year-old child?

[Answer: Dosage = 8 mg]

SELF-ASSESSMENT QUESTIONS

30a. **Based on Fried's rule, what should be the dosage for a 10-month-old if the adult dose is 60 mg?**

A. 2 mg
B. 4 mg
C. 6 mg
D. 8 mg

30b. Use Fried's rule to estimate the dosage for a 15-month-old infant if the adult dose is 30 mg.

- A. 1 mg
- B. 2 mg
- C. 3 mg
- D. 4 mg

30c. According to Fried's rule, the estimated dosage for a 5-month-old infant based on an adult dose of 30 mg is:

- A. 1 mg
- B. 2 mg
- C. 3 mg
- D. 4 mg

30d. For infants and children up to two years old, the age in months may be used to estimate the drug dosage by using:

- A. Young's rule
- B. Starling's rule
- C. Clark's rule
- D. Fried's rule

30e. Fried's rule of dosage estimation is suitable for individuals under the age of:

- A. 24 months
- B. 36 months
- C. 48 months
- D. 60 months

30f. The adult oral dose for a cough syrup is 10 mL. What should be the dosage for a 24-month-old child?

- A. 1.4 mL
- B. 1.6 mL
- C. 1.8 mL
- D. 2.0 mL

30g. The normal adult dose of an over-the-counter analgesic is 100 mg. Using Fried's rule, what should be the estimated dosage for a 24-month-old child?

- A. 10 mg
- B. 12 mg
- C. 14 mg
- D. 16 mg

» Go to **rtexam.com** for more learning resources

Endotracheal Tube Size for Children

This equation is used to estimate the size of an endotracheal (ET) tube for a child more than one year of age. The calculated size should be adjusted up or down by 0.5 mm for different body sizes. The Broselow tape may also be used to estimate the endotracheal tube size for neonates, children, and adults.

Because ET tubes come in 0.5-mm increments, the estimated ID size should be rounded to the nearest whole or half size.

For neonates, the endotracheal tube size is not calculated. Rather, **Table 31-1** shows the general rule for selecting an endotracheal tube for a neonate.

EQUATION 1

$$ID = \frac{Age + 16}{4}$$

or

EQUATION 2

$$ID = \frac{Height}{20}$$

ID   : Internal diameter of endotracheal tube, in mm
Age   : Age of child over one year of age, in years
Height : Height of child, in cm

EXAMPLE 1

What is the estimated size of an endotracheal tube for a 3-year-old child?

$$ID = \frac{Age + 16}{4}$$

$$= \frac{3 + 16}{4}$$

$$= \frac{19}{4}$$

$$= 4.75 \text{ or } 5.0 \text{ mm}$$

EXAMPLE 2

What is the estimated size of an endotracheal tube for a child who is 4 ft (about 120 cm) tall?

$$ID = \frac{Height \text{ (in cm)}}{20}$$

$$= \frac{120}{20}$$

$$= 6 \text{ mm}$$

TABLE 31-1. Endotracheal Tube Size for Neonates

Body Weight	ET size (ID mm)
<1,000 g	2.5
1,000 to 2,000 g	3.0
2,000 to 3,000 g	3.5
>3,000 g	4.0

EXERCISE 1   Calculate the estimated ET tube size for a 6-year-old child.

[Answer: ID = 5.5 mm]

EXERCISE 2   Calculate the estimated ET tube size for a child 3 ft (about 90 cm) tall.

[Answer: ID = 4.5 mm]

SELF-ASSESSMENT QUESTIONS

31a. Calculate the estimated size of an endotracheal tube for a 2-year-old child.

A. 4 mm
B. 4.5 mm
C. 5 mm
D. 5.5 mm

31b. For an 8-year-old child, the calculated size of an endotracheal tube is about:

A. 5 mm
B. 5.5 mm
C. 6 mm
D. 6.5 mm

31c. Calculate the estimated size of an endotracheal tube for a child who is 3'4" (about 100 cm) tall.

A. 3.5 mm
B. 4 mm
C. 4.5 mm
D. 5 mm

31d. What should be the size of an endotracheal tube for a child who is 2 ft 8 in tall?

A. 3.5 mm
B. 4 mm
C. 4.5 mm
D. 5 mm

31e. Refer to Table 31-1. For a 900-g neonate, the estimated endotracheal tube size is:

A. 2.5 mm

B. 3.0 mm

C. 3.5 mm

D. 4.0 mm

31f. Use Table 31-1 and determine the estimated endotracheal tube size for a 2.2-kg neonate. (1 kg = 1,000 g)

A. 2.5 mm

B. 3.0 mm

C. 3.5 mm

D. 4.0 mm

31g. What is the estimated endotracheal tube size for a 3.5-kg neonate?

A. 2.5 mm

B. 3.0 mm

C. 3.5 mm

D. 4.0 mm

Go to **rtexam.com** for more learning resources

Fick's Law of Diffusion

EQUATION

$$\text{Diffusion} = \frac{A \times D \times \Delta P}{T}$$

Diffusion : Gas diffusion rate

  A : Cross-sectional area of lung membrane

In emphysema, as healthy lung tissues are obliterated, the overall cross-sectional area of the lung parenchyma is reduced. The diffusion rate measured in the pulmonary function laboratory is usually low.

  D : Diffusion coefficient of a gas

Carbon monoxide (CO) is used in gas diffusion studies because of its high diffusion rate and its ability to combine readily with hemoglobin (250 times greater than that of oxygen). CO is known as a diffusion-limited gas because its diffusion rate in the lungs is limited only by conditions in which the cross-sectional area of the lung membrane or the thickness across the lung membrane is affected.

  ΔP : Pressure gradient of a gas

Pressure gradient of a gas is the fundamental principle of gas diffusion and exchange. Gas diffusion in the lungs and in the tissues follows the basic rule of pressure gradient: from an area of high pressure to an area of low pressure. In the pulmonary circulation, oxygen diffuses from alveoli ($P_AO_2 > 100$ mm Hg) to pulmonary capillaries ($P_{\bar{v}}O_2 = 40$ mm Hg), and carbon dioxide diffuses from pulmonary capillaries ($P_{\bar{v}}CO_2 = 46$ mm Hg) to alveoli ($P_ACO_2 = 40$ mm Hg). Oxygen therapy relies on this principle by increasing the pressure gradient of oxygen between the alveoli and pulmonary capillaries. A higher oxygen diffusion gradient facilitates oxygen diffusion into the pulmonary capillaries, and oxygenation of the mixed venous blood is therefore enhanced.

  T : Thickness across lung membrane

Gas diffusion is hindered when the thickness across the lung membrane is increased. Pulmonary or interstitial edema, consolidation, and pulmonary fibrosis are some clinical conditions accompanied by an increase in thickness across the lung membrane. Oxygen therapy is not very effective in these conditions because oxygen, having a low diffusion coefficient, cannot diffuse across these lung units very well.

NOTES

Gas diffusion rate is directly related to the cross-sectional area of the lung membrane, the diffusion coefficient of gas, and the pressure gradient. It is inversely related to the thickness across the lung membrane.

SELF-ASSESSMENT QUESTIONS

32a. The diffusion rate of oxygen across the alveolar-capillary membrane is directly related to all of the following factors, *except*:

A. diffusion coefficient of oxygen
B. cross-sectional area of lung membrane
C. alveolar-capillary pressure gradient of oxygen
D. thickness across lung membrane

32b. In patients with emphysema, the diffusion rate of gases across the alveolar-capillary membrane is lower than normal primarily because of:

A. increased airflow obstruction
B. increased compliance
C. decreased cross-sectional area of lung membrane
D. decreased arterial pH

32c. In a pulmonary function laboratory, the gas diffusion rate is usually measured by using ___ because of its ___ diffusion coefficient.

A. carbon monoxide; high
B. carbon monoxide; low
C. oxygen; high
D. oxygen; low

32d. Under normal conditions, the pressure gradient of oxygen between the arterial and mixed venous blood is about ___ mm Hg, considerably ___ than the pressure gradient of carbon dioxide.

A. 60; lower
B. 60; higher
C. 40; lower
D. 40; higher

32e. A patient with pneumonia has retained a large amount of secretions. This condition hinders gas diffusion and causes hypoxemia as a result of an increase of the:

A. diffusion coefficient of oxygen
B. cross-sectional area of lung membrane
C. pressure gradient of oxygen
D. thickness across lung membrane

» Go to **rtexam.com** for more learning resources

33

F_IO_2 from Two Gas Sources

EQUATION

$$F_IO_2 = \frac{(1st\ F_IO_2 \times 1st\ flow) + (2nd\ F_IO_2 \times 2nd\ flow)}{Total\ flow}$$

F_IO_2 : Inspired oxygen concentration in %
1st F_IO_2 : Oxygen concentration of 1st gas source in %
1st flow : Flow rate of 1st gas source in L/min
2nd F_IO_2 : Oxygen concentration of 2nd gas source in %
2nd flow : Flow rate of 2nd gas source in L/min

This equation is useful when a special oxygen setup involves two gas sources, and an oxygen analyzer is not readily available.

EXAMPLE 1

What is the final F_IO_2 if 8 L/min of air is mixed with 2 L/min of oxygen?

$$F_IO_2 = \frac{(1st\ F_IO_2 \times 1st\ flow) + (2nd\ F_IO_2 \times 2nd\ flow)}{Total\ flow}$$

$$= \frac{(0.21 \times 8) + (1.00 \times 2)}{(8+2)}$$

$$= \frac{1.68 + 2}{10}$$

$$= \frac{3.68}{10}$$

$$= 0.368\ or\ 37\%$$

EXAMPLE 2

If the oxygen:air entrainment ratio is 1:10, what is the F_IO_2?

$$F_IO_2 = \frac{(1st\ F_IO_2 \times 1st\ flow) + (2nd\ F_IO_2 \times 2nd\ flow)}{Total\ flow}$$

$$= \frac{(1.00 \times 1) + (0.21 \times 10)}{(1+10)}$$

$$= \frac{1 + 2.1}{11}$$

$$= \frac{3.1}{11}$$

$$= 0.28\ or\ 28\%$$

EXAMPLE 3   Calculate the F_1O_2 when 6 L/min of 40% oxygen is mixed with 2 L/min of air.

$$F_1O_2 = \frac{\left(\text{1st } F_1O_2 \times \text{1st flow}\right) + \left(\text{2nd } F_1O_2 \times \text{2nd flow}\right)}{\text{Total flow}}$$

$$= \frac{\left(0.40 \times 6\right) + \left(0.21 \times 2\right)}{\left(6 + 2\right)}$$

$$= \frac{2.4 + 0.42}{8}$$

$$= \frac{2.82}{8}$$

$$= 0.353 \text{ or } 35\%$$

EXERCISE 1   If 3 L/min of 28% oxygen is mixed with 6 L/min of air, what is the final F_1O_2?

[Answer: $F_1O_2 = 0.233$ or 23%]

EXERCISE 2   Calculate the F_1O_2 when 6 L/min of 60% oxygen is mixed with 4 L/min of air.

[Answer: $F_1O_2 = 0.444$ or 44%]

SELF-ASSESSMENT QUESTIONS

33a. What is the oxygen concentration if 5 L/min of air is mixed with 5 L/min of oxygen?

    A. 30%
    B. 40%
    C. 50%
    D. 60%

33b. What is the approximate F_1O_2 when 6 L/min of air is mixed with 2 L/min of oxygen?

    A. 30%
    B. 35%
    C. 40%
    D. 45%

33c. Calculate the F_IO_2 when 1 L/min of oxygen is mixed with 4 L/min of air.

    A. 32%
    B. 37%
    C. 41%
    D. 46%

33d. If the oxygen : air entrainment ratio is 1:10, what is F_IO_2?

    A. 22%
    B. 24%
    C. 26%
    D. 28%

33e. Which of the following oxygen : air entrainment ratios provides an F_IO_2 of 60%?

    A. 1:1
    B. 1:2
    C. 1:3
    D. 1:4

33f. If 6 L/min of 28% oxygen is mixed with 6 L/min of room air, what is the combined F_IO_2?

    A. 23%
    B. 25%
    C. 27%
    D. 29%

33g. Calculate the final F_IO_2 when 3 L/min of 60% oxygen is mixed with 3 L/min of room air.

    A. 41%
    B. 43%
    C. 45%
    D. 47%

» Go to **rtexam.com** for more learning resources

34

F_IO_2 Needed for a Desired P_aO_2

NOTES

This two-step calculation is used to estimate the F_IO_2 needed to obtain a desired P_aO_2. This calculation is useful to estimate the F_IO_2 needed in hypoxemia caused by hypoventilation or venous admixture (V/Q mismatch). In severe intrapulmonary shunting, this method is less dependable. In addition to oxygen, positive end-expiratory pressure (PEEP) or continuous positive airway pressure (CPAP) is often needed to correct hypoxemia due to intrapulmonary shunting.

For unusual P_aCO_2 or barometric pressure (P_B), use the F_IO_2 equation below.

$$F_IO_2 = \frac{P_AO_2 \text{ needed} + (P_aCO_2 \times 1.25)}{P_B - 47}$$

EQUATION 1

$$P_AO_2 \text{ needed} = \frac{P_aO_2 \text{ desired}}{a/A \text{ ratio}^*}$$

Arterial/Alveolar Oxygen Tension (a/A) Ratio.

EQUATION 2

$$F_IO_2 = \frac{P_AO_2 \text{ needed} + 50}{713}$$

P_AO_2 needed : Alveolar oxygen tension needed for a desired P_aO_2

P_aO_2 desired : Arterial oxygen tension desired

a/A ratio : Arterial/alveolar oxygen tension ratio in %

F_IO_2 : Inspired oxygen concentration needed to get a desired P_aO_2

EXAMPLE

Given: a/A ratio = 0.55. What should be the F_IO_2 if a P_aO_2 of 100 mm Hg is desired?

(Step 1)

$$P_AO_2 \text{ needed} = \frac{P_aO_2 \text{ desired}}{a/A \text{ ratio}}$$

$$= \frac{100}{0.55}$$

$$= 182 \text{ mm Hg}$$

(Step 2)

$$F_IO_2 \text{ needed} = \frac{P_AO_2 \text{ needed} + 50}{713}$$

$$= \frac{182 + 50}{713}$$

$$= \frac{232}{713}$$

$$= 0.325 \text{ or } 33\%$$

EXERCISE

Given: a/A ratio = 0.30. What should be the F_IO_2 if a P_aO_2 of 80 mm Hg is desired?

[Answer: F_IO_2 = 0.44 or 44%]

SELF-ASSESSMENT QUESTIONS

34a. Given: a/A ratio = 0.35. What should be the F_IO_2 if a P_aO_2 of 100 mm Hg is desired?

    A. 28%
    B. 36%
    C. 40%
    D. 47%

34b. Given: a/A ratio = 0.35. What should be the F_IO_2 if a P_aO_2 of 50 mm Hg is desired?

    A. 27%
    B. 38%
    C. 47%
    D. 55%

34c. The a/A ratio of a patient is 0.80. If a P_aO_2 of 80 mm Hg is desired, what should be the F_IO_2? Is oxygen therapy necessary?

    A. 21%; not necessary
    B. 24%; necessary
    C. 28%; necessary
    D. 32%; necessary

34d. The a/A ratio of a patient is 0.60. If a P_aO_2 of 100 mm Hg is desired, what should be the F_IO_2? Is oxygen therapy necessary?

    A. 21%; not necessary
    B. 30%; necessary
    C. 35%; necessary
    D. 40%; necessary

34e. A patient's a/A ratio is 0.40. What should be the F_IO_2 for a P_aO_2 of 60 mm Hg?

    A. 24%
    B. 28%
    C. 32%
    D. 35%

Go to **rtexam.com** for more learning resources

35

F_IO_2 Needed for a Desired P_aO_2 (COPD patients)

NOTES

This calculation is used to estimate the F_IO_2 needed to obtain a low-range (50 to 60 mm Hg) P_aO_2, a value most suitable for COPD patients with uncomplicated acute exacerbation. This equation requires a recent room air P_aO_2. In this equation, the unit for P_aO_2 (mm Hg) is not used and is replaced by percent (%).

A pulse oximeter may be used to titrate the approximate amount of oxygen suitable for patients with COPD. Under normal conditions, SpO_2 reading of 90% corresponds to a P_aO_2 of 60 mm Hg.

EQUATION

$$F_IO_2 = 21\% + \left[\frac{\left(P_aO_2 \text{ desired } - \text{Room air } P_aO_2\right)}{3}\right]\%$$

F_IO_2 : Inspired oxygen concentration needed to get a desired P_aO_2, in %

P_aO_2 desired : Arterial oxygen tension desired

Room air P_aO_2 : Arterial oxygen tension on 21% oxygen

EXAMPLE

The room air P_aO_2 of a patient with COPD is 45 mm Hg. What should be the F_IO_2 if a P_aO_2 of 60 mm Hg is desired?

$$F_IO_2 = 21\% + \left[\frac{\left(P_aO_2 \text{ desired } - \text{Room air } P_aO_2\right)}{3}\right]\%$$

$$F_IO_2 = 21\% + \left[\frac{(60 - 45)}{3}\right]\%$$

$$= 21\% + \left[\frac{(60 - 45)}{3}\right]\%$$

$$= 21\% + \left[\frac{15}{3}\right]\%$$

$$= 21\% + 5\%$$

$$= 26\%$$

EXERCISE

Given: Room air P_aO_2 = 35 mm Hg. Estimate the F_IO_2 needed for a P_aO_2 of 55 mm Hg.

[Answer: F_IO_2 = 28%]

SELF-ASSESSMENT QUESTIONS

35a. The room air P_aO_2 of a patient with COPD is 40 mm Hg. What should be the F_1O_2 if a P_aO_2 of 60 mm Hg is desired?

    A. 22%
    B. 24%
    C. 26%
    D. 28%

35b. The P_aO_2 of a COPD patient is 40 mm Hg at an F_1O_2 of 21%. If a P_aO_2 of 55 mm Hg is desired, calculate the F_1O_2 needed.

    A. 22%
    B. 24%
    C. 26%
    D. 28%

35c. Given: room air P_aO_2 = 43 mm Hg. Calculate the approximate F_1O_2 needed for a P_aO_2 of 60 mm Hg.

    A. 24%
    B. 27%
    C. 31%
    D. 35%

35d. Calculate the F_1O_2 needed for a P_aO_2 of 55 mm Hg. The room air P_aO_2 for the patient with COPD is 45 mm Hg.

    A. 24%
    B. 27%
    C. 31%
    D. 35%

35e. The typical baseline P_aO_2 for COPD should be maintained between:

    A. 40 and 50 mm Hg
    B. 50 and 60 mm Hg
    C. 60 and 70 mm Hg
    D. 70 and 80 mm Hg

» Go to **rtexam.com** for more learning resources

36

Flow Rate in Mechanical Ventilation

Inadequate inspiratory flow during mechanical ventilation is one of the causes of patient-ventilator dyssynchrony. This equation is used to estimate the *minimum* flow rate required in mechanical ventilation.

The calculated flow rate should be increased when the minute ventilation is increased during SIMV or Assist Mode. In addition, a longer expiratory time would require a higher flow rate.

Unless the minute ventilation stays consistent, the flow rate should be set 10 L/min higher than the calculated flow rate.

EQUATION

Minimum flow rate $= \dot{V}_E \times$ Sum of $I:E$ ratio

Minimum flow rate : Minimum flow rate required to provide desired minute ventilation and $I:E$ ratio, in L/min

$\dot{V}_E$: Expired minute ventilation in L/min $(V_T \times f)$

Sum of $I:E$ ratio : The sum of the inspiratory : expiratory ratio

EXAMPLE

Given: V_T = 700 mL (0.7 L)
f = 16/min
$I:E$ ratio = 1:3

Calculate the minimum flow rate required for the above settings.

Minimum flow rate $= \dot{V}_E \times$ Sum of $I:E$ ratio
$= (V_T \times f) \times$ Sum of $I:E$ ratio
$= (0.7 \times 16) \times (1 + 3)$
$= 11.2 \times 4$
$= 44.8$ or 45 L/min

EXERCISE 1

Given: V_T = 800 mL (0.8 L)
f = 12/min
$I:E$ ratio = 1:3

What is the minimum flow rate needed for the above settings?

[Answer: Minimum flow rate = 38 L/min]

EXERCISE 2

Given: V_T = 600 mL
f = 16/min
$I:E$ ratio = 1:3

Calculate the minimum flow rate for these settings.

[Answer: Minimum flow rate = 38 L/min]

SELF-ASSESSMENT QUESTIONS

36a. If the expired minute ventilation is 12 L/min and an $I:E$ ratio of 1:3 is desired, what should be the *minimum* flow rate required for the above settings?

A. 40 L/min
B. 44 L/min
C. 48 L/min
D. 52 L/min

36b. The expired minute ventilation of a mechanically ventilated patient is 15 L/min. For an $I:E$ ratio of 1:3, what should be the *minimum* flow rate?

A. 45 L/min
B. 50 L/min
C. 55 L/min
D. 60 L/min

36c. The expired minute ventilation during mechanical ventilation is 15 L/min. Calculate the *minimum* flow rate for an $I:E$ ratio of 1:2.

A. 45 L/min
B. 50 L/min
C. 55 L/min
D. 60 L/min

36d. Given: V_T = 750 mL (0.75 L), f = 12/min, $I:E$ ratio = 1:3. What should be the *minimum* flow rate required for the above settings?

A. 36 L/min
B. 40 L/min
C. 44 L/min
D. 48 L/min

36e. Given: V_T = 600 mL, f = 16/min, $I:E$ ratio = 1:3. What should be the *minimum* flow rate needed for these settings?

A. 32 L/min
B. 38 L/min
C. 42 L/min
D. 48 L/min

» Go to **rtexam.com** for more learning resources

Forced Vital Capacity Tracing (FEV$_t$ and FEV$_t$%)

The method to find other FEV$_t$ and FEV$_t$% measurements is the same as shown in Examples 1 and 2. For accurate results, it is extremely important to plot the points on the graph carefully and draw straight lines with a ruler.

The FEV$_{0.5}$ and FEV$_{1.0}$ (as well as FEF$_{200-1200}$) are used to assess the flow rates and disorders relating to the large airways. In patients with large airway obstruction, these values are decreased. However, poor patient effort may also lead to lower than normal results. The FEV$_t$% values are also reduced in patients with obstructive disorders. In patients with restrictive lung disorders, FEV$_t$ measurements are decreased but the FEV$_t$% may be normal or increased because of the concurrent reduction in FEV$_t$ and FVC. When the FVC is reduced in restrictive lung disease, the amount of volume expired in a given time (t) will also be reduced. A lower FEV$_t$ and a lower FVC yields a "normal" FEV$_t$%.

EQUATION

FEV$_t$: Forced Expiratory Volume (timed), in liters (commonly expressed in 0.5 sec, 1 sec, 2 sec, or 3 sec)

FEV$_t$% : Forced Expiratory Volume (timed)/Forced Vital Capacity (FVC), in %

NORMAL VALUES FEV$_t$

$$FEV_{0.5} = 3.1 \text{ L}$$
$$FEV_1 = 4.2 \text{ L}$$
$$FEV_2 = 4.6 \text{ L}$$
$$FEV_3 = 4.8 \text{ L}$$

The FEV$_t$ normal values are based on a 70", 20-year-old male. Since the normal predicted values are based on a person's gender, age, height, weight, smoking history, and ethnic origin, an appropriate normal table should be used to match a person's physical attributes.

FEV$_t$%

$$FEV_{0.5}\% = 50\% \text{ to } 60\%$$
$$FEV_1\% = 75\% \text{ to } 85\%$$
$$FEV_2\% = 94\%$$
$$FEV_3\% = 97\%$$

FEV$_t$% expresses a person's FEV$_t$ in reference to the same person's FVC. The FEV$_t$% normal values list above are standard regardless of gender, age, height, and other physical attributes. For clinical evaluation of lung impairments, an FEV$_1$% of 65% or less is significant and diagnostic of airflow obstruction.

EXAMPLE 1

From the PFT tracing (**Figure 37-1**), find FEV$_{0.5}$.

Step 1. Along the time (x) axis, locate 0.5 sec (point A).

Step 2. From point A, draw a vertical line upward until it intersects the PFT tracing (point B).

Step 3. From point B, draw a horizontal line until it intersects the volume (y) axis (point C).

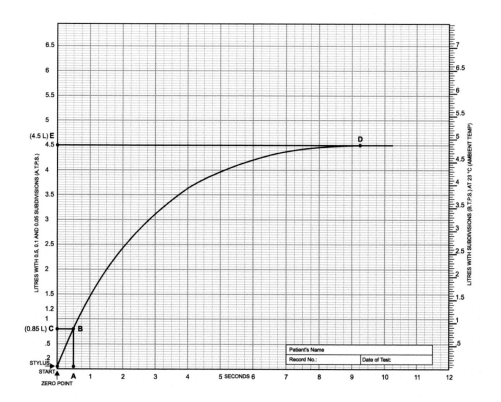

FIGURE 37-1. Examples to find FEV$_{0.5}$ and FEV$_{0.5\%}$.

Step 4. The reading at point C (0.85 L) is the volume expired during the first 0.5 sec of the FVC maneuver.

Therefore, FEV$_{0.5}$ = 0.85 L.

EXAMPLE 2

From the PFT tracing (**Figure 37-1**), find FEV$_{0.5}$%. Is the result normal?

Step 1. From the PFT tracing, locate the highest point at the end of the tracing (point D).

Step 2. From point D, draw a horizontal line until it intersects the volume (y) axis (point E).

Step 3. The reading at point E (4.5 L) represents the FVC.

$$FEV_{0.5}\% = FEV_{0.5}/FVC$$
$$= 0.85\ L/4.5\ L$$
$$= 0.1888$$
$$= 18.9\%$$

FEV$_{0.5}$% of 18.9% is below normal.

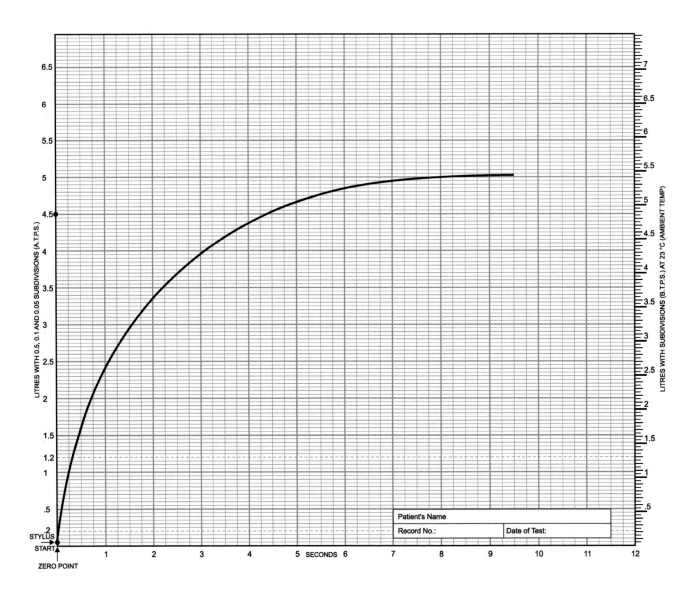

FIGURE 37–2. Exercises to find FEV$_1$ and FEV$_1$%.

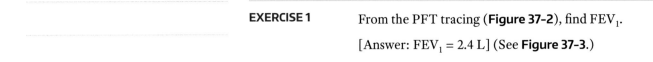

EXERCISE 1   From the PFT tracing (**Figure 37–2**), find FEV$_1$.

[Answer: FEV$_1$ = 2.4 L] (See **Figure 37–3.**)

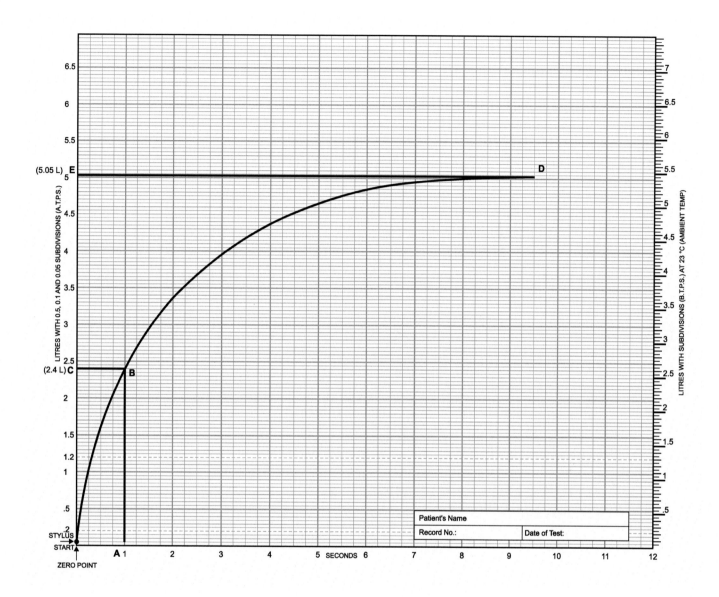

FIGURE 37-3. Solutions to Exercises 1 and 2 in **Figure 37-2**.

EXERCISE 2   From the PFT tracing (**Figure 37-2**), find FEV$_1$%. Is it normal?

[Answer: FEV$_1$% = 2.4/5.05 or 47.5%; the FEV1% is lower than predicted] (See **Figure 37-3**.)

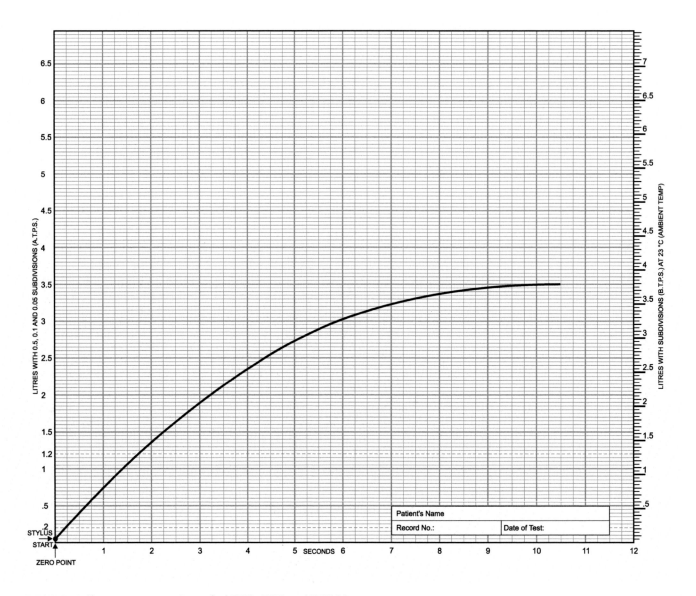

FIGURE 37-4. Self-assessment question to find FEV$_1$, FVC, and FEV$_1$%.

SELF-ASSESSMENT QUESTIONS

37a. From the PFT tracing (Figure 37-4), find FEV$_1$, FVC, and FEV$_1$%. Is the FEV$_1$% normal?

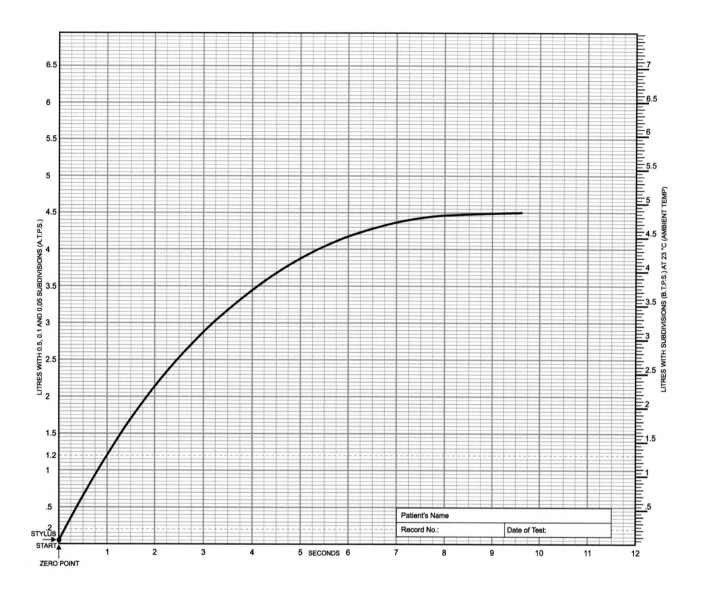

FIGURE 37-5. Self-assessment question to find FEV$_2$, FVC, and FEV$_2$%.

37b. From the PFT tracing (Figure 37-5), find FEV$_2$, FVC, and FEV$_2$%. Is the FEV$_2$% normal?

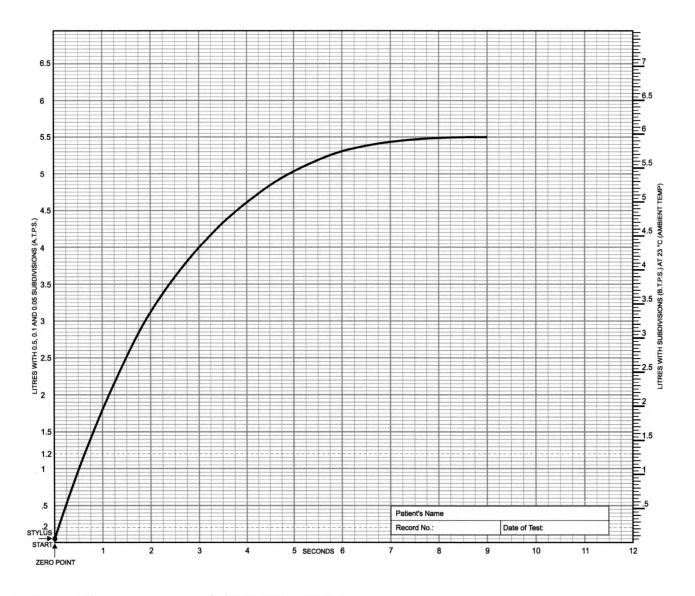

FIGURE 37-6. Self-assessment question to find FEV$_3$, FVC, and FEV$_3$%.

37c. From the PFT tracing (Figure 37-6), find FEV$_3$, FVC, and FEV$_3$%. Is the FEV$_3$% normal?

≫ Go to **rtexam.com** for more learning resources

Forced Vital Capacity Tracing ($FEF_{200-1200}$)

EQUATION

$FEF_{200-1200}$: Flow rate of the initial 200 to 1,200 mL of volume expired during the FVC maneuver, in L/sec.

NORMAL VALUE

$FEV_{200-1200} = 8.7$ L/sec

This value is based on a 70", 20-year-old male. Since the normal predicted values are based on a person's gender, age, height, weight, smoking history, and ethnic origin, an appropriate normal table should be used to match a person's physical attributes.

EXAMPLE 1

From the PFT tracing (**Figure 38-1**), find $FEV_{200-1200}$.

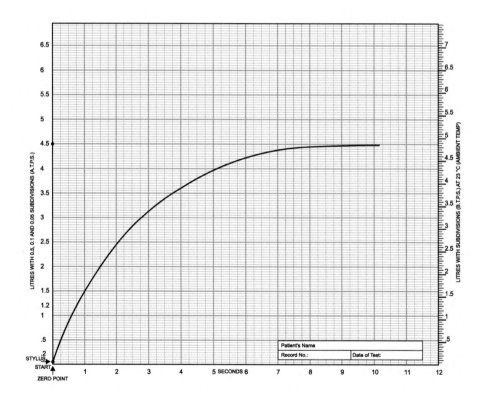

FIGURE 38-1. Example to find $FEF_{200-1200}$.

NOTES

The $FEF_{200-1200}$ measurement is dependent on the slope derived from the PFT tracing. A steep PFT tracing results in a higher $FEF_{200-1200}$ measurement. The method to plot the slopes from other PFT tracings is the same as shown in Example 1. For accurate results, it is extremely important to plot the points precisely and draw straight lines with a ruler.

The $FEF_{200-1200}$ (as well as $FEV_{0.5}$ and $FEV_{1.0}$) is used to assess flow rates and disorders relating to the large airways. In patients with large airway obstruction, the $FEF_{200-1200}$ values are usually decreased. However, poor patient effort may also lead to lower-than-normal results.

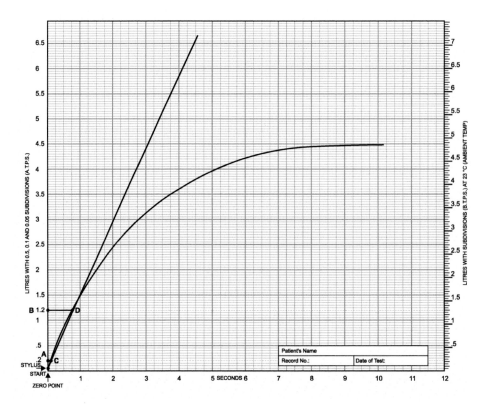

FIGURE 38-2. Locating the 0.2-L and 1.2-L markings on spirograph and determining its slope on graph paper.

Figure 38-2

Step 1. Along the volume (y) axis, locate 0.2 L (point A) and 1.2 L (point B).

Step 2. From point A, draw a horizontal line until it intersects the PFT tracing (point C). Do the same from point B until the line intersects the PFT tracing (point D).

Step 3. Use a ruler to draw a straight line connecting points C and D. Extend this straight line to top of the graph paper. This is the FEF$_{200-1200}$ flow slope.

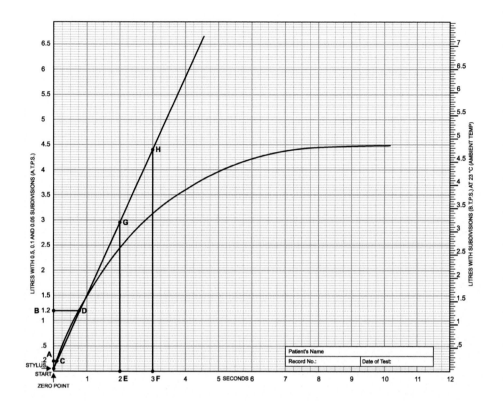

FIGURE 38-3. Determining the one-second interval on graph paper (points E, F) and spirograph tracing (points G, H).

Figure 38-3 **Step 4.** Along the time (x) axis, select two adjacent second-lines and mark them points E and F. In the example shown, the 2nd and 3rd second-lines are used. One may use the 3rd and 4th second-lines. The result would be identical as these two sets of adjacent lines intersect the same slope.

Step 5. From point E, follow the second line vertically until it intersects the slope (point G). Do the same from point F until it intersects the slope (point H).

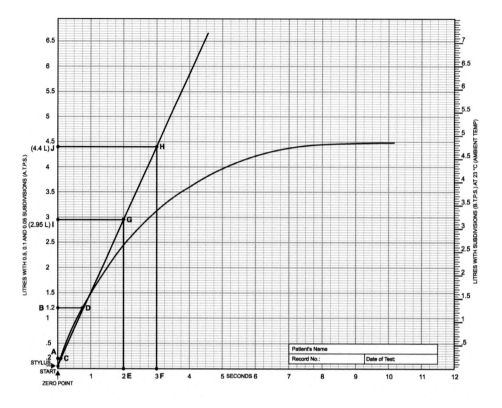

FIGURE 38-4. Determining the volume (L) that corresponds to the one-second interval (sec) on the slope. The unit of this reading is L/sec.

Figure 38-4 **Step 6.** From point G, draw a horizontal line until it intersects the volume (y) axis (point I). Do the same from point H until it intersects the volume (y) axis (point J).

Step 7. The difference between the volume readings taken at points I and J represents the flow rate of the initial 200 to 1200 mL of volume expired during the FVC maneuver.

$$FEV_{200-1200} = (4.4 \, L - 2.95 \, L)/sec$$
$$= 1.45 \, L/sec$$

EXERCISE From the PFT tracing (**Figure 38-5**), find FEF$_{200-1200}$.

[Answer: FEF$_{200-1200}$ = (6.8 L – 3.5 L)/sec or 3.3 L/sec] (See **Figure 38-6**.)

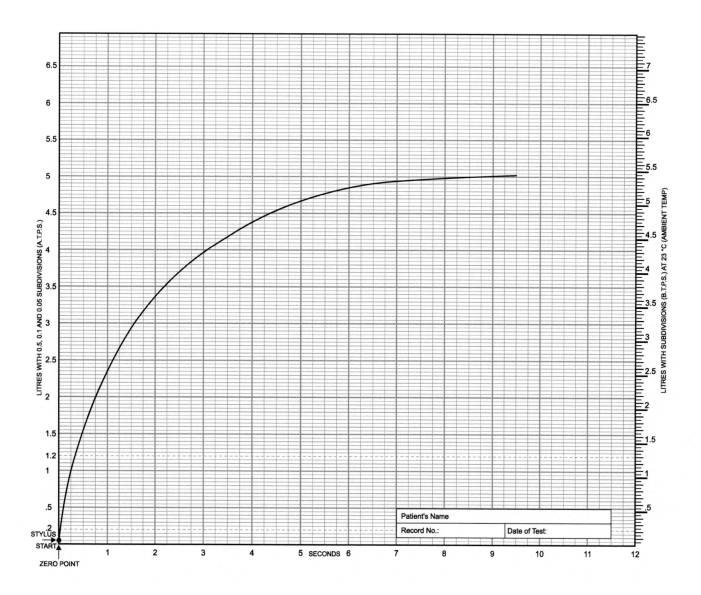

FIGURE 38-5. Exercise to find $FEF_{200-1200}$.

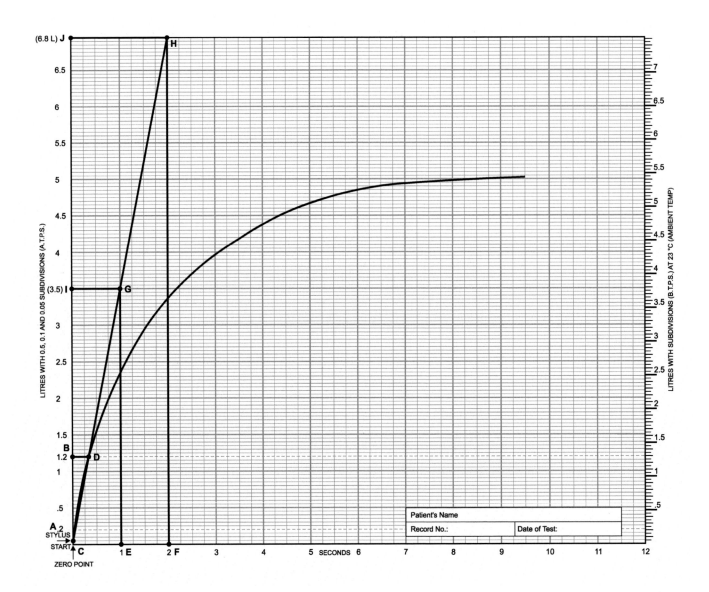

FIGURE 38-6. Solution to exercise in **Figure 38-5**.

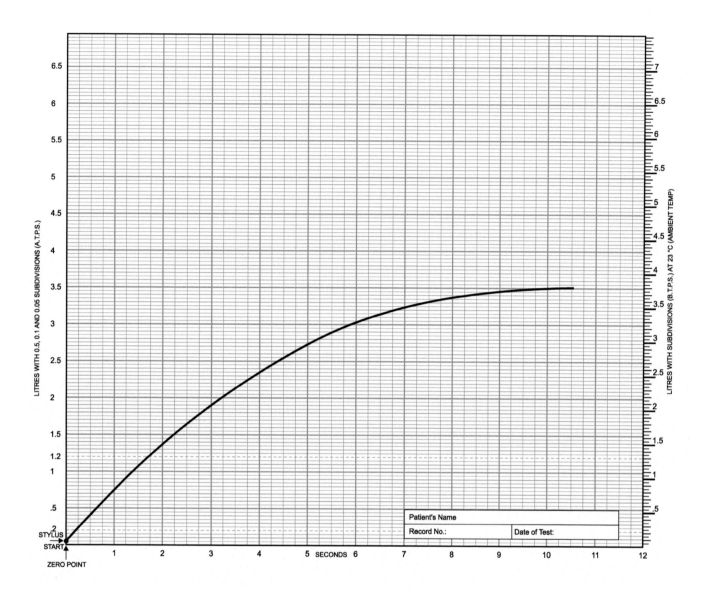

FIGURE 38-7. Self-assessment question 38a to find $FEF_{200-1200}$.

SELF-ASSESSMENT QUESTIONS

38a. From the PFT tracing (Figure 38-7), find $FEF_{200-1200}$.

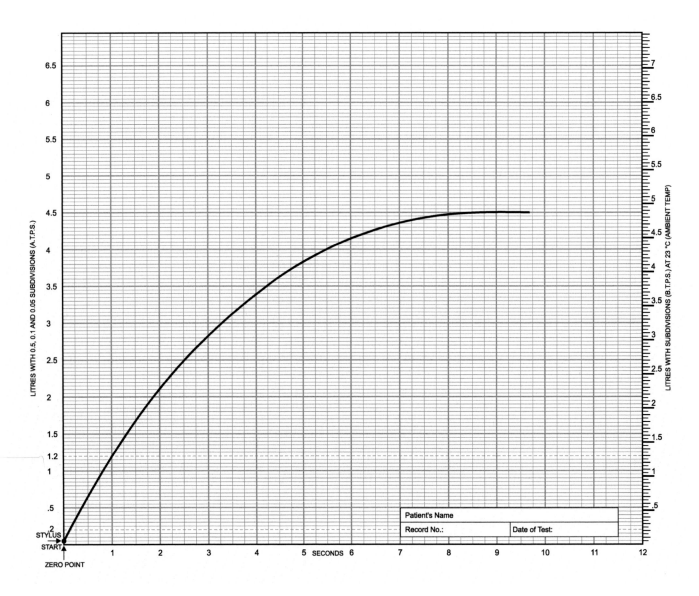

FIGURE 38-8. Self-assessment question 38b to find FEF$_{200-1200}$.

38b. From the PFT tracing (Figure 38-8), find FEF$_{200-1200}$.

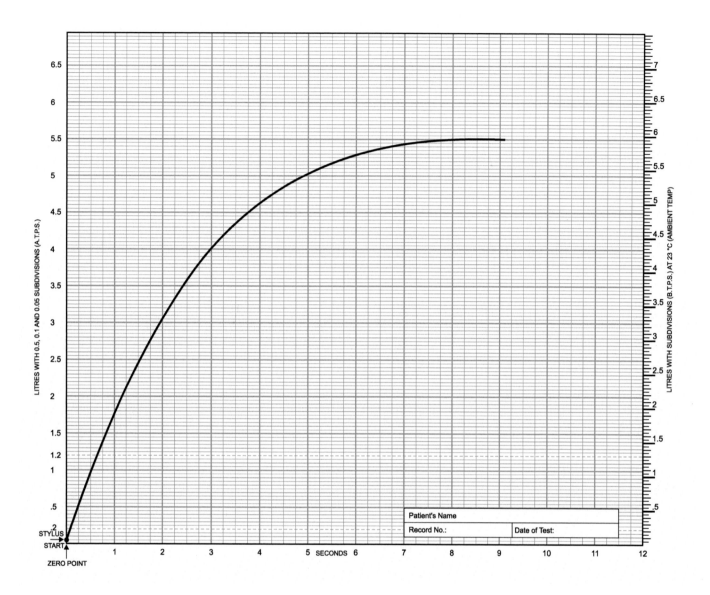

FIGURE 38-9. Self-assessment question 38c to find FEF$_{200-1200}$.

38c. From the PFT tracing (Figure 38-9), find FEF$_{200-1200}$.

Go to **rtexam.com** for more learning resources

39

Forced Vital Capacity Tracing $\left(\text{FEF}_{25-75\%}\right)$

NOTES

The method to plot the $\text{FEF}_{25-75\%}$ slopes from other PFT tracings is the same as shown in Example 1. For accurate results, it is extremely important to locate and plot the points carefully and draw straight lines using a ruler.

The $\text{FEF}_{25-75\%}$ (as well as FEV_2) is used to assess the flow rates and disorders relating to the smaller bronchi and larger bronchioles. In patients with early airway obstruction, the $\text{FEF}_{25-75\%}$ values are usually decreased. Patient effort has minimal effect on the $\text{FEF}_{25-75\%}$ measurements.

EQUATION $\text{FEF}_{25-75\%}$: Flow rate of the middle 50% of the volume expired during the FVC maneuver, in L/sec.

NORMAL VALUE $\text{FEV}_{25-75\%} = 5.2 \text{ L/sec}$

This value is based on a 70", 20-year-old male. Since the normal predicted values are based on a person's gender, age, height, weight, smoking history, and ethnic origin, an appropriate normal table should be used to match a person's physical attributes.

EXAMPLE 1   From the PFT tracing (**Figure 39-1**), find $\text{FEV}_{25-75\%}$.

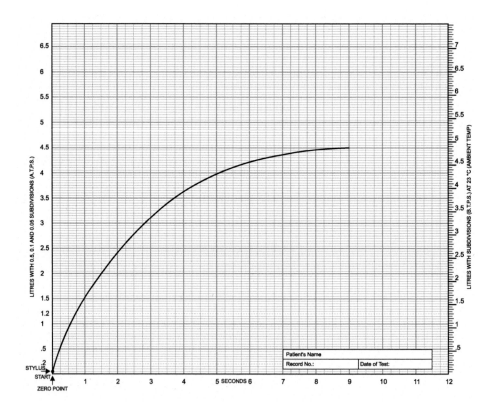

FIGURE 39-1. Example to find $\text{FEF}_{25-75\%}$.

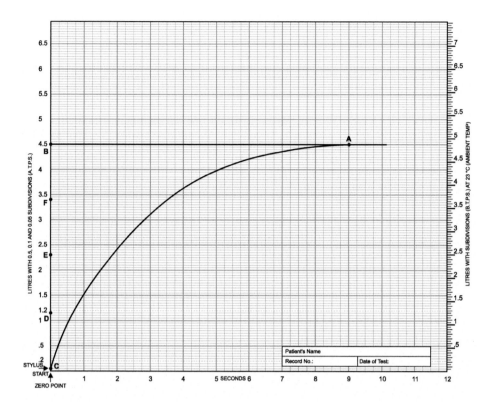

FIGURE 39-2. Determining the FVC and the four 25% segments of the FVC tracing.

Figure 39-2 **Step 1.** From the PFT tracing, locate the highest point at the end of the tracing (point A).

Step 2. From point A, draw a horizontal line until it intersects the volume (y) axis (point B).

Step 3. The difference between point B and the starting point C (4.5 L) represents the FVC.

Step 4. Divide the 4.5 L by 4 to obtain four equal segments. Plot the points D, E, F on the volume (y) axis to divide segment BC into four equal segments. The volume between points C and D represents the first 25% of the volume expired during the FVC maneuver. The volume between points D and F represents the middle 50% of the expired volume. The volume between points B and F represents the last 25% of the expired volume.

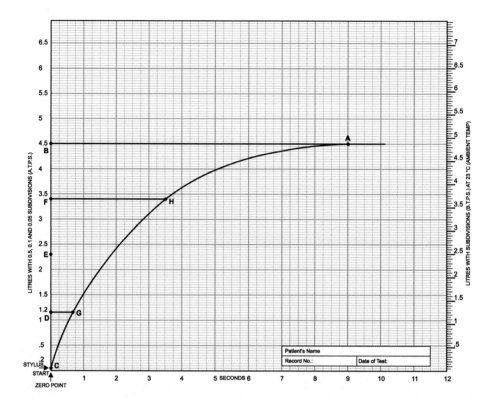

FIGURE 39-3. Determining the middle 50% of FVC on the graph paper (points D, F) and the spirograph (points G, H).

Figure 39-3   **Step 5.** From point D, draw a horizontal line until it intersects the PFT tracing (point G). Do the same from point F until the line intersects the PFT tracing (point H).

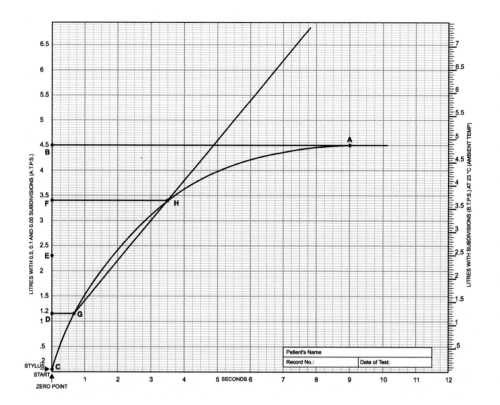

FIGURE 39-4. Determining the slope of the spirograph tracing on the graph paper.

Figure 39-4 **Step 6.** Use a ruler to draw a straight line joining points G and H. Extend this straight line to the top of the graph paper. This is the flow slope for this FEF$_{25-75\%}$ determination.

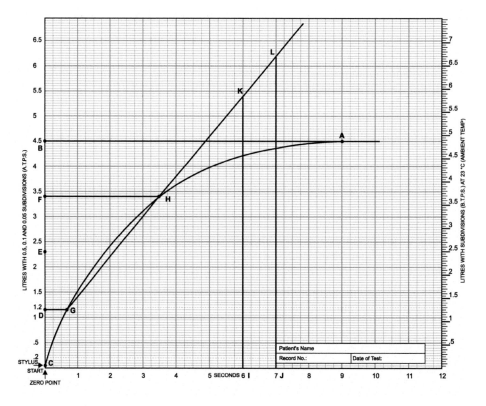

FIGURE 39-5. Determining the one-second interval on the graph paper (points I, J) and the spirograph tracing (points K, L).

Figure 39-5

Step 7. Along the time (x) axis, select two adjacent second-lines and mark them points I and J. In the example shown, the 6th and 7th second-lines are used. One may wish to use two other adjacent second-lines as long as the resulting drawings do not overlap or become too close to other existing lines.

Step 8. From point I, follow the second-line vertically until it intersects the slope (point K). Do the same from point J until it intersects the slope (point L).

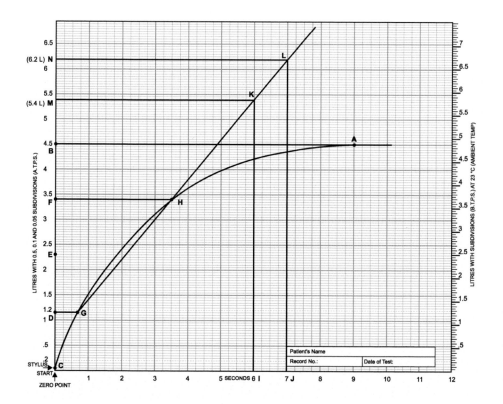

FIGURE 39-6. Determining the volume (L) that corresponds to the one-second interval (sec) on the slope. The unit of this reading is L/sec.

Figure 39-6   **Step 9.** From point K, draw a horizontal line until it intersects the volume (y) axis (point M). Do the same from point L until it intersects the volume (y) axis (point N).

Step 10. The difference between the volume readings taken at points N and M represents the flow rate of the middle 50% of volume expired during the FVC maneuver.

$$FEV_{25-75\%} = (6.2\,L - 5.4\,L)/sec$$
$$= 0.8\,L/sec$$

EXERCISE   From the PFT tracing (**Figure 39-7**), find FEF$_{25-75\%}$.

[Answer: FEF$_{25-75\%}$ = (6.3 L – 5.25 L)/sec or 1.05 L/sec] (See **Figure 39-8.**)

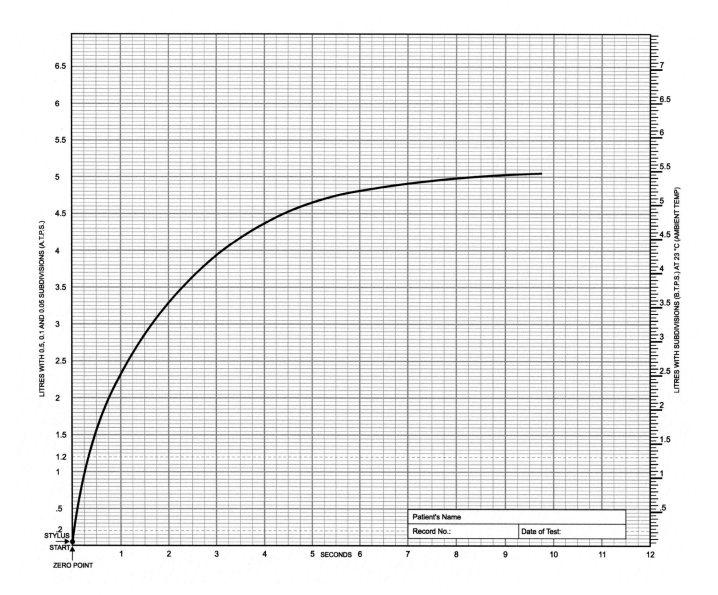

FIGURE 39-7. Exercise to find $FEF_{25-75\%}$.

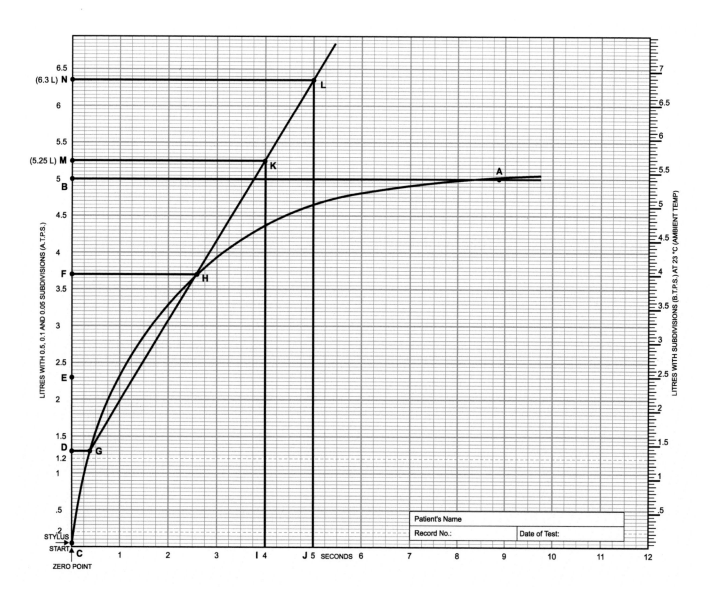

FIGURE 39–8. Solution to exercise in **Figure 39-7**.

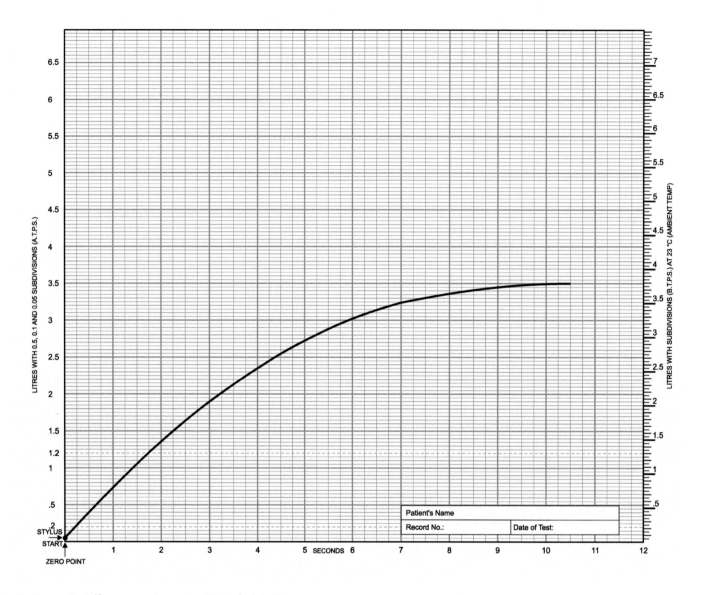

FIGURE 39-9. Self-assessment question 39a to find $FEF_{25-75\%}$.

SELF-ASSESSMENT QUESTIONS

39a. From the PFT tracing (Figure 39-9), find $FEF_{25-75\%}$.

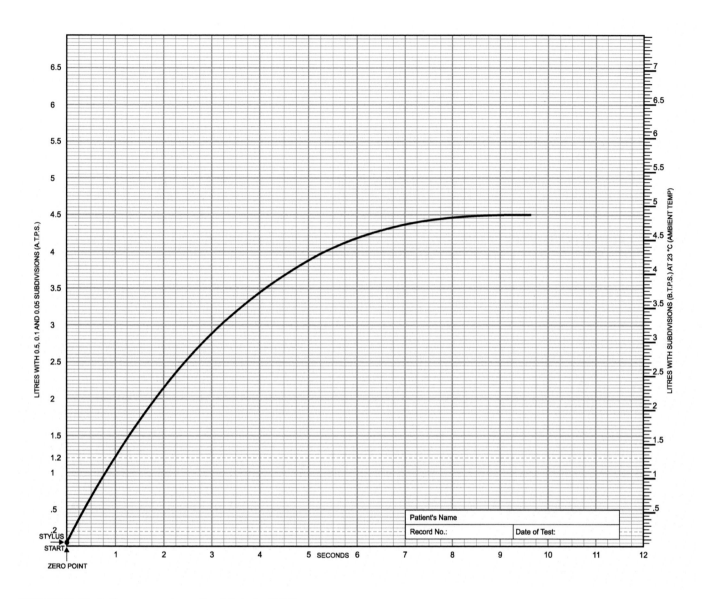

FIGURE 39-10. Self-assessment question 39b to find $\text{FEF}_{25-75\%}$.

39b. From the PFT tracing (Figure 39-10), find $\text{FEF}_{25-75\%}$.

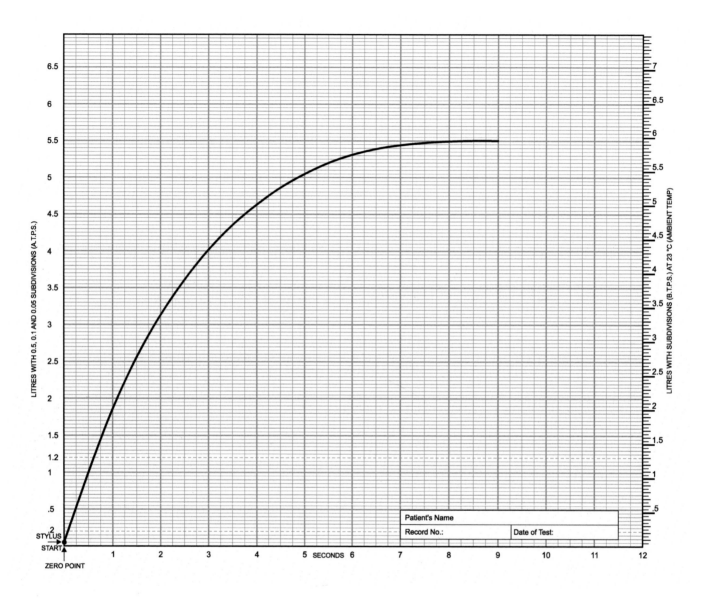

FIGURE 39-11. Self-assessment question 39c to find FEF$_{25-75\%}$.

39c. From the PFT tracing (Figure 39-11), find FEF$_{25-75\%}$.

Gas Law Equations

40

EQUATION 1	Boyle's Law: $P_1 \times V_1 = P_2 \times V_2$ (Temperature is constant)
EQUATION 2	Charles' Law: $\dfrac{V_1}{T_1} = \dfrac{V_2}{T_2}$ (Pressure is constant)
EQUATION 3	Gay-Lussac's Law: $\dfrac{P_1}{T_1} = \dfrac{P_2}{T_2}$ (Volume is constant)
EQUATION 4	Combined Gas Law: $\dfrac{P_1 \times V_1}{T_1} = \dfrac{P_2 \times V_2}{T_2}$

P : Barometric pressure in mm Hg
V : Volume in mL
T : Temperature in kelvin
1 : Original values
2 : New values

EXAMPLE See: Gas Volume Corrections.

EXERCISE

$P_1 \times V_1 = P_2 \times V_2$ is the _Boyle's_ law.

$\dfrac{P_1}{T_1} = \dfrac{P_2}{T_2}$ is the _Gay-Lussac's_ law.

$\dfrac{P_1}{T_1} = \dfrac{P_2}{T_2}$ is the _Gay-Lussac's_ law.

Write the Combined Gas Law equation: _$\dfrac{P_1 \times V_1}{T_1} = \dfrac{P_2 \times V_2}{T_2}$_

[Answer: Boyle's; Gay-Lussac's; Charles'; $\dfrac{P_1 \times V_1}{T_1} = \dfrac{P_2 \times V_2}{T_2}$]

NOTES

Boyle's law (Robert Boyle)

With constant temperature, pressure and volume are inversely related. For example, the lung volume becomes larger at high altitude (low barometric pressure) than at sea level. The inverse relationship between pressure and volume is used to measure and calculate the lung volumes and capacities.

Charles' law (Jacques Charles)

With constant pressure, the volume and absolute temperature (in kelvins) are directly related. Charles' law is most commonly used in respiratory care to "temperature-correct" lung volumes and flow rates from room to body temperature.

Gay-Lussac's law (Joseph Gay-Lussac)

With constant volume, the pressure and temperature are directly related. For example, the air pressure in a car tire increases as the ambient temperature increases, and vice versa.

Combined Gas Law

This is also called the modified Ideal Gas Law. The Combined Gas Law accounts for all three variables (P, V, T) affecting gas behaviors. This equation is especially useful when precise measurements are required.

SELF-ASSESSMENT QUESTIONS

MATCHING: Match the gas laws with the respective equations.
Use only *three* of the answers in Column II.

Column I	Column II

40a. Gas-Lussac's law *D*   A. $P_1 \times V_1 = P_2 \times V_2$

40b. Charles' law *C*   B. $\dfrac{P_1}{V_1} = \dfrac{P_2}{V_2}$

40c. Boyle's law *A*   C. $\dfrac{V_1}{T_1} = \dfrac{V_2}{T_2}$

D. $\dfrac{P_1}{T_1} = \dfrac{P_2}{T_2}$

40d. $P_1 \times V_1 = P_2 \times V_2$ **is which of the following gas laws?**

   A. Boyle's
   B. Charles'
   C. Gay-Lussac's
   D. Combined

40e. **Charles' law is represented by the equation:**

   A. $P_1 \times V_1 = P_2 \times V_2$

   B. $\dfrac{P_1}{T_1} = \dfrac{P_2}{T_2}$

   C. $\dfrac{V_1}{T_1} = \dfrac{V_2}{T_2}$

   D. $\dfrac{P_1}{V_1} = \dfrac{P_2}{V_2}$

40f. **Gay-Lussac's law is represented by the equation:**

   A. $P_1 \times V_1 = P_2 \times V_2$

   B. $\dfrac{P_1}{T_1} = \dfrac{P_2}{T_2}$

   C. $\dfrac{V_1}{T_1} = \dfrac{V_2}{T_2}$

   D. $\dfrac{P_1}{V_1} = \dfrac{P_2}{V_2}$

40g. According to Charles' law, at constant ___, the gas volume varies ____ with the temperature.

    A. flow; directly
    B. flow; indirectly
    C. pressure; directly
    D. pressure; indirectly

40h. Corrections of lung volumes and flow rates from ATPS to BTPS is based on:

    A. Gay-Lussac's law
    B. Charles' law
    C. Boyle's law
    D. Bohr effect

40i. In using the gas law equations, the temperature must first be converted to:

    A. degrees Celsius
    B. degrees Fahrenheit
    C. degrees Centigrade
    D. kelvins

40j. Which gas law states that at a constant temperature the gas volume varies inversely with the pressure?

    A. Charles' law
    B. Boyle's law
    C. Dalton's law
    D. Gay-Lussac's law

40k. Which gas law states that at a constant pressure the gas volume varies directly with the temperature?

    A. Charles' law
    B. Boyle's law
    C. Dalton's law
    D. Gay-Lussac's law

40l. Which gas law states that at a constant volume the gas pressure varies directly with the temperature?

    A. Charles' law
    B. Boyle's law
    C. Dalton's law
    D. Gay-Lussac's law

» Go to **rtexam.com** for more learning resources

41

Gas Volume Corrections

NOTES

Before using these equations for gas volume corrections, the temperature must be converted to the kelvin (K) temperature scale.

For gas volume correction problems involving *dry* gas, omit P_{H_2O} and use only P_B.

For gas correction problems involving the same pressure, omit P_1 and P_2 from the Combined Gas Law equation, and it becomes Charles' law.

Charles' law: $\dfrac{V_1}{T_1} = \dfrac{V_2}{T_2}$

To find new volume (V_2) or new temperature (T_2):

$$V_2 = \frac{V_1 \times T_2}{T_1} \text{ or } T_2 = \frac{V_2 \times T_1}{V_1}$$

For gas correction problems involving the same temperature, omit T_1 and T_2 from the Combined Gas Law equation, and it becomes Boyle's law.

Boyle's law: $P_1 \times V_1 = P_2 \times V_2$

To find new volume (V_2) or new pressure (P_2):

$$V_2 = \frac{P_1 \times V_1}{P_2} \text{ or } P_2 = \frac{P_1 \times V_1}{V_2}$$

For gas correction problems involving the same volume, omit V_1 and V_2 from the Combined Gas Law equation, and it becomes Gay-Lussac's law.

Gay-Lussac's law: $\dfrac{P_1}{T_1} = \dfrac{P_2}{T_2}$

To find new pressure (P_2) or new temperature (T_2):

$$P_2 = \frac{P_1 \times T_2}{T_1} \text{ or } T_2 = \frac{P_2 \times T_1}{P_1}$$

EQUATION

Since $\dfrac{P_1 \times V_1}{T_1} = \dfrac{P_2 \times V_2}{T_2}$ (Combined Gas Law),

$$V_2 = \frac{P_1 \times V_1 \times T_2}{T_1 \times P_2}$$

V_2 : New gas volume in mL
P_1 : Original pressure $(P_B - P_{H_2O})$
V_1 : Original gas volume in mL
T_2 : New temperature in kelvins (K)
T_1 : Original temperature in kelvins (K)
P_2 : New pressure $(P_B - P_{H_2O})$

EXAMPLE 1

Given: 100 mL of gas volume measured at 25°C and 750 mm Hg. Find the new gas volume measured at 37°C and 760 mm Hg.

At 25°C, $P_{H_2O} = 23.8$ mm Hg

$P_1 = P_B 1 - P_{H_2O} = (750 - 23.8)$ mm Hg $= 726.2$ mm Hg

At 37°C, $P_{H_2O} = 47$ mm Hg

$P_2 = P_B 2 - P_{H_2O} = (760 - 47)$ mm Hg $= 713$ mm Hg

$V_1 = 100$ mL

$T_1 = 25°C = (25 + 273)K = 298$ K

$T_2 = 37°C = (37 + 273)K = 310$ K

$$V_2 = \frac{P_1 \times V_1 \times T_2}{T_1 \times P_2}$$

$$= \frac{726.2 \times 100 \times 310}{298 \times 713}$$

$$= \frac{22,512,200}{212,474}$$

$$= 105.95 \text{ or } 106 \text{ mL}$$

EXAMPLE 2

A tidal volume of 500 mL was measured at 24°C and 750 mm Hg. Find the corrected tidal volume at 37°C and 760 mm Hg.

Given: At 24°C, P_{H_2O} = 22.4 mm Hg

At 37°C, P_{H_2O} = 47 mm Hg

Since at 24°C, P_{H_2O} = 22.4 mm Hg,

$P_1 = P_B1 - P_{H_2O} = (750 - 22.4)$ mm Hg = 727.6 mm Hg

Since at 37°C, P_{H_2O} = 47 mm Hg,

$P_2 = P_B2 - P_{H_2O} = (760 - 47)$ mm Hg = 713 mm Hg

V_1 = 500 mL

$T_1 = 24°C = (24 + 273)K = 297$ K

$T_2 = 37°C = (37 + 273)K = 310$ K

$$V_2 = \frac{P_1 \times V_1 \times T_2}{T_1 \times P_2}$$

$$= \frac{727.6 \times 500 \times 310}{297 \times 713}$$

$$= \frac{112,778,000}{211,761}$$

$$= 532.6 \text{ or } 533 \text{ mL}$$

EXERCISE 1

Given: 100 mL of dry gas volume measured at 28°C and 760 mm Hg. Find the dry gas volume measured at 37°C and 760 mm Hg. (Note: for dry gas volume, omit P_{H_2O})

[Answer: P_1 = 760 mm Hg P_2 = 760 mm Hg

T_1 = 301 K T_2 = 310 K

V_1 = 100 mL V_2 = 102.99 or 103 mL]

EXERCISE 2

A total lung capacity (TLC) of 2,500 mL was measured at 27°C and 755 mm Hg. Find the new TLC corrected to 37°C and 758 mm Hg.

Given: At 27°C, P_{H_2O} = 26.7 mm Hg

At 37°C, P_{H_2O} = 47 mm Hg

[Answer: P_1 = 728.3 mm Hg P_2 = 711 mm Hg

T_1 = 300 K T_2 = 310 K

V_1 = 2,500 mL V_2 = *Corrected*

TLC = 2,646 mL]

SELF-ASSESSMENT QUESTIONS

41a. Given:

$P_1 = 760$ mm Hg $P_2 = 755$ mm Hg
$T_1 = 300$ K $T_2 = 310$ K
$V_1 = 800$ mL

Find V_2 using the Combined Gas Law.

A. 809 mL
B. 814 mL
C. 825 mL
D. 832 mL

41b. A gas sample of 1,000 mL was measured at 28°C and 750 mm Hg. Find the new gas volume corrected to 37°C and 760 mm Hg. (At 28°C, P_{H_2O} = 28.3 mm Hg; at 37°C, P_{H_2O} = 47 mm Hg.)

A. 1,042 mL
B. 1,016 mL
C. 995 mL
D. 987 mL

41c. The vital capacity (FVC) measured at 26°C and 760 mm Hg is 3,000 mL. Find the corrected FVC at 37°C and 758 mm Hg. (At 26°C, P_{H_2O} = 25.2 mm Hg; at 37°C, P_{H_2O} = 47 mm Hg.)

A. 3,119 mL
B. 3,161 mL
C. 3,214 mL
D. 3,268 mL

41d. Given: tidal volume (V_T) = 670 mL measured at 27°C and 758 mm Hg. Calculate the corrected V_T at 37°C and 760 mm Hg. (At 27°C, P_{H_2O} = 26.7 mm Hg; at 37°C, P_{H_2O} = 47 mm Hg.)

A. 690 mL
B. 710 mL
C. 730 mL
D. 750 mL

41e. A vital capacity of 4,800 was measured at 27°C and 700 mm Hg. Calculate the corrected vital capacity at 37°C and 760 mm Hg. (At 27°C, P_{H_2O} = 26.7 mm Hg; at 37°C, P_{H_2O} = 47 mm Hg.)

A. 4,684 mL
B. 4,718 mL
C. 4,763 mL
D. 4,850 mL

41f. A tidal volume of 600 mL was measured at 28°C and 750 mm Hg. Calculate the corrected tidal volume at 37°C and 760 mm Hg. (At 28°C $P_{H_2O} = 28.3$ mm Hg; at 37°C, $P_{H_2O} = 47$ mm Hg.)

    A. 568 mL
    B. 584 mL
    C. 625 mL
    D. 641 mL

41g. At Mount Everest (altitude 29,028 ft above sea level), a dry gas volume of 500 mL was measured at 20°C and 235 mm Hg. Calculate the corrected dry gas volume at 37°C and 760 mm Hg. (Note: For dry gas volume, omit P_{H_2O}.)

    A. 143 mL
    B. 164 mL
    C. 189 mL
    D. 215 mL

42

Graham's Law of Diffusion Coefficient

NOTES

In 1833, the Scottish inorganic and physical chemist Thomas Graham proposed Graham's law, which states that the rate of gas diffusion is inversely proportional to the square root of its gram molecular weight. The solubility coefficient in the equation is added for calculation of diffusion coefficient.

In pulmonary disorders that impair the lung's diffusion rate, hypoxia is usually a more difficult situation to correct due to low diffusion coefficient of oxygen.

EQUATION

$$D = \frac{\text{Sol. Coeff.}}{\sqrt{\text{gmw}}}$$

D : Diffusion coefficient of gas
Sol. Coeff. : Solubility coefficient of gas
$\sqrt{\text{gmw}}$: Square root of gram molecular weight of gas

EXAMPLE

The diffusion coefficient of carbon dioxide is 19 times $\left(\dfrac{0.077}{0.004}\right)$ greater than that of oxygen. The diffusion coefficient of each gas is shown below.

$$D_{\text{carbon dioxide}} = \frac{0.510}{\sqrt{44}} \qquad D_{\text{oxygen}} = \frac{0.023}{\sqrt{32}}$$

$$= \frac{0.510}{6.633} \qquad\qquad = \frac{0.023}{5.657}$$

$$= 0.077 \qquad\qquad = 0.004$$

The difference in diffusion coefficient between carbon dioxide and oxygen explains why a small carbon dioxide pressure gradient of 6 mm Hg ($P_{\bar{v}}CO_2$ 46 mm Hg $- P_ACO_2$ 40 mmHg) across the alveolar-capillary membrane is sufficient for carbon dioxide elimination. On the other hand, a pressure gradient of 60 mm Hg (P_AO_2 100 mm Hg $- P_{\bar{v}}O_2$ 40 mmHg) is needed for oxygen uptake across the alveolar-capillary membrane.

SELF-ASSESSMENT QUESTIONS

42a. The diffusion coefficient of a gas is based on:

A. Charles' law
B. Gay-Lussac's law
C. Graham's law
D. Henry's law

42b. The diffusion coefficient of a gas is ___ its solubility coefficient and ___ related to the square root of its gram molecular weight.

A. directly; inversely
B. directly; directly
C. inversely; inversely
D. inversely; directly

42c. The diffusion coefficient of carbon dioxide is about ___ times higher than that of oxygen. For this reason, hypoxia is ___ to treat than hypercapnia.

A. 30; more difficult
B. 30; easier
C. 19; easier
D. 19; more difficult

42d. The solubility coefficient and gram molecular weight of carbon monoxide (CO) are 0.018 and 28, respectively. What is the diffusion coefficient of CO?

A. 0.034
B. 0.0034
C. 0.053
D. 0.0053

42e. Nitrogen (N_2) has a solubility coefficient of 0.012 and a gram molecular weight of 28. Calculate the diffusion coefficient of N_2.

A. 0.023
B. 0.0023
C. 0.034
D. 0.0034

42f. Helium (He) has a solubility coefficient of 0.008 and a gram molecular weight of 4. What is its diffusion coefficient?

A. 0.001
B. 0.002
C. 0.004
D. 0.008

Helium/Oxygen (He/O$_2$) Flow Rate Conversion

43

NOTES

A conversion factor (e.g., 1.8 or 1.6) is needed when an oxygen flow meter is used to deliver a helium/oxygen gas mixture (e.g., Heliox). This factor provides an accurate flow rate because the density of a helium/oxygen mixture is lower than that of oxygen.

The conversion factors are 1.8 for an 80%He/20%O$_2$ mixture and 1.6 for a 70%He/30%O$_2$ mixture.

Heliox is an alternative to oxygen therapy for patients with airflow obstruction. This is because a helium/oxygen mixture has a lower density and a higher diffusion rate than oxygen or air alone. Because of the high diffusion rate of a helium/oxygen mixture, a closely fitted oxygen device (e.g., non-rebreathing mask) should be used.

EQUATION 1 (80/20 Heliox)

Actual flow rate of 80%He/20%O$_2$ = Flow rate × 1.8

Flow rate : Flow rate on oxygen flowmeter
1.8 : Conversion factor for 80%He/20%O$_2$ mixture

EQUATION 2 (70/30 Heliox)

Actual flow rate of 70%He/30%O$_2$ = Flow rate × 1.6

Flow rate : Flow rate on oxygen flowmeter
1.6 : Conversion factor for 70%He/30%O$_2$ mixture

EXAMPLE 1

A gas mixture of 70%He/30%O$_2$ is running at a flow rate of 10 L/min with an oxygen flow meter. What is the actual flow rate of this He/O$_2$ gas mixture?

Actual flow rate of 70%He/30%O$_2$ = Flow rate × 1.6
= 10 L/min × 1.6
= 16 L/min

EXAMPLE 2

The physician wants to deliver 14 L/min of 70%He/30%O$_2$ to a patient with airflow obstruction. What should be the set flow rate on the oxygen flow meter?

Since actual flow rate of 70%He/30%O$_2$ = Flow rate × 1.6
Flow rate = Actual flow rate of 70%He/30%O$_2$ / 1.6
= 14 L/min / 1.6
= 8.75 L/min or 9 L/min

EXERCISE

Given: An oxygen flow meter is being used to administer 8 L/min of an 80%He/20%O$_2$ gas mixture. What is the actual flow rate of this gas mixture?

[Answer: Actual flow rate = 14.4 L/min]

SELF-ASSESSMENT QUESTIONS

43a. Given: a gas mixture of 70%He/30%O_2 is running at a flow rate of 5 L/min on an oxygen flow meter. What is the actual flow rate of this gas mixture?

A. 4 L/min
B. 6 L/min
C. 7 L/min
D. 8 L/min

43b. An oxygen flow meter is being used to regulate a gas mixture of 70%He/30%O_2. If the flow rate is set at 8 L/min, what is the approximate flow rate of this He/O₂ gas mixture?

A. 8 L/min
B. 11 L/min
C. 13 L/min
D. 15 L/min

43c. Calculate the actual flow rate if an 80%He/20%O_2 gas mixture is running at 5 L/min on an oxygen flow meter.

A. 6 L/min
B. 7 L/min
C. 8 L/min
D. 9 L/min

43d. A 80% Heliox (80%He/20%O_2) is running at a flow rate of 9 L/min with an oxygen flow meter. What is the actual flow rate of this He/O₂ gas mixture?

A. 16 L/min
B. 17 L/min
C. 18 L/min
D. 19 L/min

43e. An oxygen flow meter is used to deliver 15 L/min of 80% Heliox. The therapist should set the flow rate on the oxygen flow meter at about:

A. 7 L/min
B. 8 L/min
C. 9 L/min
D. 10 L/min

43f. The physician order reads "10 L/min of 70% Heliox via a non-rebreathing mask." What should be the approximate flow rate on the oxygen flow meter?

A. 6 L/min
B. 7 L/min
C. 8 L/min
D. 9 L/min

43g. A patient is to receive 14 L/min of 80% Heliox via a non-rebreathing mask. The therapist should set flow rate on the oxygen flow meter at about:

A. 6 L/min
B. 7 L/min
C. 8 L/min
D. 9 L/min

44

Humidity Deficit

EQUATION

HD = Capacity – Content

HD : Humidity deficit in mg/L

Capacity : Maximum amount of water the alveolar air can hold at body temperature (43.9 mg/L at 37°C). Also known as maximum absolute humidity

Content : Humidity content of inspired air; actual humidity or absolute humidity

EXAMPLE

Calculate the humidity deficit at body temperature if the inspired air has a humidity content of 26 mg/L. The humidity capacity at body temperature is 43.9 mg/L

HD = Capacity – Content
   = 43.9 mg/L – 26 mg/L
   = 17.9 or 18 mg/L

EXERCISE

Calculate the humidity deficit if the humidity content is 34 mg/L and capacity is 43.9 mg/L.

[Answer: HD = 9.9 or 10 mg/L]

SELF-ASSESSMENT QUESTIONS

44a. What is the approximate humidity deficit at body temperature if the humidity content of inspired air is 22 mg/L? (Humidity capacity at 37°C = 43.9 mg/L.)

A. 10.9 or 11 mg/L
B. 21.9 or 22 mg/L
C. 29.9 or 30 mg/L
D. 36.9 or 37 mg/L

44b. Calculate the humidity deficit at body temperature if the inspired air has a humidity content of 27 mg/L and the humidity capacity at 37°C is 43.9 mg/L.

    A. 16.9 or 17 mg/L
    B. 26.9 or 27 mg/L
    C. 31.9 or 32 mg/L
    D. 36.9 or 37 mg/L

44c. Which of the following is the most efficient device to reduce the humidity deficit?

    A. heat and moisture exchanger
    B. cool aerosol
    C. cool vaporizer
    D. heated humidifier

44d. Given: humidity content = 16 mg/L, humidity capacity at body temperature = 43.9 mg/L. Calculate the humidity deficit.

    A. 23.9 mg/L or 24 mg/L
    B. 25.9 mg/L or 26 mg/L
    C. 27.9 mg/L or 28 mg/L
    D. 29.9 mg/L or 30 mg/L

44e. Which of the following is true in regard to humidity capacity?

    A. humidity capacity = (humidity content + humidity deficit) mg/L
    B. humidity capacity = (humidity content – humidity deficit) mg/L
    C. humidity capacity = (humidity content + 43.9) mg/L
    D. humidity capacity = (43.9 – humidity content) mg/L

44f. Which of the following statements is true in regard to humidity?

    A. The humidity capacity at 37°C is 43.9 mg.
    B. The humidity capacity at 37°C is 43.9 mg/L.
    C. The humidity content at room temperature is 26 mg.
    D. The humidity content at room temperature is 26 mg/L.

44g. Which of the following humidity contents has the *lowest* humidity deficit at body temperature?

    A. 26 mg/L
    B. 28 mg/L
    C. 30 mg/L
    D. 32 mg/L

» Go to **rtexam.com** for more learning resources

45

$I{:}E$ Ratio

EXAMPLE 1

When the I time and E time are known:

What is the $I{:}E$ ratio if the inspiratory time is 0.4 sec and the expiratory time is 1.2 sec?

$$I{:}E \; = \; \left(\frac{I \text{ time}}{I \text{ time}}\right) : \left(\frac{E \text{ time}}{I \text{ time}}\right)$$

$$= \left(\frac{0.4}{0.4}\right) : \left(\frac{1.2}{0.4}\right)$$

$$= \; 1{:}3$$

NOTES

When the inspiratory time is longer than the expiratory time, divide both I time and E time by the expiratory time to get a reverse $I{:}E$ ratio.

$$I{:}E = \left(\frac{I \text{ time}}{I \text{ time}}\right) : \left(\frac{E \text{ time}}{I \text{ time}}\right)$$

See Exercise 1 for reverse $I{:}E$ ratio.

EXERCISE 1

What is the $I{:}E$ ratio if the inspiratory time is 0.6 sec and the expiratory time is 0.4 sec?

[Answer: $I{:}E = 1.5{:}1$]

EXAMPLE 2

When the I time % is known:

What is the $I{:}E$ ratio if the inspiratory time ratio is 25% or 0.25?

$$I{:}E \; = \; \left(\frac{I \text{ time \%}}{I \text{ time \%}}\right) : \left(\frac{1 - I \text{ time \%}}{I \text{ time \%}}\right)$$

$$= \left(\frac{0.25}{0.25}\right) : \left(\frac{1 - 0.25}{0.25}\right)$$

$$= \; 1 : \left(\frac{0.75}{0.25}\right)$$

$$= \; 1{:}3$$

EXERCISE 2

What is the $I{:}E$ ratio if the inspiratory time ratio is 33% or 0.33?

[Answer: $I{:}E = 1{:}2$]

EXAMPLE 3

When the *I* time and *f* are known:

What is the *I:E* ratio if the inspiratory time is 1.5 sec and the frequency is 15/min?

$$I \text{ time} = 1.5 \text{ sec}$$

$$E \text{ time} = \frac{60}{f} - I \text{ time}$$

$$= \frac{60}{15} - 1.5$$

$$= 4 - 1.5$$

$$= 2.5 \text{ sec}$$

$$I{:}E = I \text{ time} : E \text{ time}$$

$$= 1.5 : 2.5$$

$$= \left(\frac{1.5}{1.5}\right) : \left(\frac{2.5}{1.5}\right)$$

$$= 1 : 1.67$$

EXERCISE 3

What is the *I:E* ratio if the inspiratory time is 0.6 sec and the frequency is 20/min?

[Answer: *I:E* = 1:4]

EXAMPLE 4

When the minute volume ($\dot{V}_E$) and flow rate are known:

Given: V_T = 800 mL (0.8 L)
f = 12/min
Flow rate = 40 L/min

What is the *I:E* ratio?

$$I{:}E \text{ ratio} = (\text{Minute volume}) : (\text{Flow rate} - \text{Minute volume})$$

$$= (V_T \times f) : \text{Flow rate} - (V_T \times f)$$

$$= (0.8 \times 12) : 40 - (0.8 \times 12)$$

$$= 9.6 : 40 - 9.6$$

$$= 9.6 : 30.4 \text{ [divide both sides of this ratio by 9.6]}$$

$$= 1 : 3.2$$

EXERCISE 4

Given: V_T = 600 mL (0.6 L)
f = 15/min
Flow rate = 50 L/min

What is the *I:E* ratio?

[Answer: *I:E* = 1:4.6]

SELF-ASSESSMENT QUESTIONS

45a. Calculate the *I:E* ratio if the inspiratory time is 0.4 sec and the expiratory time is 0.6 sec.

    A. 1.5:1
    B. 1:1
    C. 1:1.5
    D. 1:2

45b. What is the *I:E* ratio if the inspiratory time is 0.5 sec and the expiratory time is 1.5 sec?

    A. 1:1
    B. 1:2
    C. 1:3
    D. 2:1

45c. Calculate the *I:E* ratio when the inspiratory time is 1.8 sec and the expiratory time is 1.2 sec. Is this an inverse *I:E* ratio?

    A. 1:1.5; no
    B. 1:2; no
    C. 1.5:1; yes
    D. 2:1; yes

45d. Which of the following sets of inspiratory time (*I* time) and expiratory time (*E* time) does not have an *I:E* ratio of 1:2?

	I time (sec)	*E* time (sec)
A.	2.0	4.0
B.	1.5	3.0
C.	0.8	1.6
D.	2.0	1.0

45e. Calculate the *I:E* ratio when the inspiratory time ratio is 25%.

    A. 4:1
    B. 3:1
    C. 1:3
    D. 1:4

45f. What is the *I:E* ratio if the inspiratory time ratio is 40% or 0.4?

    A. 1:1.5
    B. 1:2
    C. 1:2.5
    D. 1:3

45g. The inspiratory time is set at 30% of one complete respiratory cycle. The *I:E* ratio is about:

A. 1:2.3
B. 1:1.3
C. 1:0.7
D. 1:0.3

45h. Calculate the *I:E* ratio when the inspiratory time on a ventilator is set at 20% of one complete respiratory cycle.

A. 1:3
B. 1:4
C. 3:1
D. 4:1

45i. Which of the following inspiratory time percent (%) settings would give an *I:E* ratio of 1:3?

A. 20%
B. 25%
C. 30%
D. 40%

45j. What is the *I:E* ratio if the inspiratory time is 0.5 sec and the frequency is 30/min?

A. 1:3
B. 1:4
C. 1:5
D. insufficient information to calculate answer

45k. Calculate the *I:E* ratio for the following settings: inspiratory time = 1 sec, frequency = 20/min.

A. 1:1
B. 1:2
C. 1:3
D. 1:4

45l. Given: inspiratory time = 1.5 sec, frequency = 16/min. Find the expiratory time. What is the *I:E* ratio at these settings?

A. 1.75 sec; 1:0.5
B. 1.75 sec; 1:1
C. 2.25 sec; 1:1.5
D. 2.25 sec; 1:1.75

45m. A mechanically ventilated patient has an inspiratory time of 1.2 sec and a ventilator frequency of 25/min. What are the expiratory time and *I:E* ratio at these settings?

A. 0.96 sec; 1 : 0.8
B. 1.2 sec; 1 : 1
C. 1.44 sec; 1 : 1.2
D. 1.68 sec; 1 : 1.4

45n. Which of the following settings would *not* produce an *I:E* ratio of about 1 : 0.5?

	I time (sec)	*f*
A.	2.0	20
B.	1.6	25
C.	1.33	30
D.	3	15

45o. Given: V_T = 600 mL (0.6 L), f = 15/min, flow rate = 45 L/min. What is the *I:E* ratio?

A. 1 : 2
B. 1 : 3
C. 1 : 4
D. 2 : 1

45p. Given: V_T = 700 mL (0.7 L), f = 12/min, flow rate = 40 L/min. The calculated *I:E* ratio is about:

A. 1 : 3.8
B. 1 : 3.3
C. 1 : 3
D. 1 : 2

45q. Which of the following settings has a calculated *I:E* ratio of 1 : 4?

	V_T (mL)	*f*	Flow rate
A.	800	15	40
B.	800	15	45
C.	800	15	50
D.	800	15	60

45r. A patient on the ventilator has a tidal volume of 850 mL (0.85 L), frequency of 16/min, and flow rate of 50 L/min. Based on these settings, what is the *I:E* ratio? If the flow rate is increased to 60 L/min, will the *E* ratio be longer or shorter?

A. 1 : 2.7; *E* ratio will be longer (1 : 3.4)
B. 1 : 2.7; *E* ratio will be shorter (1 : 2.4)
C. 1 : 2.4; *E* ratio will be shorter (1 : 1.7)
D. 1 : 2.1; *E* ratio will be shorter (1 : 1.4)

45s. A patient has the following settings on a mechanical ventilator: $V_T = 750$ mL (0.75 L), $f = 16$/min, flow rate = 50 L/min. Calculate the *I:E* ratio based on these settings. If a *longer E* ratio is desired, should the flow rate be increased or decreased?

A. 1 : 1.6; flow rate should be increased
B. 1 : 2.4; flow rate should be increased
C. 1 : 2.4; flow rate should be decreased
D. 1 : 3.2; flow rate should be increased

45t. The following settings are found on a mechanical ventilator: $V_T = 650$ mL (0.65 L), $f = 14$/min, flow rate = 45 L/min. What is the calculated *I:E* ratio based on these settings? If a *shorter E* ratio is desired, what should be done to the flow rate?

A. 1 : 3.1; flow rate should be increased
B. 1 : 3.1; flow rate should be decreased
C. 1 : 3.9; flow rate should be increased
D. 1 : 3.9; flow rate should be decreased

45u. An *I:E* ratio of 1.5 : 1 is the same as:

A. 1 : 0.5
B. 1 : 0.67
C. 1 : 0.8
D. 1 : 1.5

» Go to **rtexam.com** for more learning resources

Lung Volumes and Capacities

46

EQUATION 1

$$TLC = IRV + V_T + ERV + RV$$
$$TLC = VC + RV$$
$$TLC = IC + FRC$$

EQUATION 2

$$VC = IRV + V_T + ERV$$
$$VC = IC + ERV$$
$$VC = TLC - RV$$

EQUATION 3

$$IC = IRV + V_T$$
$$IC = TLC - FRC$$
$$IC = VC - ERV$$

EQUATION 4

$$FRC = ERV + RV$$
$$FRC = TLC - IC$$

TLC : Total lung capacity
VC : Vital capacity
IC : Inspiratory capacity
FRC : Functional residual capacity
IRV : Inspiratory reserve volume
V_T : Tidal volume
ERV : Expiratory reserve volume
RV : Residual volume

NOTES

There are four lung volumes and four lung capacities. Lung volumes are distinct measurements that do not overlap each other. Lung capacities are measurements containing two or more lung volumes (**Figure 46-1**).

Residual volume, functional residual capacity, and total lung capacity cannot be measured directly. They are measured indirectly by one of the following methods: helium dilution, nitrogen washout, body plethysmograph, or radiologic estimation. Changes in lung volumes/capacities are used to interpret restrictive and obstructive lung impairments. In general, restrictive impairments show reduction in lung volumes and capacities. Due to chronic air trapping and hyperinflation, obstructive lung impairments typically have increased residual volume, functional residual capacity and total lung capacity (**Figure 46-2**).

NORMAL VALUES Normal values depend on a person's gender, age, ethnic origin, height, weight, and smoking history. The traditional adult normal values are listed below to show calculation of lung volumes and capacities.

Lung volumes

IRV = 3,100 mL, V_T = 500 mL, ERV = 1,200 mL, RV = 1,200 mL

Lung capacities

$$IC = (IRV + V_T) = 3,600 \text{ mL}$$
$$FRC = (ERV + RV) = 2,400 \text{ mL}$$
$$VC = (IRV + V_T + ERV) = 4,800 \text{ mL}$$
$$TLC = (IRV + V_T + ERV + RV) = 6,000 \text{ mL}$$

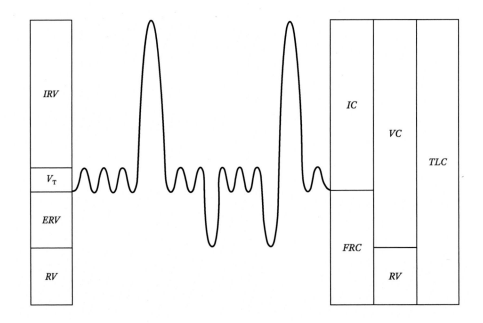

FIGURE 46-1. Spirogram showing the distribution of lung volumes and capacities.

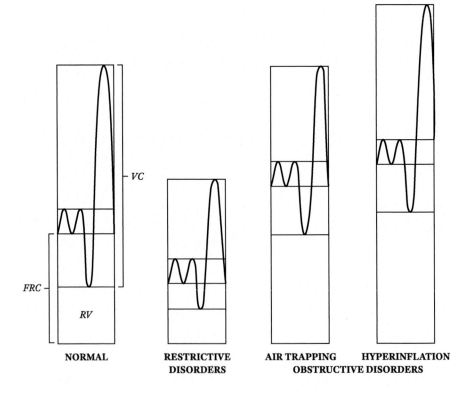

FIGURE 46-2. Spirogram showing the alteration of lung volumes and capacities with restrictive and obstructive lung disorders.

EXAMPLE 1   What is the calculated residual volume if the total lung capacity is 5,800 mL and the vital capacity is 4,950 mL?

$$TLC = VC + RV \text{ (See Equation 1)}$$
$$
\begin{aligned}
RV &= TLC - VC \\
&= 5,800 - 4,950 \\
&= 850 \text{ mL}
\end{aligned}
$$

EXAMPLE 2   Given: Total lung capacity   = 6,400 mL
                        Functional residual capacity = 2,600 mL

What is the calculated inspiratory capacity?

$$
\begin{aligned}
IC &= TLC - FRC \text{ (See Equation 3)} \\
&= 6,400 - 2,600 \\
&= 3,800 \text{ mL}
\end{aligned}
$$

EXERCISE 1   Given: inspiratory capacity 3,900 mL and tidal volume 620 mL. Calculate the inspiratory reserve volume.

[Answer: IRV = 3,280 mL]

EXERCISE 2   Calculate the functional residual capacity if the expiratory reserve volume and residual volume are 1,100 mL and 1,500 mL, respectively.

[Answer: FRC = 2,600 mL]

EXERCISE 3   What is the calculated tidal volume if the inspiratory capacity is 3,450 mL and the inspiratory reserve volume is 2,950 mL?

[Answer: V_T = 500 mL]

SELF-ASSESSMENT QUESTIONS

46a. The sum of IRV and V_T equals to:

A. VC
B. TLC
C. IC
D. FRC

46b. A patient's vital capacity can be calculated by the equation:

A. VC = IRV + ERV
B. VC = TLC − IRV
C. VC = IRV + V_T
D. VC = TLC − RV

46c. The following lung volumes and capacities *cannot* be measured directly by simple spirometry:

A. RV, FRC, TLC
B. TLC, FRC, V_T
C. IRV, RV, FRC
D. FRC, TLC, ERV

46d. A patient's vital capacity (VC) can be calculated by:

I.   TLC − RV
II. IC + FRC
III. IRV + V_T + ERV
IV. FRC + V_T
V.   IC + ERV

A. I, III, and V only
B. I and V only
C. II, III and IV only
D. II, IV and V only

46e. Which of the following *cannot* be used to calculate the total lung capacity (TLC)?

A. IRV + V_T + ERV + RV
B. VC + RV
C. IC + FRC
D. IRV + V_T + ERV

46f. Which of the following equations *cannot* be used to calculate the vital capacity (VC)?

A. VC = IRV + V_T + ERV
B. VC = IRV + V_T
C. VC = IC + ERV
D. VC = IC + FRC − RV

46g. All of the following equations are correct with the *exception* of:

A. IC = IRV + V_T
B. TLC = IC + FRC
C. RV = VC − IC
D. V_T = IC − IRV

Use the lung volumes provided below and match the lung capacities in Column I with the respective values in Column II.

Given: IRV = 3,100 mL, V_T = 500 mL, ERV = 1,200 mL, RV = 1,200 mL

	Column I	Column II
46h.	VC	A. 6,000 mL
46i.	FRC	B. 4,800 mL
46j.	IC	C. 3,600 mL
46k.	TLC	D. 2,400 mL

46l. A pulmonary function study shows the following: IRV = 1,200 mL, V_T = 500 mL, ERV = 1,000 mL. Based on these values, the patient's TLC is:

A. 2,700 mL
B. 2,700 mL + RV
C. 2,700 mL − RV
D. 2,700 mL + FRC

46m. The pulmonary function results show IRV = 1,600 mL, V_T = 500 mL, ERV = 1,000 mL. Based on these data, the patient's TLC is:

A. 2,100 mL minus RV
B. 2,600 mL plus RV
C. 3,100 mL
D. 3,100 mL plus RV

46n to 46q: use the following lung volumes to calculate the lung capacities:

IRV = 3,000 mL, V_T = 650 mL, ERV = 1,100 mL, RV = 1,150 mL

46n. Total lung capacity (TLC) is:

A. 2,900 mL
B. 3,650 mL
C. 4,800 mL
D. 5,900 mL

46o. Vital capacity (VC) is:

A. 4,355 mL
B. 4,750 mL
C. 4,900 mL
D. 5,450 mL

46p. Inspiratory capacity (IC) is:

A. 3,450 mL
B. 3,650 mL
C. 3,850 mL
D. 4,050 mL

46q. Functional residual capacity (FRC) is:

A. 2,250 mL
B. 2,900 mL
C. 3,650 mL
D. 4,750 mL

46r. Calculate the expiratory reserve volume with total lung capacity of 6,200 mL, vital capacity of 4,900 mL, and functional residual capacity of 2,300 mL.

A. 1,000 mL
B. 1,100 mL
C. 1,200 mL
D. 1,300 mL

46s. Given: inspiratory reserve volume = 2,600 mL, total lung capacity = 5,500 mL, functional residual capacity = 2,300 mL. Calculate the inspiratory capacity (IC) and tidal volume (V_T).

A. IC = 3,000 mL; V_T = 700 mL
B. IC = 3,200 mL; V_T = 600 mL
C. IC = 3,300 mL; V_T = 700 mL
D. IC = 3,400 mL; V_T = 600 mL

46t. Given: total lung capacity 5,800 mL, expiratory reserve volume 1,200 mL, inspiratory capacity 3,200 mL and tidal volume 500 mL. Calculate the inspiratory reserve volume (IRV) and residual volume (RV).

A. IRV = 2,700 mL; RV = 1,400 mL
B. IRV = 2,700 mL; RV = 1,500 mL
C. IRV = 2,800 mL; RV = 1,400 mL
D. IRV = 2,800 mL; RV = 1,500 mL

47

Mean Airway Pressure ($\bar{P}aw$)

EQUATION

$$\bar{P}aw = \left[\frac{f \times I \text{ time}}{60}\right] \times (PIP - PEEP) + PEEP$$

(Pressure-controlled or constant pressure ventilation)

$$\bar{P}aw = 0.5 \left[\frac{f \times I \text{ time}}{60}\right] \times (PIP - PEEP) + PEEP$$

(Constant flow ventilation)

$\bar{P}aw$: Mean airway pressure in cm H_2O
f : Frequency/min
I time : Inspiratory time in sec
PIP : Peak inspiratory pressure in cm H_2O
$PEEP$: Positive end-expiratory pressure in cm H_2O

NORMAL VALUE   <30 cm H_2O during mechanical ventilation

EXAMPLE 1

When PEEP is used:

Given: f = 45/min
I time = 0.5 sec
PIP = 35 cm H_2O
PEEP = 5 cm H_2O

Calculate the mean airway pressure.

$$\bar{P}aw = \left[\frac{f \times I \text{ time}}{60}\right] \times (PIP - PEEP) + PEEP$$

$$= \left[\frac{45 \times 0.5}{60}\right] \times (35 - 5) + 5$$

$$= \left[\frac{22.5}{60}\right] \times 30 + 5$$

$$= [0.375] \times 30 + 5$$

$$= 11.25 + 5$$

$$= 16.25 \text{ or } 16 \text{ cm } H_2O$$

NOTES

The mean airway pressure is the average pressure in the airways over a series of breathing cycles during mechanical ventilation. $\bar{P}aw$ is directly related to the frequency, inspiratory time, and peak inspiratory pressure. $\bar{P}aw$ is also increased when expiratory resistance (hold), pressure support, or PEEP is applied during mechanical ventilation.

An increase in $\bar{P}aw$ may cause the cardiac output to fall, particularly in patients with unstable hemodynamic status. An increase in $\bar{P}aw$ may also cause an increase in intracranial pressure. Therefore, $\bar{P}aw$ should be kept at the lowest possible level by limiting the factors listed above, particularly the I time and PEEP. According to the ARDSNet, the plateau pressure (a static measurement) during mechanical ventilation should be kept below 30 cm H_2O to prevent lung injuries. It stands to reason that the mean airway pressure (a dynamic measurement) should also be kept below 30 cm H_2O.

In constant flow ventilation, the ascending pressure curve yields about 50% of the pressure under pressure-controlled (constant pressure) ventillation.

EXAMPLE 2　　When PEEP is not used (same PIP as in Example 1):

Given:　f　　= 45/min
　　　　　I time = 0.5 sec
　　　　　PIP　= 35 cm H_2O
　　　　　PEEP = 0 cm H_2O

Calculate the mean airway pressure.

$$\bar{P}\text{aw} = \left[\frac{f \times I \text{ time}}{60}\right] \times (PIP - PEEP) + PEEP$$

$$= \left[\frac{45 \times 0.5}{60}\right] \times (35 - 0) + 0$$

$$= \left[\frac{22.5}{60}\right] \times 35 + 0$$

$$= [0.375] \times 35 + 0$$

$$= 13.13 + 0$$

$$= 13.13 \text{ or } 13 \text{ cm } H_2O$$

EXERCISE 1　　When PEEP is used:

Given:　f　　= 16/min
　　　　　I time = 1 sec
　　　　　PIP　= 40 cm H_2O
　　　　　PEEP = 10 cm H_2O

Calculate the mean airway pressure.

[Answer: $\bar{P}$aw = 18 cm H_2O]

EXERCISE 2　　When PEEP is not used (same PIP as in Exercise 1):

Given:　f　　= 16/min
　　　　　I time = 1 sec
　　　　　PIP　= 40 cm H_2O
　　　　　PEEP = 0 cm H_2O

Calculate the mean airway pressure.

[Answer: $\bar{P}$aw = 10.67 or 11 cm H_2O]

SELF-ASSESSMENT QUESTIONS

47a. Given: f = 20/min, I time = 0.5 sec, PIP = 40 cm H_2O, PEEP = 5 cm H_2O. Calculate the mean airway pressure.

    A. 11 cm H_2O
    B. 13 cm H_2O
    C. 15 cm H_2O
    D. 17 cm H_2O

47b. Given: f = 26/min, I time = 1.0 sec, PIP = 65 cm H_2O, PEEP = 15 cm H_2O. Calculate the approximate mean airway pressure ($\bar{P}$aw).

    A. 23 cm H_2O
    B. 31 cm H_2O
    C. 37 cm H_2O
    D. 42 cm H_2O

47c. A mechanically ventilated patient has the following data: f = 16/min, I time = 1.5 sec, PIP = 50 cm H_2O, PEEP = 0 cm H_2O. What is the calculated mean airway pressure ($\bar{P}$aw)?

    A. 16 cm H_2O
    B. 20 cm H_2O
    C. 24 cm H_2O
    D. 30 cm H_2O

47d. Positive end-expiratory pressure (PEEP) of 10 cm H_2O is added to the patient in the preceding question. The new data are f = 16/min, I time = 1.5 sec, PIP = 60 cm H_2O, PEEP = 10 cm H_2O. What is the calculated mean airway pressure?

    A. 24 cm H_2O
    B. 26 cm H_2O
    C. 28 cm H_2O
    D. 30 cm H_2O

47e. A neonate is being mechanically ventilated via pressure-controlled mode. The settings are f = 36/min, I time = 0.5 sec, PIP = 35 cm H_2O, PEEP = 5 cm H_2O. Based on this information, calculate the mean airway pressure.

    A. 9 cm H_2O
    B. 14 cm H_2O
    C. 20 cm H_2O
    D. 30 cm H_2O

47f. An infant ventilator has these settings: $f = 30/\text{min}$, I time $= 0.5$ sec, PIP $= 25$ cm H_2O, PEEP $= 6$ cm H_2O. What is the approximate mean airway pressure ($\bar{P}$aw)? If the I time is increased to 0.6 sec, would the $\bar{P}$aw be higher or lower if other parameters remain unchanged?

A. 9 cm H_2O; higher (10 cm H_2O)
B. 11 cm H_2O; lower (10 cm H_2O)
C. 11 cm H_2O; higher (12 cm H_2O)
D. 13 cm H_2O; lower (11 cm H_2O)

47g. A recent ventilator round in the NICU shows the following ventilator settings: $f = 40/\text{min}$, I time $= 0.4$ sec, PIP $= 30$ cm H_2O, PEEP $= 0$ cm H_2O. What is the neonate's approximate mean airway pressure? If PEEP of 5 cm H_2O is added to the ventilator settings, what will be the new mean airway pressure if other parameters remain unchanged?

A. 7 cm H_2O; 9 cm H_2O
B. 7 cm H_2O; 11 cm H_2O
C. 8 cm H_2O; 10 cm H_2O
D. 8 cm H_2O; 12 cm H_2O

48

Mean Arterial Pressure (MAP)

EQUATION

$$MAP = \frac{BP_{systolic} + 2\,BP_{diastolic}}{3}$$

MAP : Mean arterial pressure in mm Hg
$BP_{systolic}$: Systolic blood pressure in mm Hg
$BP_{diastolic}$: Diastolic blood pressure in mm Hg

NORMAL VALUE   >60 mm Hg

EXAMPLE

Given: $BP_{systolic}$ = 120 mm Hg
         $BP_{diastolic}$ = 80 mm Hg

Calculate the mean arterial pressure.

$$MAP = \frac{BP_{systolic} + 2\,BP_{diastolic}}{3}$$

$$= \frac{120 + 2 \times 80}{3}$$

$$= \frac{120 + 160}{3}$$

$$= \frac{280}{3}$$

$$= 93 \text{ mm Hg}$$

EXERCISE

Given: Systolic blood pressure = 110 mm Hg
         Diastolic blood pressure = 50 mm Hg

Calculate the MAP.

[Answer: MAP = 70 mm Hg]

NOTES

This equation calculates the mean (average) arterial blood pressure in the systemic circulation. A normal value of 60 mm Hg is considered the minimum MAP needed to maintain adequate tissue or cerebral perfusion pressure.

MAP is directly related to the systolic and diastolic blood pressures. It is also directly related to the systemic vascular resistance (SVR) and the cardiac output (CO):

$$MAP = SVR \times CO$$

In patients whose systemic vascular resistance is low (e.g., loss of venous tone) or whose cardiac output is low (e.g., CHF), the MAP will be low. The MAP is increased in patients with systemic hypertension.

This equation uses $2 \times BP_{diastolic}$ because the diastolic phase is estimated to be twice as long as the systolic phase. When the heart rate is greater than 120/min, this equation loses its accuracy.

SELF-ASSESSMENT QUESTIONS

48a. Given: systolic blood pressure = 100 mm Hg, diastolic blood pressure = 60 mm Hg. Calculate the mean arterial pressure (MAP).

A. 60 mm Hg
B. 73 mm Hg
C. 80 mm Hg
D. 100 mm Hg

48b. Given: systolic blood pressure = 110 mm Hg, diastolic blood pressure = 70 mm Hg. Calculate the mean arterial pressure (MAP).

A. 35 mm Hg
B. 60 mm Hg
C. 70 mm Hg
D. 83 mm Hg

48c. A patient has a systemic blood pressure reading of 90/60 mm Hg. The calculated mean arterial pressure (MAP) is:

A. 50 mm Hg
B. 60 mm Hg
C. 70 mm Hg
D. 75 mm Hg

48d. The mean arterial pressure is directly related to the:

A. systemic vascular resistance
B. cardiac output
C. systolic and diastolic pressures
D. All of the above

48e. A patient's vital sign measurements are HR 110/min, BP 106/72 mm Hg, SpO_2 95% on room air. What is the calculated mean arterial pressure?

A. 83 mm Hg
B. 90 mm Hg
C. 97 mm Hg
D. 104 mm Hg

48f. Mr. Jones has a blood pressure measurement of 140/90 mm Hg. The calculated mean arterial pressure (MAP) is:

A. 107 mm Hg
B. 115 mm Hg
C. 120 mm Hg
D. 126 mm Hg

>> Go to **rtexam.com** for more learning resources

49

Minute Ventilation

EQUATION 1
Expired Minute Ventilation

$$\dot{V}_E = V_T \times f$$

EQUATION 2
Alveolar Minute Ventilation

$$\dot{V}_A = (V_T - V_D) \times f$$

EQUATION 3
Minute Ventilation in IMV

$$\dot{V}_E = (V_T\,\text{mech} \times f\,\text{mech}) + (V_T \times f)$$

$\dot{V}_E$: Expired minute ventilation in L/min
$\dot{V}_A$: Alveolar minute ventilation in L/min
V_T : Spontaneous tidal volume in mL
$V_T\,\text{mech}$: Ventilator tidal volume in mL
f : Spontaneous frequency/min
$f\,\text{mech}$: Ventilator frequency/min
V_D : Deadspace volume in mL

EXAMPLE 1
(Expired and Alveolar Minute Ventilation)

Given: V_T = 600 mL
V_D = 150 mL
f = 12/min

Calculate the expired minute ventilation $\dot{V}_E$ and the alveolar minute ventilation $\dot{V}_A$.

$$
\begin{aligned}
\dot{V}_E &= V_T \times f \\
&= 600 \times 12 \\
&= 7{,}200 \text{ mL/min or } 7.2 \text{ L/min} \\
\dot{V}_A &= (V_T - V_D) \times f \\
&= (600 - 150) \times 12 \\
&= 450 \times 12 \\
&= 5{,}400 \text{ mL/min or } 5.4 \text{ L/min}
\end{aligned}
$$

NOTES

Minute ventilation equations are used to calculate the expired minute ventilation (Equations 1 and 2) or alveolar minute ventilation (Equation 3). In Equation 1, the expired minute ventilation ($\dot{V}_E$) estimates a patient's ventilation effort (i.e., spontaneous tidal volume and frequency) (**Figure 49-1**). Equation 2 shows the minute ventilation during Intermittent Mandatory Ventilation [IMV or synchronized IMV (SIMV)]. IMV ventilation consists of two parts — mechanical ventilation and spontaneous ventilation. In Equation 3, the alveolar minute ventilation ($\dot{V}_A$) reflects the effective ventilation (alveolar ventilation) — the portion of ventilation capable of taking part in gas exchange (**Figure 49-2**).

Under normal condition, the estimated anatomic deadspace is 1 mL/lb ideal body weight. If the physiologic deadspace is significant (i.e., ↓ pulmonary perfusion as in pulmonary embolism), the V_D should be measured $[\frac{V_D}{V_T} = \frac{(P_aCO_2 - P_ECO_2)}{P_aCO_2}]$.

In mechanical ventilation, the V_T should be the corrected tidal volume.

**EXAMPLE 2
(Minute Ventilation in IMV)**

The average mechanical tidal volume and frequency are 500 mL and 6/min, respectively. During this period, the patient has an average spontaneous tidal volume and frequency of 240 mL and 10/min, respectively. Calculate the expired minute ventilation during IMV.

$$\dot{V}_E = (V_T \text{ mech} \times f\text{mech}) + (V_T \text{ spon} \times f\text{spon})$$
$$= (500 \times 6) \text{ mL/min} + (240 \times 10) \text{ mL/min}$$
$$= 3{,}000 \text{ mL/min} + 2{,}400 \text{ mL/min}$$
$$= 5{,}400 \text{ mL/min or } 5.4 \text{ L/min}$$

EXERCISE 1

Given: $V_T = 550$ mL
$V_D = 100$ mL
$f = 12$/min

Calculate the $\dot{V}_E$ and the $\dot{V}_A$.

[Answer: $\dot{V}_E = 6.6$ L/min, $\dot{V}_A = 5.4$ L/min]

EXERCISE 2

Given the following data during SIMV:

Average mechanical tidal volume = 550 mL
Mechanical frequency = 8/min
Average spontaneous tidal volume = 180 mL
Spontaneous frequency = 16/min

Calculate the expired minute ventilation during SIMV.

[Answer: $\dot{V}_E = 7.28$ L/min]

SELF-ASSESSMENT QUESTIONS

49a. The anatomic deadspace can be estimated to be:

A. 1 mL/kg of ideal body weight
B. 1 mL/lb of ideal body weight
C. 10 mL/kg of ideal body weight
D. 10 mL/lb of ideal body weight

49b. A 130-lb patient has a tidal volume of 600 mL and a respiratory frequency of 12/min. What is the expired minute ventilation and estimated alveolar minute ventilation?

A. 6.3 L/min; 4.8 L/min
B. 6.5 L/min; 5.0 L/min
C. 6.8 L/min; 5.2 L/min
D. 7.2 L/min; 5.6 L/min

49c to 49e: $V_T = 550$ mL, $V_D = 150$ mL, $f = 16$/min

49c. What is the expired minute ventilation?

A. 8.4 L/min
B. 8.6 L/min
C. 8.8 L/min
D. 9.0 L/min

49d. What is the alveolar tidal volume?

A. 380 mL
B. 400 mL
C. 420 mL
D. 440 mL

49e. The alveolar minute ventilation can be calculated by:

A. $[(550 + 150) / 16]$ L/min
B. $[(550 + 150) \times 16]$ L/min
C. $[(550 - 150) / 16]$ L/min
D. $[(550 - 150) \times 16]$ L/min

49f. A patient has an average spontaneous tidal volume of 530 mL and a spontaneous frequency of 16/min. What is the estimated alveolar minute ventilation if the patient weighs 140 lb?

A. 6.24 L/min
B. 6.52 L/min
C. 6.88 L/min
D. 7.25 L/min

49g. Exhaled volumes are collected from a patient over one minute. During this period, 18 breaths are recorded. If the total expired volume is 10 L, the average tidal volume is about:

A. 540 mL
B. 556 mL
C. 572 mL
D. 600 mL

49h. Given: $V_T = 630$ mL, $V_D = 130$ mL, $f = 16$/min. Calculate the approximate expired minute ventilation $\dot{V}_E$ and alveolar minute ventilation $\dot{V}_A$.

A. 9 L/min; 6 L
B. 9 L/min; 7 L/min
C. 10 L/min; 7 L/min
D. 10 L/min; 8 L/min

49i. A patient weighing 130 lb has an average V_T of 610 mL and frequency of 16/min. What is the estimated deadspace volume (V_D)? What is the calculated alveolar minute ventilation $\dot{V}_A$?

A. 100 mL; 6.10 L
B. 100 mL; 7.68 L
C. 130 mL; 7.68 L
D. 130 mL; 9.76 L

49j. Which of the following measurements provide the largest alveolar minute ventilation?

	V_T (mL)	V_D (mL)	f
A.	800	110	15
B.	750	130	18
C.	760	140	14
D.	690	120	16

49k. Based on the equation $\dot{V}_A = (V_T - V_D) \times f$, the alveolar minute ventilation $\dot{V}_A$ may be increased by:

A. increasing the V_T or f
B. decreasing the V_T
C. increasing the V_D
D. decreasing the V_T or f

49l. Given the following data during SIMV: ventilator $V_T = 700$ mL, $f = 6$/min, spontaneous $V_T = 200$ mL, $f = 12$/min. Calculate the expired minute ventilation during SIMV.

A. 2.4 L/min
B. 4.2 L/min
C. 6.6 L/min
D. 9.0 L/min

49m. Which of the following sets of SIMV data produces the *highest* expired minute ventilation?

SIMV	V_T mech	f mech	V_T spon	f spon
A.	550 mL	8/min	200 mL	12/min
B.	600 mL	6/min	250 mL	10/min
C.	650 mL	6/min	200 mL	10/min
D.	700 mL	4/min	250 mL	14/min

Go to **rtexam.com** for more learning resources

50

Oxygen : Air (O_2 : Air) Entrainment Ratio and Total Flow

NOTES

This equation calculates the O_2:air entrainment ratio at any F_IO_2 between 21% and 99%. There is no air entrainment for 100% F_IO_2.

In the equation shown, the 100 represents the fraction of oxygen and 21 represents the oxygen fraction of room air. The 21 should not be rounded off to 20 in calculations with F_IO_2 less than 30% because rounding to 20 can cause erroneous results.

To find the total flow of an O_2:air entrainment device, simply add the O_2:air ratio and multiply the sum by the oxygen flow rate. For example, the O_2:air ratio for 28% oxygen is 1:10. Therefore, the total flow for a 28% O_2:air entrainment device running at 4 L/min of oxygen is $(1 + 10) \times 4 = 11 \times 4 =$ or 44 L/min.

EQUATION 1

O_2:Air Entrainment Ratio

$$O_2:air = 1 : \frac{100 - F_IO_2}{F_IO_2 - 21}$$

O_2 : air : Oxygen : air entrainment ratio

F_IO_2 : Fraction (concentration) of inspired oxygen in %

EQUATION 2

Total Flow of O_2:Air Entrainment Device

Total Flow = Sum of I:E Ratio × Oxygen Flow

Total flow   : Oxygen flow + Air entrained

Sum of I:E ratio : $I + E$

Oxygen flow   : Oxygen flow on the O_2 : air entrainment device

EXAMPLE 1

Find the O_2 : air ratio of a 28% O_2 : air entrainment device.

$$O_2 : air = 1 : \frac{100 - 28}{28 - 21}$$

$$= 1 : \frac{72}{7}$$

$$= 1 : 10.3 \text{ or } 1 : 10$$

On a 28% O_2 : air entrainment device, every 1 unit (L/min) of oxygen is combined with 10 units (L/min) of air. See **Figure 50-1** for the progression of a "tick-tack-toe" method to solve this problem.

21 — 100 — F_IO_2 — — — —	21 — 100 — 28 — — — —	21 — 100 — 28 — 72 / −7 = 10.3
Set up tick-tack-toe as above.	To find O_2:air ratio for 28% oxygen, write 28% in the F_IO_2 block.	Subtract the numbers diagonally. Divide the resulting numbers (72/7). The ratio is 1:10.3 or 1:10. [Disregard the minus sign]

FIGURE 50-1. A "tick-tack-toe" method to solve for O_2:air entrainment ratio of 28% oxygen. The number 21 represents the percentage of oxygen in room air, and 100 represents the percentage of oxygen from a pure oxygen source.

EXAMPLE 2   Find the O_2 : air ratio of a 70% O_2 : air entrainment device.

$$O_2 : air = 1 : \frac{100 - 70}{70 - 21}$$

$$= 1 : \frac{30}{49}$$

$$= 1 : 0.61 \text{ or } 1 : 0.6$$

On a 70% O_2 : air entrainment device, every 1 unit of oxygen is mixed with 0.6 units of air. See **Figure 50-2** for the progression of another "tick-tack-toe" method to solve this problem.

21 — 100 — F_1O_2 — — — —	21 — 100 — 70 — — — —	21 — 100 — 70 — 30 / —49 = 0.61
Set up tick-tack-toe as above.	To find O_2 : air ratio for 70% oxygen, write 70% in the F_1O_2 block.	Subtract the numbers diagonally. Divide the resulting numbers (30/49). The ratio is 1 : 0.61 or 1 : 0.6. [Disregard the minus sign]

FIGURE 50-2. A "tick-tack-toe" method to solve for O_2 : air entrainment ratio of 70% oxygen. The number 21 represents the percentage of oxygen in room air, and 100 represents the percentage of oxygen from a pure oxygen source.

EXAMPLE 3   What is the total flow of an 40% O_2 : air entrainment device (O_2 : air ratio = 1:3) running at 6 L/min of oxygen?

$$\text{Total Flow} = \text{Sum of } I : E \text{ Ratio} \times \text{Oxygen Flow}$$
$$= (1 + 3) \times 6 \text{ L/min}$$
$$= 4 \times 6 \text{ L/min}$$
$$= 24 \text{ L/min}$$

EXERCISE 1   Find the O_2 : air ratio of a 24% O_2 : air entrainment device.

[Answer: O_2 : air = 1 : 25.33 or 1 : 25]

EXERCISE 2   What is the total flow of this 24% O_2 : air entrainment device if an oxygen flow rate of 4 L/min is used? (Use O_2 : air ratio of 1 : 25)

[Answer: Total flow = 104 L/min]

SELF-ASSESSMENT QUESTIONS

50a. The oxygen : air entrainment ratio for 60% oxygen is:

A. 1 : 0.7
B. 1 : 1
C. 1 : 3
D. 1 : 5

50b. Calculate the O_2 : air ratio of a 30% O_2 : air entrainment device.

A. 1 : 7.8
B. 1 : 8.1
C. 1 : 8.9
D. 1 : 10

50c. An oxygen flow rate of 12 L/min is used on a 60% O_2 : air entrainment mask. What is the O_2 : air entrainment ratio and total flow?

A. 1 : 0.5; 12 L/min
B. 1 : 0.5; 24 L/min
C. 1 : 1; 12 L/min
D. 1 : 1; 24 L/min

50d. What is the approximate total flow of a 40% O_2 : air entrainment mask running at 6 L/min of oxygen?

A. 20 L/min
B. 22 L/min
C. 24 L/min
D. 26 L/min

50e. If a patient is using a 40% O_2 : air entrainment mask and a total flow of 36 L/min is needed, what should be the minimum oxygen flow rate?

A. 6 L/min
B. 7 L/min
C. 8 L/min
D. 9 L/min

50f. An O_2 : air entrainment aerosol unit is used to deliver 50% oxygen with aerosol to a patient. What is the approximate O_2 : air ratio and total flow at 6 L/min of oxygen flow?

A. 1 : 1.7; 16 L/min
B. 1 : 1.7; 19 L/min
C. 1 : 2.1; 16 L/min
D. 1 : 2.1; 19 L/min

50g. Which of the following O_2:air entrainment device and flow setting provide the *highest* total flow?

	O_2:Air Entrainment Device	Oxygen Flow	Total Flow
A.	24% O_2:air entrainment mask	3 L/min	
B.	30% O_2:air entrainment large volume aerosol nebulizer	6 L/min	
C.	50% O_2:air entrainment mask	8 L/min	
D.	80% O_2:air entrainment large volume aerosol nebulizer	15 L/min	

50h. Which of the following O_2:air entrainment device and flow setting provide the *lowest* total flow?

	O_2:Air Entrainment Device	Oxygen Flow	Total Flow
A.	24% O_2:air entrainment mask	3 L/min	
B.	30% O_2:air entrainment large volume aerosol nebulizer	6 L/min	
C.	50% O_2:air entrainment mask	8 L/min	
D.	80% O_2:air entrainment large volume aerosol nebulizer	15 L/min	

51

Oxygen Consumption ($\dot{V}O_2$) and Index ($\dot{V}O_2$ index)

EQUATION 1

$$\dot{V}O_2 = \dot{Q}_T \times C(a-\bar{v})O_2$$

EQUATION 2

$$\dot{V}O_2 \text{ index} = \frac{\dot{V}O_2}{BSA}$$

$\dot{V}O_2$: Oxygen consumption in mL/min; same as oxygen uptake

$\dot{V}O_2$ index : Oxygen consumption index in L/min/m²

$\dot{Q}_T$: Total perfusion; same as cardiac output (CO) in L/min

$C(a-\bar{v})O_2$: Arterial-mixed venous oxygen content difference in vol%

BSA : Body surface area in m²

NORMAL VALUES

$\dot{V}O_2$ = 200 to 350 mL/min

$\dot{V}O_2$ index = 125 to 165 mL/min/m²

EXAMPLE

Given: $\dot{Q}_T$ = 5 L/min

         $C(a-\bar{v})O_2$ = 4 vol%

         BSA   = 1.4 m² (patient 1) and

         BSA   = 2 m² (patient 2)

Calculate the oxygen consumption and oxygen consumption indices for both patients.

$$\dot{V}O_2 = \dot{Q}_T \times C(a-\bar{v})O_2$$

$$= 5 \text{ L/min} \times 4 \text{ vol\%}$$

$$= 5 \text{ L/min} \times 0.04$$

$$= 0.2 \text{ L/min}$$

$$= 200 \text{ mL/min}$$

$$\dot{V}O_2 \text{ index for patient 1} = \frac{\dot{V}O_2}{BSA \text{ of patient 1}}$$

$$= \frac{200}{1.4}$$

$$= 143 \text{ mL/min/m}^2$$

The example shows that with a cardiac output ($\dot{Q}_T$) of 5 L/min and an arterial mixed venous oxygen content difference [$C(a-\bar{v})O_2$] of 4 vol%, the oxygen consumption is 200 mL of oxygen per minute. Under normal conditions, oxygen consumption ($\dot{V}O_2$) is directly related to $\dot{Q}_T$ and $C(a-\bar{v})O_2$.

Conditions leading to higher oxygen consumption (e.g., exercise, fever) cause the cardiac output ($\dot{Q}_T$) to increase. If the cardiac output fails to keep up with oxygen consumption, the $C(a-\bar{v})O_2$ gradient increases. Some factors that increase oxygen consumption are listed in **Table 51-1**.

Conditions leading to lower oxygen consumption (e.g., skeletal relaxation, hypothermia) cause the cardiac output to decrease. If the cardiac output remains unchanged, the $C(a-\bar{v})O_2$ gradient decreases. Some factors that decrease oxygen consumption are listed in **Table 51-2**.

Oxygen consumption index ($\dot{V}O_2$ index) is used to normalize oxygen consumption measurements among patients with different body sizes. The examples show that a $\dot{V}O_2$ index of 143 mL/min/m² is within normal range for an average-sized person (BSA = 1.4 m²) but low ($\dot{V}O_2$ index = 100 mL/min/m²) for a larger person (BSA = 2 m²).

$$\dot{V}O_2 \text{ index for patient 2} = \frac{\dot{V}O_2}{BSA \text{ of patient 2}}$$

$$= \frac{200}{2}$$

$$= 100 \text{ mL/min/m}^2$$

EXERCISE Given: $\dot{Q}_T$ = 4.5 L/min
$C(a-\bar{v})O_2$ = 5 vol%
BSA = 1.2 m²

Calculate the oxygen consumption and oxygen consumption indices. Are they within normal limits?

[Answer: $\dot{V}O_2$ = 225 mL/min/m², normal;
$\dot{V}O_2$ index = 187.5 mL/min/m², abnormal]

TABLE 51-1. Factors that increase oxygen consumption

Exercise
Seizures
Shivering in postoperative patient
Hyperthermia
Increase in metabolic rate

TABLE 51-2. Factors that decrease oxygen consumption

Skeletal relaxation (e.g., induced by drugs)
Peripheral shunting (e.g., sepsis, trauma)
Certain poisons (e.g., cyanide prevents cellular metabolism)
Hypothermia
Decrease in metabolic rate

SELF-ASSESSMENT QUESTIONS

51a. Oxygen consumption ($\dot{V}O_2$) in mL/min, is calculated by:

A. $\dot{Q}_T \times C(a-\bar{v})O_2$

B. $\dfrac{\dot{Q}_T}{C(a-\bar{v})O_2}$

C. $\dot{Q}_T + C(a-\bar{v})O_2$

D. $\dot{Q}_T - C(a-\bar{v})O_2$

51b. The normal oxygen consumption ($\dot{V}O_2$) rate for an adult is between:

A. 80 and 120 mL/min

B. 120 and 200 mL/min

C. 200 and 350 mL/min

D. 350 and 500 mL/min

51c. Given: cardiac output $\dot{Q}_T$ = 5.0 L/min, arterial–mixed venous oxygen content difference $C(a-\bar{v})O_2$ = 3.5 vol%, body surface area (BSA) = 1.6 m². Calculate the oxygen consumption rate.

A. 130 mL/min

B. 145 mL/min

C. 160 mL/min

D. 175 mL/min

51d. A patient whose body surface area is 1.4 m² has a measured oxygen consumption ($\dot{V}O_2$) of 200 mL/min. What is the calculated oxygen consumption index ($\dot{V}O_2$ index)?

A. 130 mL/min

B. 143 mL/min

C. 130 mL/min/m²

D. 143 mL/min/m²

51e. Given: cardiac output $\dot{Q}_T$ = 3.6 L/min, arterial–mixed venous oxygen content difference $C(a-\bar{v})O_2$ = 4.0 vol%, body surface area (BSA) = 1.2 m². Calculate the oxygen consumption ($\dot{V}O_2$) and its index ($\dot{V}O_2$ index).

A. 132 mL/min; 110 mL/min/m²

B. 144 mL/min; 120 mL/min/m²

C. 150 mL/min; 125 mL/min/m²

D. 165 mL/min; 138 mL/min/m²

51f. Which of the following measurements has the *highest* oxygen consumption rate?

	$\dot{Q}_T$ (L/min)	$C(a-\bar{v})O_2$ (vol%)
A.	5.5	3.9
B.	3.9	4.9
C.	3.2	5.0
D.	4.7	4.1

51g. Which of the following measurements has the *lowest* oxygen consumption index?

	$\dot{Q}_T$ (L/min)	$C(a-\bar{v})O_2$ (vol%)	Body surface area (m^2)
A.	3.4	5.3	1.6
B.	3.9	4.9	1.5
C.	4.7	4.1	1.9
D.	4.2	5.0	1.7

51h. The oxygen consumption index is used to normalize the oxygen consumption rate according to a person's:

A. age
B. body size
C. gender
D. medical history

52

Oxygen Content: Arterial (C_aO_2)

EQUATION

$C_aO_2 = (\text{Hb} \times 1.34 \times S_aO_2) + (P_aO_2 \times 0.003)$

C_aO_2 : Arterial oxygen content in vol%
Hb : Hemoglobin content in g%
1.34 : Amount of oxygen in 1 g of fully saturated hemoglobin
S_aO_2 : Arterial oxygen saturation in %
P_aO_2 : Arterial oxygen tension in mm Hg
0.003 : Amount of dissolved oxygen for 1 mm Hg of P_aO_2 in vol%

NORMAL VALUE

16 to 20 vol%

EXAMPLE

Given: Hb = 15 g%
S_aO_2 = 98%
P_aO_2 = 100 mm Hg

Calculate the arterial oxygen content.

$C_aO_2 = (\text{Hb} \times 1.34 \times S_aO_2) + (P_aO_2 \times 0.003)$
$= (15 \times 1.34 \times 98\%) + (100 \times 0.003)$
$= 19.70 + 0.3$
$= 20$ vol%

EXERCISE

Given: Hb = 10 g%
S_aO_2 = 80%
P_aO_2 = 60 mm Hg

Calculate the C_aO_2.

[Answer: C_aO_2 = 10.9 vol%]

NOTES

C_aO_2 reflects the overall oxygen-carrying capacity of arterial blood. The major determinants of oxygen content are the hemoglobin (Hb) level and the oxygen saturation (S_aO_2). In normal arterial blood gases, the amount of dissolved O_2 contributes only about 0.3 vol% to the oxygen content of 20 vol% (**Figure 52-1**). A low Hb level (e.g., anemia) or a low O_2 saturation (e.g., hypoxia) significantly lowers the arterial oxygen content. On the other hand, a high Hb level (e.g., polycythemia) or high O_2 saturation (e.g., hyperoxia) raises the arterial oxygen content.

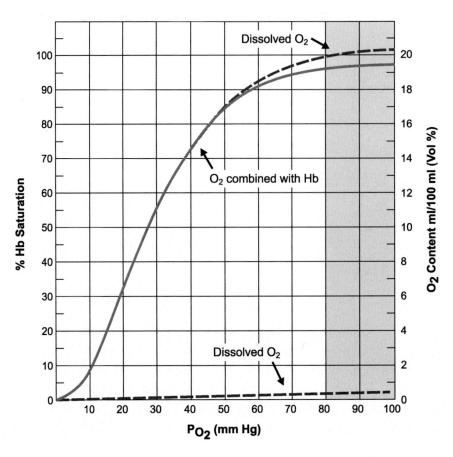

FIGURE 52-1. Oxygen dissociation curve.

SELF-ASSESSMENT QUESTIONS

52a. When the P_aO_2 is 50 mm Hg, the amount of oxygen dissolved in 100 mL of blood is about:

A. 0.05 mL
B. 0.10 mL
C. 0.15 mL
D. 0.20 mL

52b. The amount of oxygen bound to the hemoglobin (Hb) is normally calculated by using the equation:

A. $Hb \times 1.34 + P_aO_2 \times 0.003$
B. $Hb \times 1.34$
C. $Hb \times 1.34 \times S_aO_2$
D. $Hb \times S_aO_2$

52c. In 100 mL of blood, 1 g of fully saturated hemoglobin can carry:

A. 100 mL of oxygen
B. 40 mL of oxygen
C. 47 mL of oxygen
D. 1.34 mL of oxygen

52d. The sum of the oxygen attached to hemoglobin and that dissolved in plasma is called:

A. oxygen content
B. oxygen tension
C. oxygen concentration
D. oxygen saturation

52e. What is the arterial oxygen content of an individual who has a P_aO_2 of 300 mm Hg, oxygen saturation of 99%, and hemoglobin of 16 g%?

A. 21.6 vol%
B. 22.1 vol%
C. 22.9 vol%
D. 23.6 vol%

52f. Given: Hb = 10 g%, S_aO_2 = 95%, P_aO_2 = 60 mm Hg. The calculated C_aO_2 is:

A. 11.1 vol%.
B. 12.9 vol%.
C. 14.6 vol%.
D. 15.3 vol%.

52g. Given: Hb = 15 g%. What is the estimated C_aO_2 under normal conditions?

A. 17 vol%
B. 18 vol%
C. 19 vol%
D. 20 vol%

52h. What is the arterial oxygen content (C_aO_2) of a patient who has a P_aO_2 of 100 mm Hg, oxygen saturation of 98%, and a hemoglobin of 12 g%?

A. 16 vol%
B. 17 vol%
C. 18 vol%
D. 19 vol%

52i. Given: Hb = 10 g%, S_aO_2 = 90%, P_aO_2 = 80 mm Hg. Calculate the arterial oxygen content (C_aO_2).

A. 10.2 vol%

B. 11.1 vol%

C. 12.3 vol%

D. 13.4 vol%

52j. A polycythemic patient has the following blood gas values: Hb 17 g%, S_aO_2 90%, P_aO_2 60 mm Hg. Based on these results, what is the calculated arterial oxygen content (C_aO_2)?

A. 19.4 vol%

B. 19.6 vol%

C. 20.5 vol%

D. 20.7 vol%

52k. Which of the following blood gas measurements has the *lowest* calculated arterial oxygen content (C_aO_2)?

	Hb (g%)	S_aO_2 (%)	P_aO_2 (mm Hg)
A.	13	98	100
B.	15	70	55
C.	16	80	76
D.	14	85	82

52l. The blood gas measurements of a patient recovering from massive blood loss are as follows: Hb = 8 g%, S_aO_2 = 98%, P_aO_2 = 100 mm Hg. What is the calculated C_aO_2? Is it normal?

A. 10.8 vol%; normal

B. 10.8 vol%; abnormal

C. 11.6 vol%; normal

D. 11.6 vol%; abnormal

52m. Given: Hb = 13 g%, S_aO_2 = 90%, P_aO_2 = 60 mm Hg. Calculate the C_aO_2.

A. 13.7 vol%

B. 14.6 vol%

C. 15.9 vol%

D. 16.5 vol%

52n. What is the amount of oxygen carried by 15 g% of 100% saturated hemoglobin?

A. 17 vol%

B. 18 vol%

C. 19 vol%

D. 20.1 vol%

52o. Calculate the C_aO_2 of a patient with the following blood gas data: P_aO_2 90 mm Hg, oxygen saturation of 98%, and a hemoglobin of 14 g%?

    A. 16.4 vol%
    B. 17.3 vol%
    C. 18.7 vol%
    D. 19.5 vol%

52p. Given: Hb = 12 g%, S_aO_2 = 100%, P_aO_2 = 100 mm Hg. Calculate the C_aO_2.

    A. 15.1 vol%
    B. 16.4 vol%
    C. 17.5 vol%
    D. 18.4 vol%

52q. The blood gas data of an anemic patient are as follows: Hb 7 g%, S_aO_2 80%, P_aO_2 80 mm Hg. What is the calculated arterial oxygen content (C_aO_2)?

    A. 7.7 vol%
    B. 8.8 vol%
    C. 9.3 vol%
    D. 10.2 vol%

53

Oxygen Content: End-Capillary (C_cO_2)

NOTES

C_cO_2 is a calculated value representing the best oxygen content possible at the pulmonary end-capillary level. C_cO_2 is used in other calculations such as the shunt equation.

End-capillary oxygen content reflects the optimal oxygen-carrying capacity of the cardiopulmonary system. The oxygen saturation is assumed to be 100%. The major determinant of C_cO_2 is the hemoglobin (Hb) level. A low Hb level (e.g., anemia) significantly lowers the end-capillary oxygen content.

EQUATION

$$C_cO_2 = (Hb \times 1.34 \times S_aO_2) + (P_AO_2 \times 0.003)$$

C_cO_2 : End-capillary oxygen content in vol%
Hb : Hemoglobin content in g%
1.34 : Amount of oxygen in 1 g of fully saturated hemoglobin
S_aO_2 : Arterial oxygen saturation in % (100%)
P_AO_2 : Alveolar oxygen tension in mm Hg, used in place of end-capillary PO_2 (P_cO_2)
0.003 : Amount of dissolved oxygen for 1 mm Hg of P_aO_2

NORMAL VALUE

Varies according to the hemoglobin level and the F_IO_2.

EXAMPLE

Given: Hb = 15 g%
F_IO_2 = 21% [P_AO_2 = 100 mm Hg]

Calculate the end-capillary oxygen content (C_cO_2).

$$
\begin{aligned}
C_cO_2 &= (Hb \times 1.34 \times S_aO_2) + (P_AO_2 \times 0.003) \\
&= (15 \times 1.34 \times 100\%) + (100 \times 0.003) \\
&= 20.1 + 0.3 \\
&= 20.4 \text{ vol}\%
\end{aligned}
$$

EXERCISE

Given: Hb = 10 g%
F_IO_2 = 40% [P_AO_2 = 235 mm Hg]

Calculate the C_cO_2.

[Answer: C_cO_2 = 14.1 vol%]

SELF-ASSESSMENT QUESTIONS

53a. Which of the following calculations requires a P_AO_2 value?

A. $C_{\bar{v}}O_2$

B. C_aO_2

C. C_cO_2

D. $\dfrac{V_D}{V_T}$

53b. Given: Hb = 14 g%, F_IO_2 = 21% (P_AO_2 = 100 mm Hg). Calculate the end-capillary oxygen content (C_cO_2).

A. 18.8 vol%

B. 19.1 vol%

C. 20.1 vol%

D. 21 vol%

53c. Given: Hb = 15 g%; F_IO_2 = 100% (P_AO_2 = 673 mm Hg). Calculate the end-capillary oxygen content (C_cO_2).

A. 19.3 vol%

B. 20.1 vol%

C. 21.4 vol%

D. 22.1 vol%

53d. Which of the following measurements has the *highest* calculated end-capillary oxygen content (C_cO_2)?

	Hb (g%)	F_IO_2 (%)	P_AO_2 (mm Hg)
A.	15	21	100
B.	12	80	530
C.	11	100	673
D.	14	40	235

53e. A polycythemic patient who is recovering from coronary artery bypass surgery has the following measurements: Hb = 17 g%, F_IO_2 = 30% (P_AO_2 = 164 mm Hg). What is the calculated C_cO_2 for this patient?

A. 20.1 vol%

B. 21.9 vol%

C. 22.8 vol%

D. 23.3 vol%

53f. Given: Hb = 15 g%, P_AO_2 = 435 mm Hg). Calculate the end-capillary oxygen content (C_cO_2).

A. 19.1 vol%
B. 19.7 vol%
C. 20.5 vol%
D. 21.4 vol%

53g. Which of the following sets of data has the *lowest* calculated C_cO_2?

	Hb (g%)	P_AO_2 (mm Hg)
A.	12	640
B.	13	100
C.	14	260
D.	15	128

53h. An anemic patient in the Surgical ICU suffering from massive blood loss has the following data: Hb = 8 g%, F_IO_2 = 30% (P_AO_2 = 164 mm Hg). What is the calculated C_cO_2?

A. 11.2 vol%
B. 12.9 vol%
C. 13.6 vol%
D. 14.4 vol%

53i. A patient in the hyperbaric chamber is undergoing treatment at 3 atmospheric pressure (P_B = 2,280 mm Hg). The P_AO_2 on room air (21% O_2) is about 420 mm Hg. If the hemoglobin is 10 g%, what is the calculated C_cO_2?

A. 11.3 vol%
B. 13.1 vol%
C. 14.7 vol%
D. 15.8 vol%

53j. Which of the following set of data (F_IO_2 = 21% O_2) has the *lowest* calculated end-capillary oxygen content (C_cO_2)?

	Hb (g%)	P_B (mm Hg)	P_AO_2 (mm Hg)
A.	9	2,280	420
B.	10	1,520	260
C.	11	760	100
D.	12	380	20

Oxygen Content: Mixed Venous $(C_{\bar{v}}O_2)$

EQUATION

$$C_{\bar{v}}O_2 = (Hb \times 1.34 \times S_{\bar{v}}O_2) + (P_{\bar{v}}O_2 \times 0.003)$$

$C_{\bar{v}}O_2$: Mixed venous oxygen content in vol%
Hb : Hemoglobin content in g%
1.34 : Amount of oxygen in 1 g of fully saturated hemoglobin
$S_{\bar{v}}O_2$: Mixed venous oxygen saturation in %
$P_{\bar{v}}O_2$: Mixed venous oxygen tension in mm Hg
0.003 : Amount of dissolved oxygen for 1 mm Hg of $P_{\bar{v}}O_2$

NORMAL VALUE   12 to 15 vol%

EXAMPLE

Given: Hb $= 15$ g%
$S_{\bar{v}}O_2 = 70\%$
$P_{\bar{v}}O_2 = 35$ mm Hg

Calculate the mixed venous oxygen content $(C_{\bar{v}}O_2)$.

$$C_{\bar{v}}O_2 = (Hb \times 1.34 \times S_{\bar{v}}O_2) + (P_{\bar{v}}O_2 \times 0.003)$$
$$= (15 \times 1.34 \times 70\%) + (35 \times 0.003)$$
$$= 14.07 + 0.11$$
$$= 14.18 \text{ vol\%}$$

EXERCISE

Given: Hb $= 12$ g%
$S_{\bar{v}}O_2 = 75\%$
$P_{\bar{v}}O_2 = 40$ mm Hg

Calculate the $C_{\bar{v}}O_2$.

[Answer: $C_{\bar{v}}O_2 = 12.18$ vol%]

TABLE 54-1. Factors that decrease $C_{\bar{v}}O_2$

Low hemoglobin
Low O_2 saturation
Decreased cardiac output
Increased metabolic rate

SELF-ASSESSMENT QUESTIONS

54a. Given: Hb = 13 g%, $S_{\bar{v}}O_2$ = 70%, $P_{\bar{v}}O_2$ = 40 mm Hg. Calculate the mixed venous oxygen content $(C_{\bar{v}}O_2)$.

    A. 12.3 vol%
    B. 12.9 vol%
    C. 13.6 vol%
    D. 14.2 vol%

54b. A sample obtained from the pulmonary artery has the following results: Hb = 14 g%, $S_{\bar{v}}O_2$ = 75%, $P_{\bar{v}}O_2$ = 40 mm Hg. Calculate the $C_{\bar{v}}O_2$. Is it normal?

    A. 14.2 vol%; abnormal
    B. 14.2 vol%; normal
    C. 15.8 vol%; abnormal
    D. 15.8 vol%; normal

54c. Which of the following blood gas measurements has the *lowest* mixed venous oxygen content $(C_{\bar{v}}O_2)$?

	Hb (g%)	$S_{\bar{v}}O_2$ (%)	$P_{\bar{v}}O_2$ (mm Hg)
A.	13	74	30
B.	15	66	34
C.	14	75	38
D.	14	72	36

54d. An anemic patient who is admitted for shortness of breath has the following mixed venous blood data: Hb = 9 g%, $S_{\bar{v}}O_2$ = 73%, $P_{\bar{v}}O_2$ = 38 mm Hg. What is the calculated $C_{\bar{v}}O_2$ for this patient? Is it normal?

    A. 8.9 vol%; normal
    B. 8.9 vol%; abnormal
    C. 12.1 vol%; normal
    D. 12.1 vol%; abnormal

54e. Given the mixed venous blood data below: Hb = 8 g%, $S_{\bar{v}}O_2$ = 70%, $P_{\bar{v}}O_2$ = 40 mm Hg. Calculate the mixed venous oxygen content $(C_{\bar{v}}O_2)$. Is it normal?

    A. 6.9 vol%; normal
    B. 6.9 vol%; abnormal
    C. 7.6 vol%; normal
    D. 7.6 vol%; abnormal

54f. The normal range for mixed venous oxygen content is:

A. 8 to 11 vol%
B. 10 to 12 vol%
C. 12 to 15 vol%
D. 14 to 16 vol%

54g. The mixed venous oxygen saturation and partial pressure are 60% and 30 mm Hg, respectively. Hemoglobin is 15 g%. Calculate the mixed venous oxygen content.

A. 9.7 vol%
B. 10.3 vol%
C. 11.6 vol%
D. 12.2 vol%

54h. Which of the following sets of data has the *lowest* mixed venous oxygen content?

	Hb (g%)	$S_{\bar{v}}O_2$ (%)	$P_{\bar{v}}O_2$ (mm Hg)
A.	10	76	38
B.	10	72	46
C.	10	74	44
D.	10	70	42

54i. Which of the following sets of data has the *highest* mixed venous oxygen content?

	Hb (g%)	$S_{\bar{v}}O_2$ (%)	$P_{\bar{v}}O_2$ (mm Hg)
A.	14	70	40
B.	14	75	45
C.	15	75	40
D.	15	70	45

54j. A polycythemic patient has the following mixed venous data: Hb = 17 g%, $S_{\bar{v}}O_2$ = 75%, $P_{\bar{v}}O_2$ = 40 mm Hg. What is the calculated mixed venous oxygen content? Is it within normal range?

A. 17.2 vol%; outside normal range
B. 17.2 vol%; within normal range
C. 14.6 vol%; within normal range
D. 14.6 vol%; outside normal range

» Go to **rtexam.com** for more learning resources

55

Oxygen Duration of E Cylinder

NOTES

In this type of oxygen duration calculation, it is essential to remember the conversion factor (0.28) for the E oxygen cylinder. This conversion factor (0.28 L/psig) is derived from dividing the volume of oxygen (622 L) by the gauge pressure (2,200 psig) of a full E cylinder (622 L/2,200 psig = 0.283 L/psig).

The 622 L comes from 22 ft³ × 28.3 L/ft³ as an E cylinder holds about 22 ft³ of compressed oxygen and each ft³ of compressed oxygen gives 28.3 L of gaseous oxygen.

To change minutes to hours and minutes, simply divide the minutes by 60. The whole number represents the hours, and the remainder is the minutes.

When a calculator is used, the number in front of the decimal is the hours. The number after the decimal, including the decimal point, should be multiplied by 60 to obtain minutes.

EQUATION

$$\text{Duration of E} = \frac{0.28 \times \text{psig}}{\text{Liter flow}}$$

Duration of E : Duration of oxygen remaining in an E cylinder in minutes

psig : Gauge pressure, in pounds per square inch (psi)

Liter flow : Oxygen flow rate in L/min

EXAMPLE

Given: E oxygen cylinder with 2,000 psig
Oxygen flow rate = 5 L/min

A. Calculate how long the cylinder will last until empty (0 psig).

$$\begin{aligned} \text{Duration} &= \frac{0.28 \times \text{psig}}{\text{Liter flow}} \\ &= \frac{0.28 \times 2,000}{5} \\ &= \frac{560}{5} \\ &= 112 \text{ min or 1 hr 52 min} \end{aligned}$$

B. Calculate how long the cylinder will last until the pressure reaches 500 psig.

$$\begin{aligned} \text{Duration to 500 psig} &= \frac{0.28 \times (\text{psig} - 500)}{\text{Liter flow}} \\ &= \frac{0.28 \times (2,000 - 500)}{5} \\ &= \frac{0.28 \times 1,500}{5} \\ &= \frac{420}{5} \\ &= 84 \text{ min or 1 hr 24 min} \end{aligned}$$

EXERCISE 1

Given: E oxygen cylinder with 2,200 psig
Oxygen flow rate = 2 L/min

How long will the oxygen remain in this cylinder at this flow rate until the cylinder reaches 0 psig?

[Answer: Duration = 308 min or 5 hr 8 min]

EXERCISE 2   Given: E oxygen cylinder with 1,600 psig
                            Oxygen flow rate = 1 L/min

What is the duration of oxygen until empty (0 psig). How long will it last until 200 psig?

[Answer: Duration until empty = 448 min or 7 hr 28 min
            Duration to 200 psig = 392 min or 6 hr 32 min]

SELF-ASSESSMENT QUESTIONS

55a. The conversion factor for calculating the oxygen duration of a size "E" cylinder is:

A. 0.18
B. 0.28
C. 3.14
D. 4.56

55b. Given: E oxygen cylinder with 2,000 psig, oxygen flow = 2 L/min. Calculate the duration until the pressure reaches 0 psig at this flow rate.

A. 3 hr 55 min
B. 4 hr 5 min
C. 4 hr 20 min
D. 4 hr 40 min

55c. An E oxygen cylinder is full at 2,200 psig. If a flow rate is set at 2 L/min, how long will this cylinder last until it reaches a gauge pressure of 200 psig?

A. 1 hr 20 min
B. 3 hr 30 min
C. 4 hr 40 min
D. 5 hr 10 min

55d. An E oxygen cylinder with 1,400 psig is available for patient transport. At an oxygen flow rate of 2 L/min, what is the maximum travel time the patient can rely on until this cylinder reaches 500 psig?

A. 2 hr 6 min
B. 2 hr 20 min
C. 2 hr 40 min
D. 3 hr

55e. An E oxygen cylinder with 1,800 psig is running at a flow rate of 3 L/min. How long will the cylinder last until empty? Until 200 psig?

A. 2 hr 48 min; 2 hr 29 min
B. 2 hr 48 min; 2 hr 35 min
C. 3 hr 20 min; 3 hr 14 min
D. 3 hr 20 min; 3 hr 42 min

55f. Given: E oxygen cylinder with 2,000 psig, oxygen flow = 1 L/min. Calculate the duration until the 500 psig at this flow rate.

A. 5 hr
B. 6 hr
C. 7 hr
D. 8 hr

55g. An E oxygen cylinder is full at 2,100 psig. If a flow rate is set at 1 L/min, how long will this cylinder last until empty?

A. 8 hr 17 min
B. 9 hr 48 min
C. 10 hr 20 min
D. 11 hr 55 min

55h. An E oxygen cylinder with 2,000 psig is being used for a CT scan procedure. At an oxygen flow rate of 2 L/min, what is the maximum time until the cylinder becomes empty?

A. 3 hr 50 min
B. 4 hr
C. 4 hr 20 min
D. 4 hr 40 min

55i. An E oxygen cylinder with 2,000 psig is being used at a flow rate of 5 L/min. How long will the cylinder last until the pressure reaches 0 psig? Until 100 psig?

A. 1 hr 52 min; 1 hr 42 min
B. 1 hr 52 min; 1 hr 46 min
C. 2 hr 20 min; 2 hr 5 min
D. 2 hr 20 min; 2 hr 12 min

55j. A neonate is being transported to the nursery at an oxygen flow of 0.5 L/min via the nasal cannula. If the cylinder has a pressure of 500 psig, what is the duration until 200 psig?

A. 2 hr 10 min
B. 2 hr 25 min
C. 2 hr 48 min
D. 3 hr 10 min

55k. Which of the following E cylinder set up provides the longest duration of oxygen until empty?

	psig	Flow (L/min)
A.	500	1
B.	700	1.5
C.	800	2
D.	900	2.5

55l. At its respective psig and flow rate, which of the E cylinders empties (to 0 psig) first?

	psig	Flow (L/min)
A.	700	1
B.	800	1.5
C.	900	2
D.	1,000	2.5

Go to **rtexam.com** for more learning resources

56

Oxygen Duration of H or K Cylinder

NOTES

In this type of oxygen duration calculation, it is essential to remember the conversion factor (3.14) for the H or K oxygen cylinder. This conversion factor (3.14 L/psig) is derived from dividing the volume of oxygen (6,900 L) by the gauge pressure (2,200 psig) of a full H or K cylinder:

$$\frac{6,900 \text{ L}}{2,200 \text{ psig}} = 3.136 \text{ L/psig}$$

The 6900 L comes from 224 ft³ × 28.3 L/ft³ because H and K cylinders hold about 244 ft³ of compressed oxygen, and each ft³ of compressed oxygen gives 28.3 L of gaseous oxygen.

To change minutes to hours and minutes, simply divide the minutes by 60. The whole number represents the hours, and the remainder is the minutes.

When a calculator is used to divide, the number in front of the decimal is the hours. The number after the decimal, including the decimal point, should be multiplied by 60 to obtain minutes.

EQUATION

$$\text{Duration of H or K} = \frac{3.14 \times \text{psig}}{\text{Liter flow}}$$

Duration of H or K : Duration of oxygen remaining in an H or K cylinder in minutes

psig : Gauge pressure, in pounds per square inch (psi)

Liter flow : Oxygen flow rate in L/min

EXAMPLE

Given: Size H oxygen cylinder with 1,000 psig
Oxygen flow rate = 5 L/min

A. Calculate how long the cylinder will last until empty (0 psig).

$$\text{Duration of H or K} = \frac{3.14 \times \text{psig}}{\text{Liter flow}}$$

$$= \frac{3.14 \times 1,000}{5}$$

$$= \frac{3,140}{5}$$

$$= 628 \text{ min or } 10 \text{ hr } 28 \text{ min}$$

B. Calculate how long the cylinder will last until the pressure reaches 200 psig.

$$\text{Duration to 200 psig} = \frac{3.14 \times (\text{psig} - 200)}{\text{Liter flow}}$$

$$= \frac{3.14 \times (1,000 - 200)}{5}$$

$$= \frac{3.14 \times 800}{5}$$

$$= \frac{2,512}{5}$$

$$= 502 \text{ min or } 8 \text{ hr } 22 \text{ min}$$

EXERCISE

Given: Size K oxygen cylinder with 2,200 psig
Oxygen flow rate = 2 L/min

Calculate the duration of oxygen remaining in this cylinder until empty (0 psig). How long will the cylinder last until it reaches 200 psig?

[Answer: Duration to 0 psig = 3,454 min or 57 hr 34 min;
Duration to 200 psig = 3,140 min or 52 hr 20 min]

SELF-ASSESSMENT QUESTIONS

56a. An H oxygen cylinder has a gauge pressure of 1,600 psig and is running at a flow rate of 5 L/min. How long will the pressure reach 0 psig at this flow rate?

A. 12 hr 10 min
B. 14 hr 20 min
C. 16 hr 45 min
D. 18 hr 55 min

56b. Given: K oxygen cylinder with 2,200 psig, oxygen flow = 5 L/min. Calculate the duration until the pressure reaches 0 psig at this flow rate.

A. 20 hr
B. 21 hr
C. 22 hr
D. 23 hr

56c. Given: H oxygen cylinder with 1,200 psig, oxygen flow rate = 2 L/min. Calculate the duration of oxygen remaining in this cylinder until it reaches 200 psig.

A. 26 hr 10 min
B. 27 hr 15 min
C. 28 hr 30 min
D. 29 hr 40 min

56d. A K oxygen cylinder has a gauge reading of 1,700 psig. At a flow rate of 2 L/min, how long will this cylinder last until 500 psig?

A. 30 hr 16 min
B. 31 hr 24 min
C. 32 hr 10 min
D. 33 hr 42 min

56e. An H oxygen cylinder with 2,000 psig is running at a flow rate of 3 L/min. How long will the cylinder last until empty (0 psig)? Until 500 psig?

A. 29 hr 35 min; 18 hr 8 min
B. 29 hr 35 min; 21 hr 12 min
C. 34 hr 53 min; 24 hr 26 min
D. 34 hr 53 min; 26 hr 10 min

56f. During the last oxygen rounds at 10 p.m., an H oxygen cylinder has a gauge reading of 800 psig and the oxygen flow was set at 5 L/min. At this oxygen flow rate, about what time the next morning will the gauge reading reach 500 psig?

A. 1 a.m.
B. 2 a.m.
C. 3 a.m.
D. 6 a.m.

56g. A size H oxygen cylinder with 1,800 psig is running at a flow rate of 1 L/min. Calculate the duration of oxygen until the pressure reaches 200 psig.

A. 76 hr 10 min or 3 d 4 hr 10 min
B. 83 hr 44 min or 3 d 11 hr 44 min
C. 88 hr 30 min or 3 d 16 hr 30 min
D. 91 hr 22 min or 3 d 19 hr 22 min

56h. A size K oxygen cylinder has a gauge reading of 2,100 psig. At a flow rate of 4 L/min, how long will the pressure reach 300 psig?

A. 21 hr 17 min
B. 22 hr 24 min
C. 23 hr 33 min
D. 24 hr 42 min

56i. During the oxygen rounds at 7 a.m. on Monday an H oxygen cylinder has a gauge pressure of 1,900 psig. At an oxygen flow of 3 L/min, about what time the next morning (Tuesday) will the gauge reading reach 400 psig?

A. 8 a.m.
B. 9 a.m.
C. 10 a.m.
D. 11 a.m.

56j. Which of the following H cylinders would have the *longest* duration of oxygen until empty at its respective oxygen flow rate?

	psig	Flow (L/min)
A.	600	2
B.	700	2.5
C.	800	3
D.	900	3.5

Go to **rtexam.com** for more learning resources

57

Oxygen Duration of Liquid System

When the liquid weight is known

EQUATION 1

$$\text{Duration} = \frac{344 \times \text{Liquid weight}}{\text{Flow}}$$

Duration	:	Duration of oxygen remaining in a *liquid* O_2 cylinder, in min
344	:	A conversion factor from liquid to gaseous oxygen, in L/lb
Liquid weight	:	The net weight of liquid oxygen in lb
Flow	:	Oxygen flow rate in L/min

EXAMPLE 1

If the net weight of liquid oxygen in a cylinder is 2 lb and the patient is using the contents at 1 L/min, how long will the liquid oxygen last?

$$\text{Duration} = \frac{344 \times \text{Liquid weight}}{\text{Flow}}$$

$$= \frac{344 \times 2}{1}$$

$$= \frac{688}{1}$$

$$= 688 \text{ min or } 11 \text{ hr } 28 \text{ min}$$

EXERCISE

If the net weight of liquid oxygen in a cylinder is 2.5 lb, how long will the liquid oxygen last if the oxygen flow is running at 2 L/min?

[Answer: Duration = 430 min or 7 hr 10 min]

NOTES

When the liquid weight is known

In this type of oxygen duration calculation, it is essential to remember the conversion factor (344 L/lb) for the liquid oxygen cylinders. This conversion factor comes from 860/2.5 = 344 (**Figure 57-1**). Each lb of liquid oxygen expands to 344 L of gaseous oxygen.

If the net weight of liquid oxygen is not shown, one can compute it by weighing the cylinder with liquid oxygen and subtracting the weight of the empty cylinder. To change minutes to hours and minutes, manually divide minutes by 60. The whole number represents the hours, and the remainder is the minutes.

When a calculator is used to divide, the number in front of the decimal is the hours. The number after the decimal, including the decimal point, should be multiplied by 60 to obtain minutes.

The calculated duration does not account for the amount of liquid oxygen lost due to normal evaporation and leakage. The evaporative rate of liquid oxygen ranges from 1 to 1.8 lb (0.4 to 0.72 liquid liters or 344 to 619 gaseous liters) per day.

NOTES

When the gauge fraction is known

One liter of liquid oxygen expands to about 860 L of gaseous oxygen (**Figure 57-2**). Therefore, the liquid capacity is converted to gaseous capacity by multiplying the liquid capacity by 860.

To change minutes to hours and minutes, (manually) divide minutes by 60. The whole number represents the hours, and the remainder is the minutes.

When a calculator is used to divide, the number in front of the decimal is the hours. The number after the decimal, including the decimal point, should be multiplied by 60 to obtain minutes.

The calculated duration does not account for the amount of liquid oxygen due to normal evaporation and leakage. The evaporative rate of liquid oxygen ranges from 1 to 1.8 lb (0.4 to 0.72 liquid liters of 344 to 619 gaseous liters) per day.

When the gauge fraction is known

EQUATION 2

$$\text{Duration} = \frac{\text{Capacity} \times 860 \times \text{Gauge fraction}}{\text{Flow}}$$

Duration : Duration of oxygen remaining in a *liquid* O_2 cylinder, in min

Capacity : Capacity of liquid oxygen in cylinder, in L

860 : Factor to convert liquid to gaseous oxygen, in L

Gauge fraction : Fractional reading of cylinder content

Flow : Oxygen flow rate in L/min

EXAMPLE 2

A portable liquid oxygen cylinder has a liquid capacity of 0.60 L. What is the gaseous oxygen capacity?

$$\begin{aligned}\text{Gaseous capacity} &= \text{Liquid capacity} \times 860 \\ &= 0.60 \times 860 \\ &= 516 \text{ L}\end{aligned}$$

EXAMPLE 3

If the capacity of a liquid oxygen cylinder is 2.0 L and the gauge reading of the cylinder indicates it is $\frac{1}{3}$ full, how long will the liquid oxygen last if the flow is at 2 L/min?

$$\begin{aligned}\text{Duration} &= \frac{\text{Capacity} \times 860 \times \text{Gauge fraction}}{\text{Flow}} \\ &= \frac{2 \times 860 \times \frac{1}{3}}{2} \\ &= \frac{1{,}720 \times \frac{1}{3}}{2} \\ &= \frac{573}{2} \\ &= 287 \text{ min or } 4 \text{ hr } 47 \text{ min}\end{aligned}$$

EXERCISE

If the capacity of a liquid oxygen cylinder is 1.8 L and the gauge reading indicates it is $\frac{1}{2}$ full, how long will the liquid oxygen last if the oxygen flow is at 1 L/min?

[Answer: Duration = 774 min or 12 hr 54 min]

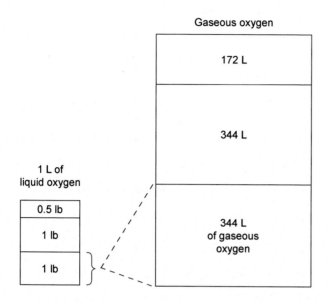

FIGURE 57-1. Volume relationship of liquid and gaseous oxygen. One liter of liquid oxygen weighs about 2.5 lbs. One pound of liquid oxygen equals 344 L of gaseous oxygen.

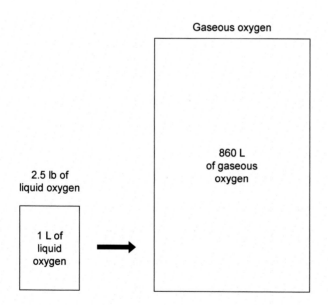

FIGURE 57-2. Volume relationship of liquid and gaseous oxygen. One liter of liquid oxygen weighs about 2.5 lbs and is equal to 860 L of gaseous oxygen.

SELF-ASSESSMENT QUESTIONS

57a. One pound of liquid oxygen equals how many liters of gaseous oxygen?

A. 2.5 L
B. 344 L
C. 500 L
D. 860 L

57b. One liter of liquid oxygen weighs ___ pounds, and each liter equals ___ L of gaseous oxygen.

A. 2 lb; 100 L
B. 2 lb; 344 L
C. 2.5 lb; 500 L
D. 2.5 lb; 860 L

57c. Given: net weight of liquid oxygen in a cylinder = 4 lb. How long will the liquid oxygen last if the oxygen flow rate is 2 L/min?

A. 9 hr 33 min
B. 10 hr 12 min
C. 11 hr 28 min
D. 12 hr 47 min

57d. The net weight of liquid oxygen in a cylinder is 3 lb. If a patient is using 2 L/min of oxygen on a continuous basis, how long will the liquid oxygen last?

A. 7 hr 43 min
B. 8 hr 36 min
C. 9 hr 22 min
D. 10 hr 15 min

57e. A portable liquid oxygen cylinder has a net weight of 1.5 lb. At a flow rate of 1.5 L/min of oxygen, how long will it last until the portable system needs refilling?

A. 3 hr 23 min
B. 4 hr 45 min
C. 5 hr 44 min
D. 6 hr 55 min

57f. The net weight of liquid oxygen in a stationary liquid system is 10 lb. The patient is using it 8 hr per day during sleep at a flow rate of 1 L/min. Based on this usage, about how many days will this liquid oxygen system last? [Hint: After finding the duration remaining in hours, divide by 8 (from 8 hr per day) to obtain days of usage.]

A. 6 days
B. 7 days
C. 8 days
D. 9 days

57g. If the capacity of a full liquid oxygen cylinder is 0.42 L, approximately how many hours will the liquid oxygen last at a flow rate of 2 L/min?

A. 3 hr
B. 4 hr
C. 5 hr
D. 6 hr

57h. A portable liquid oxygen cylinder has a liquid capacity of 0.49 L. What is the gaseous capacity?

A. 319 L
B. 387 L
C. 403 L
D. 421 L

57i. The capacity of a portable liquid oxygen cylinder is 2 L, and the gauge reading indicates it is full. If a patient is using 2 L/min of oxygen on a continuous basis, how long will the liquid oxygen last until empty?

A. 14 hr 20 min
B. 14 hr 45 min
C. 15 hr 20 min
D. 15 hr 45 min

57j. The capacity of a stationary home liquid oxygen system is 25.5 L, and it is full. If a patient is using 1.5 L/min of oxygen on a continuous basis, about how many hours will the liquid system become empty?

A. 214 hr
B. 227 hr
C. 236 hr
D. 243 hr

» Go to **rtexam.com** for more learning resources

58

Oxygen Extraction Ratio (O_2ER)

NOTES

Oxygen extraction ratio (O_2ER) is also called oxygen utilization ratio or oxygen coefficient ratio. In the O_2ER equation, C_aO_2 represents the total amount of oxygen available for peripheral tissue utilization, and $C_aO_2 - C_{\bar{v}}O_2$ reflects the amount of oxygen extracted or consumed by the peripheral tissues.

The O_2ER provides a useful indication of a patient's oxygen transport status. Factors that cause a low C_aO_2 or a high $C(a-\bar{v})O_2$ lead to a high O_2ER value. On the other hand, factors that contribute to a high C_aO_2 or a low $C(a-\bar{v})O_2$ result in a low O_2ER value. **Tables 58-1** and **58-2** summarize the major factors that affect the oxygen extraction ratio.

EQUATION

$$O_2ER = \frac{C_aO_2 - C_{\bar{v}}O_2}{C_aO_2}$$

O_2ER : Oxygen extraction ratio in %
C_aO_2 : Arterial oxygen content in vol%
$C_{\bar{v}}O_2$: Mixed venous oxygen content in vol%

NORMAL VALUE   20 to 28%

EXAMPLE

Given: $C_aO_2 = 20$ vol%
 $C_{\bar{v}}O_2 = 16$ vol%

What is the calculated oxygen extraction ratio (O_2ER)?

$$O_2ER = \frac{C_aO_2 - C_{\bar{v}}O_2}{C_aO_2}$$

$$= \frac{20 - 16}{20}$$

$$= \frac{4}{20}$$

$$= 0.2 \text{ or } 20\%$$

EXERCISE

What is the oxygen extraction ratio (O_2ER) for a patient with C_aO_2 of 19 vol% and $C_{\bar{v}}O_2$ of 16 vol%?

[Answer: $O_2ER = 15.8\%$]

TABLE 58-1. Factors that increase the O_2ER

Decreased cardiac output
Periods of increased oxygen consumption
   Increase in metabolism (e.g., exercise)
   Seizures
   Shivering in postoperative patient
   Hyperthermia (e.g., fever)
Anemia
Decreased arterial oxygenation

TABLE 58–2. Factors that decrease the O_2ER

Increased cardiac output
Peripheral shunting (e.g., sepsis, trauma)
Certain poisons (e.g., cyanide prevents cellular metabolism)
Hypothermia (slows cellular metabolism)
Polycythemia ($\uparrow$ hemoglobin)
Increased arterial oxygenation

SELF-ASSESSMENT QUESTIONS

58a. In the oxygen extraction ratio equation, $C_aO_2 - C_{\bar{v}}O_2$ represents:

A. amount of oxygen remaining after tissue consumption
B. oxygen consumption
C. arterial oxygen content
D. mixed venous oxygen content

58b. The oxygen extraction ratio is *increased* in conditions of:

A. increased metabolism
B. sepsis
C. hypothermia
D. polycythemia

58c. The oxygen extraction ratio is *decreased* in conditions of:

A. fever
B. exercise
C. sepsis
D. anemia

58d. Given: $C_aO_2 = 18$ vol%, $C_aO_2 - C_{\bar{v}}O_2 = 4.5$ vol%. What is the oxygen extraction ratio?

A. 23%
B. 24%
C. 25%
D. 26%

58e. With an arterial oxygen content (C_aO_2) of 19% and an arterial-mixed venous oxygen content difference ($C_aO_2 - C_{\bar{v}}O_2$) of 4.5 vol%. Calculate the oxygen extraction ratio.

A. 16%
B. 20%
C. 24%
D. 28%

58f. The oxygen content measurements of a patient with anemia are as follows: $C_aO_2 = 15$ vol%, $C_aO_2 - C_{\bar{v}}O_2 = 5$ vol%. What is the oxygen extraction ratio?

A. 15%
B. 28%
C. 30%
D. 33%

58g. Given: $C_aO_2 = 21$ vol%, , $C_{\bar{v}}O_2 = 15.6$ vol%. Calculate the oxygen extraction ratio (O_2ER).

A. 19%
B. 21%
C. 23%
D. 26%

58h. Which of the following pairs of oxygen content measurements has the *highest* oxygen extraction ratio?

	C_aO_2 (vol%)	$C_{\bar{v}}O_2$ (vol%)
A.	21	16
B.	21	17
C.	20	16
D.	20	17

58i. Which of the following pairs of oxygen content measurements has the *lowest* oxygen extraction ratio?

	C_aO_2 (vol%)	$C_{\bar{v}}O_2$ (vol%)
A.	18.5	13.8
B.	18.5	14.2
C.	19.3	14.2
D.	19.3	15.5

59

P/F Index

EQUATION

$$P/F = P_aO_2/F_IO_2$$

P/F : P_aO_2/F_IO_2 index (ratio) in mm Hg

P_aO_2 : Partial pressure of oxygen in arterial blood, in mm Hg

F_IO_2 : Inspired oxygen concentration in %

NORMAL VALUE >300 mm Hg

EXAMPLE

What is the *P/F* index for P_aO_2 of 60 mm Hg while on an F_IO_2 of 40% (0.4)? If PEEP is ≥5 cm H_2O, classify the severity of ARDS if other criteria for ARDS are met.

$$P/F = P_aO_2/F_IO_2$$
$$= 60 \text{ mm Hg}/0.4$$
$$= 150 \text{ mm Hg}$$

[Answer: *P/F* = 150 mm Hg; moderate ARDS]

EXERCISE

A mechanically ventilated patient has the following data: P_aO_2 70 mm Hg, F_IO_2 80%, PEEP 10 cm H_2O. Calculate the *P/F* index and classify the severity of ARDS.

[Answer: *P/F* = 88 mm Hg; severe ARDS]

NOTES

P_aO_2/F_IO_2 (*P/F*) index describes the relationship between P_aO_2 and its respective F_IO_2. It evaluates a person's oxygenation status (P_aO_2) relative to the amount of oxygen required to achieve this P_aO_2. Patients with intrapulmonary shunting (e.g., ARDS) typically have refractory hypoxemia (type of hypoxemia that responds poorly to oxygen therapy). Refractory hypoxemia has a persistently low P_aO_2 in spite of high F_IO_2. The *P/F* is therefore lower than normal.

In 2012, the Berlin definition of ARDS uses *P/F* index extensively in the classification of ARDS severity (**Table 59-1**).

TABLE 59-1. Berlin definition of acute respiratory distress syndrome

Onset	Within one week of a known clinical condition or new or worsening respiratory symptoms
Chest radiograph	Bilateral opacities not fully explained by effusions, atelectasis or nodules
Pulmonary edema	Respiratory failure not fully explained by heart failure or fluid overload
Mild ARDS	P_aO_2/F_IO_2 200 mm Hg to ≤300 mm Hg with PEEP or CPAP ≥5 cm H_2O
Moderate ARDS	P_aO_2/F_IO_2 100 mm Hg to ≤200 mm Hg with PEEP or CPAP ≥5 cm H_2O
Severe ARDS	P_aO_2/F_IO_2 ≤100 mm Hg with PEEP ≥5 cm H_2O

SELF-ASSESSMENT QUESTIONS

59a. Given: P_aO_2 100 mm Hg, F_IO_2 30% (0.3). What is the *P/F* index? Is it normal?

   A. 111 mm Hg; abnormal
   B. 222 mm Hg; abnormal
   C. 333 mm Hg; normal
   D. 444 mm Hg; normal

59b. Given: P_aO_2 50 mm Hg, F_IO_2 40% (0.4). What is the *P/F* index? Is it normal?

   A. 125 mm Hg; normal
   B. 125 mm Hg; abnormal
   C. 200 mm Hg; normal
   D. 200 mm Hg; abnormal

59c. A mechanically ventilated patient has a P_aO_2 of 70 mm Hg and F_IO_2 55% (0.55). Calculate the *P/F*. If the patient meets all criteria for ARDS, classify the severity of ARDS.

   A. 39 mm Hg; moderate ARDS
   B. 39 mm Hg; severe ARDS
   C. 127 mm Hg; mild ARDS
   D. 127 mm Hg; moderate ARDS

59d. A patient has a P_aO_2 of 65 mm Hg on an F_IO_2 of 40% while using 8 cm H_2O *CPAP*. Calculate the *P/F*. If the patient meets all criteria for ARDS, classify the severity of ARDS.

   A. 163 mm Hg; moderate ARDS
   B. 196 mm Hg; moderate ARDS
   C. 251 mm Hg; mild ARDS
   D. 324 mm Hg; normal

59e. Which of the following sets of data has the *highest P/F* index?

	P_aO_2 (mm Hg)	F_IO_2 (%)
A.	75	60
B.	80	45
C.	60	50
D.	95	70

59f. Which of the following sets of data has the *lowest P/F* index?

	P_aO_2 (mm Hg)	F_IO_2 (%)
A.	58	40
B.	60	55
C.	72	60
D.	88	45

59g. Assuming all 4 patients below have met the criteria for ARDS, which patient has *mild* ARDS?

	Patient	P_aO_2 (mm Hg)	F_IO_2 (%)
A.	John	87	40
B.	Jane	45	50
C.	Kate	66	60
D.	Kerry	72	45

59h. All 4 patients below have met the criteria for ARDS, which patient has *moderate* ARDS?

	Patient	P_aO_2 (mm Hg)	F_IO_2 (%)
A.	Arlene	108	45
B.	Aaron	48	55
C.	Pam	76	60
D.	Paul	87	40

59i. All patients below may be classified as having *severe* ARDS *except*:

	Patient	P_aO_2 (mm Hg)	F_IO_2 (%)
A.	Chi	60	65
B.	Hero	48	50
C.	Tang	77	55
D.	Lo	54	60

60

Partial Pressure of a Dry Gas

NOTES

Dalton's law states that the partial pressures of all gases in a gas mixture equal the total pressure exerted by the gas mixture. There-fore, the partial pressure of a gas can be determined by multiplying the barometric pressure (P_B) by the percentage of the gas in the mixture (%g).

At high altitude, the P_B decreases. Consequently the partial pressures of all gases also decrease. For exam-ple, at an altitude of 26,000 ft above sea level (P_B = 270 mm Hg), PO_2 = 270 mm Hg × 0.21 = 56.7 mm Hg. On the other hand, hyperbaric conditions (e.g., below sea level, hyperbaric chambers) increase the barometric pressure and partial pres-sures of all gases. At a depth of 66 ft below sea level (P_B = 2,280 mm Hg), PO_2 = 2,280 mm Hg × 0.21 = 478.8 mm Hg.

The purpose of oxygen therapy is to increase the partial pressure of oxygen in the inspired gas mixture. There are two methods to increase the partial pressure of oxygen – by increasing the F_IO_2 or the baromet-ric pressure. In most clinical settings, the F_IO_2 is increased by using nasal cannula, oxygen mask, or mechani-cal ventilator. In special conditions such as wound care or treatment of bends (air bubbles in blood), the barometric pressure is increased (i.e., hyperbaric chamber) to raise the partial pressure of oxygen.

EQUATION

$$P_g = P_B \times \%g$$

P_g : Partial pressure of a dry gas
P_B : Barometric pressure in mm Hg
%g : Percent of gas in the mixture

EXAMPLE

What is the partial pressure of (a) nitrogen and (b) oxygen in an air sample at a barometric pressure of 720 mm Hg?

Since nitrogen comprises 78% of room air:

A. $PN_2 = P_B \times \%N_2$
   $= 720 \times 78\%$
   $= 561.6$ mm Hg

Since oxygen comprises 21% of room air:

B. $PO_2 = P_B \times \%O_2$
   $= 720 \times 21\%$
   $= 151.2$ mm Hg

EXERCISE 1

Calculate the partial pressure of oxygen in a dry air sample at 40,000 ft above sea level (P_B = 141 mm Hg). (Note: the F_IO_2 at 40,000 ft above sea level is same as at sea level = 21%.)

[Answer: PO_2 = 29.6 mm Hg]

SELF-ASSESSMENT QUESTIONS

60a. Given: P_B = 760 mm Hg, F_IO_2 21%. What is the partial pressure of oxy-gen in a dry, ambient gas sample?

A. 100 mm Hg
B. 130 mm Hg
C. 160 mm Hg
D. 190 mm Hg

60b. At two atmospheric pressures, the P_B is 1,520 mm Hg. On an F_IO_2 of 21%, what is the partial pressure of oxygen in a dry, ambient gas sample?

A. 100 mm Hg
B. 146 mm Hg
C. 278 mm Hg
D. 319 mm Hg

60c. Given: P_B = 760 mm Hg, F_ICO_2 0.03%. What is the partial pressure of carbon dioxide in a dry, ambient gas sample?

A. 0.228 mm Hg
B. 2.28 mm Hg
C. 22.8 mm Hg
D. 228 mm Hg

60d. Given: P_B = 760 mm Hg, F_IO_2 40% via air entrainment mask. What is the partial pressure of oxygen in a dry gas sample?

A. 160 mm Hg
B. 286 mm Hg
C. 304 mm Hg
D. 413 mm Hg

60e. At sea level (P_B = 760 mm Hg), a patient is receiving 3 L/min via nasal cannula with an estimated F_IO_2 of about 32%. What is the partial pressure of oxygen in the inspired dry gas sample?

A. 243 mm Hg
B. 265 mm Hg
C. 277 mm Hg
D. 291 mm Hg

60f. At 2,000 ft above sea level (P_B = 707), a patient is being mechanical ventilated on an F_IO_2 of 60%. What is the partial pressure of oxygen in the inspired dry gas sample?

A. 386 mm Hg
B. 424 mm Hg
C. 457 mm Hg
D. 473 mm Hg

60g. At 6,000 ft above sea level (Denver, CO), the P_B is 609 mm Hg. What is the partial pressure of oxygen (PO_2) in a dry, ambient air sample at this altitude? How much lower is it than the calculated PO_2 at sea level (P_B = 760 mm Hg)? Note: the F_IO_2 at sea level and at 6,000 ft above sea level is 21%.

A. 100 mm Hg; 60 mm Hg lower
B. 128 mm Hg; 32 mm Hg lower
C. 140 mm Hg; 20 mm Hg lower
D. 160 mm Hg; same as sea level

60h. At 66 ft below sea level (P_B = 2,280 mm Hg), what is the partial pressure of oxygen of a diver's inspired air (21% oxygen)?

A. 311 mm Hg
B. 346 mm Hg
C. 423 mm Hg
D. 479 mm Hg

60i. Calculate the partial pressure of oxygen in a dry air sample at 14,000 ft (Mt. Elbert, CO) above sea level. The P_B is 446 mm Hg at this altitude.

A. 80 mm Hg
B. 94 mm Hg
C. 110 mm Hg
D. 122 mm Hg

60j. Nitrogen makes up about 78% of ambient air. Calculate its partial pressure in a dry air sample at sea level (P_B = 760 mm Hg).

A. 554 mm Hg
B. 575 mm Hg
C. 593 mm Hg
D. 617 mm Hg

61

pH (Henderson-Hasselbalch)

EQUATION 1

$$pH = 6.1 + \log\left[\frac{HCO_3^-}{H_2CO_3}\right]$$

EQUATION 2

$$pH = 6.1 + \log\left[\frac{HCO_3^-}{PCO_2 \times 0.03}\right]$$

pH   : Puissance hydrogen, negative logarithm of H^+ ion concentration
HCO_3^- : Serum bicarbonate concentration in mEq/L
H_2CO_3 : Carbonate acid in mEq/L
PCO_2 : Carbon dioxide tension in mm Hg

NORMAL VALUE

Arterial pH   = 7.40 (7.35 to 7.45)
Mixed venous pH = 7.36

EXAMPLE

Given: H_2CO_3 : 24 mEq/L
         PCO_2 : 40 mm Hg

Calculate the pH.

$$pH = 6.1 + \log\left[\frac{HCO_3^-}{PCO_2 \times 0.03}\right]$$

$$= 6.1 + \log\left[\frac{24}{40 \times 0.03}\right]$$

$$= 6.1 + \log\left[\frac{24}{1.2}\right]$$

$$= 6.1 + \log 20$$

(From a scientific calculator or common logarithms table in Appendix J, log 20 = 1.301)

pH = 6.1 + 1.301
     = 7.401 or 7.40

EXERCISE 1

Given: HCO_3^- : 30 mEq/L
         PCO_2 : 50 mm Hg
         log 20 : 1.301

Calculate the pH.

[Answer: pH = 7.401 or 7.40]

NOTES

The pH is directly related to the bicarbonate (HCO_3^-) level and inversely related to the carbonic acid (H_2CO_3) or the carbon dioxide tension (PCO_2) level.

Unless there is compensation, the pH will be higher than 7.40 with an increase of HCO_3^- (metabolic alkalosis) or a decrease of PCO_2 (respiratory alkalosis). If the $HCO_3^- : H_2CO_3$ ratio is higher than 20:1, the pH will be higher than 7.40.

On the other hand, the pH will be lower than 7.40 with a decrease of HCO_3^- (metabolic acidosis) or an increase of PCO_2 (respiratory acidosis). If the $HCO_3^- : H_2CO_3$ ratio is lower than 20:1, the pH will be lower than 7.40.

It is essential to note that the pH will be 7.40 as long as the $HCO_3^- : H_2CO_3$ ratio is 20:1. The Example and Exercise 1 illustrate this compensatory effect even though the HCO_3^- and PCO_2 values are quite different in these two examples.

EXERCISE 2

Given: HCO_3^- : 16 mEq/L
PCO_2 : 32 mm Hg

Use the Henderson-Hasselbalch equation and common logarithms table (Appendix J) to calculate the pH.

[Answer: pH = 7.32 (log 16.67 = 1.222)]

SELF-ASSESSMENT QUESTIONS

61a. Based on the Henderson Hasselbach equation, when the bicarbonate to carbonic acid (HCO_3^- : H_2CO_3) ratio in blood is 20 : 1, the calculated pH is always:

A. 7.20
B. 7.30
C. 7.40
D. 7.50

61b. The pH is lower than 7.40 when the bicarbonate to carbonic acid ratio is:

A. 20 : 1
B. 1 : 20
C. higher than 20 : 1
D. lower than 20 : 1

61c. Given: HCO_3^- = 30 mEq/L, PCO_2 = 50 mm Hg. The calculated carbonic acid is:

A. 1.2 mEq/L
B. 12 mEq/L
C. 1.5 mEq/L
D. 15 mEq/L

61d. Given: HCO_3^- 18 mEq/L, PCO_2 30 mm Hg. Calculate the HCO_3^- : H_2CO_3 ratio and pH.

A. 19 : 1; 7.40
B. 19 : 1; 7.38
C. 20 : 1; 7.40
D. 20 : 1; 7.38

61e. Given: HCO_3^- 34 mEq/L, PCO_2 56.7 mm Hg. What are the approximate HCO_3^- : H_2CO_3 ratio and pH?

A. 20:1; 7.40
B. 20:1; 7.38
C. 22:1; 7.40
D. 22:1; 7.44

61f. Given: HCO_3^- 12 mEq/L, PCO_2 20 mm Hg. What are the approximate HCO_3^- : H_2CO_3 ratio and pH?

A. 20:1; 7.38
B. 20:1; 7.40
C. 16:1; 7.30
D. 16:1; 7.40

61g. A patient has the following blood gas results: pH 7.40, HCO_3^- 12 mEq/L, PCO_2 20 mm Hg. What is the calculated pH? Is the measured pH consistent with the calculated pH?

A. calculated pH = 7.40; measured pH is consistent with the calculated pH
B. calculated pH = 7.50; measured pH is not consistent with the calculated pH
C. calculated pH = 7.33; measured pH is not consistent with the calculated pH
D. calculated pH = 7.20; measured pH is not consistent with the calculated pH

61h. Given the following blood gas data: pH 7.33, HCO_3^- 30 mEq/L, PCO_2 50 mm Hg. What is the calculated pH? Is the measured pH consistent with the calculated pH?

A. calculated pH = 7.33; measured pH is consistent with the calculated pH
B. calculated pH = 7.40; measured pH is not consistent with the calculated pH
C. calculated pH = 7.50; measured pH is not consistent with the calculated pH
D. calculated pH = 7.26; measured pH is not consistent with the calculated pH

61i. Which of the following sets of data does *not* produce a calculated pH of 7.40? [Hint: Look for a bicarbonate : carbonate acid (HCO_3^- : H_2CO_3) ratio of 20:1 for a pH of 7.40]

	HCO_3^- (mEq/L)	PCO_2 (mm Hg)
A.	24	40
B.	28	42
C.	36	60
D.	12	20

61j. Which of the following sets of data has a calculated pH of 7.40? [Hint: Look for a bicarbonate : carbonate acid (HCO_3^- : H_2CO_3) ratio of 20 : 1 for a pH of 7.40]

	HCO_3^- (mEq/L)	PCO_2 (mm Hg)
A.	29	40
B.	18	47
C.	31	46
D.	33	55

61k. The blood gas results of a patient with severe ketoacidosis show: pH 7.33, PCO_2 30 mm Hg, HCO_3^- 10 mEq/L. The physician asks you to verify the data. Calculate the pH. Is there a technical error in the results? {Hint: Use Appendix J or a scientific calculator to find the log of $[HCO_3^- / (PCO_2 \times 0.03)]$ and then apply to the pH equation}

A. 7.15; could have a technical error
B. 7.22; could have a technical error
C. 7.33; no technical error
D. 7.42; could have a technical error

61l. The blood gas results of a patient with combined alkalosis show: pH 7.46, PCO_2 28 mm Hg, HCO_3^- 30 mEq/L. The physician asks you to verify the data. Calculate the pH. Is there a technical error in the results? {Hint: Use Appendix J or a scientific calculator to find the log of $[HCO_3^- / (PCO_2 \times 0.03)]$ and then apply to the pH equation}

A. 7.46; no technical error
B. 7.38; could have a technical error
C. 7.24; could have a technical error
D. 7.65; could have a technical error

62

Poiseuille Equation

EQUATION

$$\dot{V} = \frac{\Delta P r^4 \pi}{\mu l 8}$$

$\dot{V}$: Flow
ΔP : Driving pessure
r : Radius of airway
$\dfrac{\pi}{8}$: Constant for equation
μ : Gas viscosity
l : Length of airway

EXAMPLE

The internal radius of a size 6 endotracheal tube (ETT) is 3 mm. With this ETT, the peak inspiratory pressure (ΔP) during volume-controlled ventilation is 40 cm H_2O. If the ETT is changed to a size 7 ETT (radius 3.5 mm), calculate the ΔP needed to maintain the same settings on the ventilator.

$$\Delta P = \frac{\dot{V}}{r^4}$$

Since $\dot{V}$ is unchanged,

$$\text{(size 6) } \Delta P \times r^4 = \text{(size 7) } \Delta P \times r^4$$
$$40 \times 3^4 = \text{size 7 } \Delta P \times 3.5^4$$
$$\text{size 7 } \Delta P = \frac{40 \times 3^4}{3.5^4} \text{ cm } H_2O$$
$$= \frac{40 \times 81}{150} \text{ cm } H_2O$$
$$= 21 \text{ cm } H_2O$$

[Size 7 ETT $\Delta P = 21$ cm H_2O]

EXERCISE

With a size 8 ETT, the PIP is 60 cm H_2O. Calculate the PIP when a size 8.5 ETT is used. (Note: radius is half of the ETT size.)

[Answer: size 8.5 ETT $\Delta P = 47$ cm H_2O]

NOTES

The Poiseuille equation describes the characteristic of flow (turbulent or laminar) in the airway. The gas flow is influenced by the driving pressure difference, gas viscosity, and radius and length of the airway.

Under clinical conditions where gas viscosity (μ), length of airway (l), and $\dfrac{\pi}{8}$ remain stable and unchanged, they may be disregarded and simplified to an abbreviated equation:

$$\Delta P = \frac{\dot{V}}{r^4}$$

The abbreviated equation shows the inverse relationship between the work of breathing (ΔP) and radius of airway (r). When the radius of the airway (r) decreases by half, the driving pressure (ΔP) must increase 16 times to maintain the same gas flow. In a clinical setting, bronchoconstriction (decrease in r) can cause a significant increase in the work of breathing ($\uparrow \Delta P$). If the work of breathing cannot keep up with the bronchoconstriction, airflow ($\dot{V}$) will be decreased. In pulmonary function testing, reduction in flow rate measurements is generally indicative of airflow obstruction (e.g., bronchospasm, bronchoconstriction, secretions in airway).

SELF-ASSESSMENT QUESTIONS

62a. Which of the following is the simplified form of the Poiseuille equation that describes the relationship between work of breathing and radius of airway?

A. $\Delta P = \dot{V} \times r^2$

B. $\Delta P = \dfrac{\dot{V}}{r^2}$

C. $\Delta P = \dot{V} \times r^4$

D. $\Delta P = \dfrac{\dot{V}}{r^4}$

62b. The Poiseuille equation shows that when the radius of the airway (r) decreases by half, the driving pressure (ΔP) must increase _____ times to maintain the same flow.

A. 2

B. 4

C. 8

D. 16

62c. The driving pressure (ΔP) during volume-controlled ventilation is 20 cm H_2O for a constant flow of 50 L/min. If the radius of the endotracheal tube is reduced by 50%, calculate the ΔP needed to maintain the same ventilator settings (i.e., flow, tidal volume, frequency).

A. 32 cm H_2O

B. 52 cm H_2O

C. 320 cm H_2O

D. 360 cm H_2O

62d. The internal radius of a size 8 endotracheal tube (ETT) is 4 mm. With this ETT, the peak inspiratory pressure (ΔP) during volume-controlled ventilation is 30 cm H_2O. If the ETT is changed to a size 7 ETT (radius 3.5 mm), calculate the ΔP needed to maintain the same settings on the ventilator. (Hint: 30 cm $H_2O \times 4^4$ mm = new $\Delta P \times 3.5^4$ mm)

A. 43 cm H_2O

B. 51 cm H_2O

C. 58 cm H_2O

D. 65 cm H_2O

62e. The internal radius of a pediatric size 4 endotracheal tube (ETT) is 2 mm. With this ETT, the peak inspiratory pressure (ΔP) is 12 cm H_2O during volume-controlled ventilation. If the ETT is changed to size 4.5 (radius 2.25 mm), calculate the ΔP needed to maintain the same ventilator settings.

   A. 6.4 cm H_2O
   B. 6.8 cm H_2O
   C. 7.5 cm H_2O
   D. 8.1 cm H_2O

62f. The internal radius of a size 6 endotracheal tube (ETT) is 3 mm. The peak inspiratory pressure (ΔP) is 50 cm H_2O during volume-controlled ventilation. If the ETT is changed to a size 7 ETT (radius 3.5 mm), calculate the ΔP needed to maintain the same ventilator settings.

   A. 27 cm H_2O
   B. 33 cm H_2O
   C. 39 cm H_2O
   D. 44 cm H_2O

63

Pressure Support Ventilation Setting

NOTES

To calculate the PSV setting, the $\dot{V}_{mach}$ and $\dot{V}_{spon}$ should have the same units of measurement (L/min or mL/sec).

Pressure support ventilation reduces the work of spontaneous breathing by overcoming the airflow resistance during invasive and noninvasive ventilation. PSV is active only when spontaneous breathing is available (e.g., SIMV). During *mechanical ventilation* and in patients with measurable spontaneous breathing efforts, the calculated PSV setting is used to overcome airflow resistance imposed by the endotracheal tube, secretions, and ventilator circuit. The calculated PSV setting is used during the initial phase of PSV. The PSV setting is adjusted based on the changing airflow resistance and compliance.

For *weaning* from mechanical ventilation using a *spontaneous breathing trial*, PSV is titrated until a spontaneous frequency of 20 to 25/min or a spontaneous tidal volume of 8 to 10 mL/kg ideal body weight (IBW) is reached. A PSV of greater than 30 cm H_2O is rarely used because patients needing high level of pressure support are typically not ready for weaning. If indicated, PSV level is reduced by 2 to 4 cm H_2O increments as tolerated. Extubation can be considered when the PSV level reaches 5 to 8 cm H_2O for at least 30 minutes with no signs of respiratory distress.

EQUATION

$$\text{PSV setting} = \left[\frac{\left(\text{PIP} - P_{plat}\right)}{\dot{V}_{mach}} \right] \times \dot{V}_{spon}$$

PSV setting : Initial pressure support ventilation setting
PIP : Peak inspiratory pressure
P_{PLAT} : Plateau pressure
$\dot{V}_{mach}$: Inspiratory flow of ventilator, in L/min
$\dot{V}_{spon}$: Inspiratory flow during spontaneous breathing in L/min (obtained via flow/time graphic or estimated to be 500 mL/sec or 30 L/min)

EXAMPLE

Calculate the PSV setting for a mechanically ventilated patient with the following data: PIP = 50 cm H_2O, P_{plat} = 35 cm H_2O, $\dot{V}_{mach}$ = 50 L/min, $\dot{V}_{spon}$ = 30 L/min).

$$\text{PSV setting} = \left[\frac{\left(\text{PIP} - P_{plat}\right)}{\dot{V}_{mach}} \right] \times \dot{V}_{spon}$$

$$= \left[\frac{\left(50 \text{ cm } H_2O - 35 \text{ cm } H_2O\right)}{50 \text{ L/min}} \right] \times 30 \text{ L/min}$$

$$= \left[\frac{\left(15 \text{ cm } H_2O\right)}{50 \text{ L/min}} \right] \times 30 \text{ L/min}$$

$$= \left[\frac{\left(0.3 \text{ cm } H_2O\right)}{\text{L/min}} \right] \times 30 \text{ L/min}$$

$$= 9 \text{ cm } H_2O$$

[Answer: Initial PSV setting = 9 cm H_2O.]

EXERCISE 1

A mechanically ventilated patient has the following data: PIP = 45 cm H_2O, P_{PLAT} = 25 cm H_2O, $\dot{V}_{mach}$ = 60 L/min, $\dot{V}_{spon}$ = 30 L/min. Calculate the initial PSV setting.

[Answer: Initial PSV setting = 10 cm H_2O]

EXERCISE 2

The following data are obtained from a patient who is being mechanically ventilated on a SIMV mode: PIP = 50 cm H_2O, P_{PLAT} = 35 cm H_2O, $\dot{V}_{mach}$ = 40 L/min, $\dot{V}_{spon}$ = 20 L/min. What should be the initial PSV setting?

[Answer: Initial PSV setting = 7.5 cm H_2O]

SELF-ASSESSMENT QUESTIONS

63a. A patient is being mechanically ventilated, and the data below are obtained: PIP = 60 cm H_2O, P_{PLAT} = 40 cm H_2O, $\dot{V}_{mach}$ = 50 L/min, $\dot{V}_{spon}$ = 20 L/min. What should be the initial PSV setting?

A. 6 cm H_2O
B. 8 cm H_2O
C. 10 cm H_2O
D. 12 cm H_2O

63b. A respiratory therapist has recorded the following data from a mechanically ventilated patient: PIP = 50 cm H_2O, P_{PLAT} = 40 cm H_2O, $\dot{V}_{mach}$ = 60 L/min, $\dot{V}_{spon}$ = 30 L/min. Calculate the initial PSV setting.

A. 5 cm H_2O
B. 7 cm H_2O
C. 9 cm H_2O
D. 11 cm H_2O

63c. Since pressure support ventilation is active only during spontaneous breathing, PSV *cannot* be used during which mode of ventilation?

A. synchronized intermittent mandatory ventilation (SIMV)
B. controlled or continuous mandatory ventilation (CMV)
C. continuous positive airway pressure (CPAP)
D. intermittent mandatory ventilation (IMV)

63d. When weaning a patient from mechanical ventilation using a spontaneous breathing trial, the initial PSV level is titrated until it reaches a spontaneous:

A. frequency of 25 to 30/min
B. tidal volume of 4 to 6 mL/kg IBW
C. frequency of 20 to 25/min
D. tidal volume of 6 to 8 mL/kg IBW

63e. The physician asks a therapist to perform a spontaneous breathing trial for weaning purpose. The respiratory therapist should titrate the PSV setting until the patient achieves a:

A. spontaneous tidal volume of 6 mL/kg to 8 mL/kg IBW
B. spontaneous frequency of 30/min to 35/min
C. spontaneous frequency of 8/min to 12/min
D. spontaneous tidal volume of 8 mL/kg to 10 mL/kg IBW

63f. A mechanically ventilated patient has the following data: PIP 45 cm H_2O, P_{PLAT} 25 cm H_2O, $\dot{V}_{mach}$ 50 L/min, $\dot{V}_{spon}$ 20 L/min. Calculate the initial pressure support ventilation setting.

    A. 6 cm H_2O
    B. 7 cm H_2O
    C. 8 cm H_2O
    D. 9 cm H_2O

63g. The mechanical ventilation data are as follows: PIP 30 cm H_2O, P_{PLAT} 15 cm H_2O, $\dot{V}_{mach}$ 40 L/min, $\dot{V}_{spon}$ 20 L/min. The initial pressure support ventilation setting should be:

    A. 7.5 cm H_2O
    B. 8.5 cm H_2O
    C. 9.5 cm H_2O
    D. 10.5 cm H_2O

63h. A mechanically ventilated patient has these data: PIP 40 cm H_2O, P_{PLAT} 20 cm H_2O, $\dot{V}_{mach}$ 50 L/min, $\dot{V}_{spon}$ 30 L/min. What should be the initial pressure support ventilation setting?

    A. 6 cm H_2O
    B. 8 cm H_2O
    C. 10 cm H_2O
    D. 12 cm H_2O

63i. Given the mechanical ventilation data below: PIP 60 cm H_2O, P_{PLAT} 40 cm H_2O, $\dot{V}_{mach}$ 50 L/min, $\dot{V}_{spon}$ 40 L/min. What should be the initial pressure support ventilation setting?

    A. 12 cm H_2O
    B. 14 cm H_2O
    C. 16 cm H_2O
    D. 18 cm H_2O

63j. A mechanically ventilated patient has these data: PIP 55 cm H_2O, P_{PLAT} 20 cm H_2O, $\dot{V}_{mach}$ 50 L/min, $\dot{V}_{spon}$ 20 L/min. Calculate the initial pressure support ventilation setting.

    A. 14 cm H_2O
    B. 15 cm H_2O
    C. 16 cm H_2O
    D. 17 cm H_2O

63k. Which set of mechanical ventilation data below requires the *highest* initial PSV setting?

	PIP (cm H_2O)	P_{PLAT} (cm H_2O)	$\dot{V}_{mach}$ (L/min)	$\dot{V}_{spon}$ (L/min)
A.	40	30	50	30
B.	40	20	50	40
C.	50	30	60	30
D.	50	20	60	40

63l. Which set of mechanical ventilation data below requires the *lowest* initial PSV setting?

	PIP (cm H_2O)	P_{PLAT} (cm H_2O)	$\dot{V}_{mach}$ (L/min)	$\dot{V}_{spon}$ (L/min)
A.	45	25	40	30
B.	45	35	50	40
C.	55	25	40	30
D.	55	35	50	40

64

Relative Humidity

NOTES

Relative humidity is usually measured by a hygrometer. The examples show how humidity content and capacity are related to relative humidity. Since humidity capacity is directly related to the temperature, a higher temperature allows the air to hold more humidity (↑ capacity). If the humidity content remains constant, a higher temperature (higher humidity capacity) leads to a *lower* relative humidity. Converse is also true.

Heated aerosol therapy provides two components to respiratory care. First, the heat increases the capacity of the gas mixture to carry humidity. Second, the aerosol increases the content (actual humidity) of the inspired gas, thus lowering the humidity deficit.

EQUATION

$$RH = \frac{Content}{Capacity}$$

RH : Relative humidity in %

Content : Humidity content of a volume of gas in mg/L or mm Hg; also known as actual or absolute humidity

Capacity : Humidity capacity or maximum amount of water that air can hold at a given temperature, in mg/L or mm Hg; also known as maximum absolute humidity

NORMAL VALUE   The relative humidity is directly related to the humidity content.

EXAMPLE 1   What is the relative humidity if the content of an air sample is 12 mg/L and its capacity is 18 mg/L?

$$RH = \frac{Content}{Capacity}$$

$$= \frac{12}{18}$$

$$= 0.67 \text{ or } 67\%$$

EXAMPLE 2   Calculate the relative humidity if the content of an air sample is 16 mg/L and its capacity is 20 mg/L.

$$RH = \frac{Content}{Capacity}$$

$$= \frac{16}{20}$$

$$= 0.8 \text{ or } 80\%$$

EXERCISE   An air sample has a humidity content of 15 mg/L and a capacity of 26 mg/L. What is the calculated relative humidity?

[Answer: RH = 0.577 or 58%]

SELF-ASSESSMENT QUESTIONS

64a. What is the relative humidity if the humidity content of an air sample is 12 mg/L and the humidity capacity is 24 mg/L?

    A. 20%
    B. 40%
    C. 50%
    D. 60%

64b. Calculate the relative humidity of an air sample if its humidity content is 14 mg/L and the humidity capacity is 19 mg/L.

    A. 33%
    B. 74%
    C. 80%
    D. 85%

64c. An air sample has a humidity content of 23 mg/L and a capacity of 26 mg/L at 100% saturation. Calculate the relative humidity of this sample.

    A. 72%
    B. 76%
    C. 83%
    D. 88%

64d. Given humidity content 14 mg/L and humidity capacity 44 mg/L at 100% saturation. Calculate the relative humidity.

    A. 32%
    B. 36%
    C. 40%
    D. 44%

64e. What is the relative humidity if the humidity content and capacity are 20 mg/L and 30 mg/L, respectively?

    A. 65%
    B. 67%
    C. 69%
    D. 71%

64f. **Which set of humidity data has the *highest* relative humidity?**

	Humidity Content (mg/L)	Humidity Capacity (mg/L)
A.	20	24
B.	25	32
C.	30	35
D.	35	40

64g. **Which set of humidity data has the *lowest* relative humidity?**

	Humidity Content (mg/L)	Humidity Capacity (mg/L)
A.	21	26
B.	27	31
C.	32	37
D.	35	42

65

Reynolds Number

EQUATION

$$R_N = \frac{v \times D \times d}{\mu}$$

R_N : Reynolds number
v : Velocity of fluid (or gas)
D : Fluid density
d : Diameter of tube
μ : Viscosity of fluid (or gas)

When the Reynolds number is less than 2,000, it reflects laminar flow; when over 2,000, it reflects turbulent flow. In actuality, values between 2,000 and 4,000 provide a mixed or transitional pattern (laminar and turbulent), but most respiratory care references refer to values within this range as turbulent flow. In respiratory care, an increase in gas flow rate (v) or gas density (D) will increase the Reynolds number, thus making a turbulent flow more likely. Laminar flow may be achieved by using a lower flow rate or a gas mixture with low density. For example, helium has a low gas density and the oxygen/helium mixture may be used to promote laminar gas flow in patients with airflow obstruction.

Velocity, density, and diameters are three variables directly related to the Reynolds number. Viscosity is inversely related to the Reynolds number. An increase in airway size (d) does not increase the Reynolds number because the resulting lower flow rate (v) offsets any significant increase in the Reynolds number.

NORMAL VALUE $R_N < 2,000$

NOTES

Osborne Reynolds (1842–1912), an English scientist, developed a dimensionless number (ratio) to describe the dynamics of fluid and airflow.

SELF-ASSESSMENT QUESTIONS

65a. **The Reynolds number is used to describe the characteristic of:**

A. gas flow
B. gas density
C. lung elasticity
D. lung compliance

65b. Laminar flow is likely when the:

A. gas flow is greater than 10 L/min
B. gas flow is less than 10 L/min
C. Reynolds number is greater than 4,000
D. Reynolds number is less than 2,000

65c. Oxygen/helium mixture may be used to manage airflow obstruction because it has a_____ gas density and promotes _____ flow.

A. higher; laminar
B. higher; turbulent
C. lower; laminar
D. lower; turbulent

65d. An increase in airway size _____ the Reynolds number because the resulting _____ flow rate ($\dot{V}$) offsets any significant change in the Reynolds number.

A. increases; higher
B. decreases; higher
C. does not change; lower
D. does not change; higher

65e. Which of the following fluid or gas variables are *directly* related to the Reynolds number (R_N)?

A. velocity and density
B. velocity, density, and diameter
C. density, diameter, and viscosity
D. velocity, density, and viscosity

65f. Which of the following fluid or gas variables are *inversely* related to the Reynolds number (R_N)?

A. viscosity
B. density
C. diameter
D. velocity

Go to **rtexam.com** for more learning resources

66

Shunt Equation ($Q_{sp}/\dot{Q}_T$): Classic Physiologic

EQUATION

$$\frac{Q_{sp}}{\dot{Q}_T} = \frac{C_cO_2 - C_aO_2}{C_cO_2 - C_{\bar{v}}O_2}$$

$Q_{sp}/\dot{Q}_T$: Physiologic shunt to total perfusion ratio in %
C_cO_2　: End-capillary oxygen content in vol%
C_aO_2　: Arterial oxygen content in vol%
$C_{\bar{v}}O_2$　: Mixed venous oxygen content in vol%

NORMAL VALUE　Less than 10%

EXAMPLE

Given:　C_cO_2　= 20.4 vol%
$\qquad\quad C_aO_2$　= 19.8 vol%
$\qquad\quad C_{\bar{v}}O_2$　= 13.4 vol%

$$\frac{Q_{sp}}{\dot{Q}_T} = \frac{C_cO_2 - C_aO_2}{C_cO_2 - C_{\bar{v}}O_2}$$

$$= \frac{20.4 - 19.8}{20.4 - 13.4}$$

$$= \frac{0.6}{7}$$

$$= 0.086 \text{ or } 8.6\%$$

EXERCISE

Given:　C_cO_2　= 20.6 vol%
$\qquad\quad C_aO_2$　= 17.2 vol%
$\qquad\quad C_{\bar{v}}O_2$　= 10.6 vol%

Calculate the $Q_{sp}/\dot{Q}_T$. What is the interpretation?

[Answer: $Q_{sp}/\dot{Q}_T$ = 34%; severe shunt]

NOTES

The shunt equation calculates the portion of cardiac output not taking part in gas exchange (i.e., wasted perfusion). The classic physiologic shunt equation requires an arterial sample for C_aO_2 and a mixed venous sample for $C_{\bar{v}}O_2$.

A calculated shunt of less than 10% is considered normal in clinical settings. A shunt of 10 to 20% indicates mild intrapulmonary shunting, and a shunt of 21 to 30% indicates moderate (or significant) intrapulmonary shunting. Greater than 30% of calculated shunt reflects severe (or critical) intrapulmonary shunting. $Q_{sp}/\dot{Q}_T$ is increased in the presence of one of the following categories of shunt-producing diseases: *anatomic shunt* (e.g., congenital heart disease, intrapulmonary fistulas, vascular lung tumors); *capillary shunt* (e.g., atelectasis, alveolar fluid); *venous admixture* (e.g., hypoventilation, uneven distribution of ventilation, diffusion defects).

Modified Shunt Equation

$$\frac{Q_{sp}}{\dot{Q}_T} = \frac{(P_AO_2 - P_aO_2) \times 0.003}{(C_aO_2 - C_{\bar{v}}O_2) + (P_AO_2 - P_aO_2) \times 0.003}$$

The modified shunt equation originates from the classic physiologic shunt equation where $(P_AO_2 - P_aO_2) \times 0.003$ is used to substitute for $C_cO_2 - C_aO_2$. The equation requires an arterial PO_2 greater than 150 mm Hg. As most critically ill patients do not achieve this level of PO_2, it has limited clinical application.

SELF-ASSESSMENT QUESTIONS

66a. Normal cardiopulmonary function usually provides a calculated shunt of:

A. 10% or less
B. 20% or less
C. 30% or less
D. 40% or less

66b. The classic physiologic shunt equation is:

A. $\left(C_aO_2 - C_{\bar{v}}O_2\right) \times \left(C_cO_2 - C_aO_2\right)$

B. $\dfrac{C_aO_2 - C_{\bar{v}}O_2}{C_cO_2 - C_aO_2}$

C. $\dfrac{C_aO_2 - C_{\bar{v}}O_2}{C_cO_2 - C_{\bar{v}}O_2}$

D. $\dfrac{C_cO_2 - C_aO_2}{C_cO_2 - C_{\bar{v}}O_2}$

66c. The $\left(C_cO_2 - C_aO_2\right)$ portion of the classic physiologic shunt equation represents:

A. oxygen consumption
B. shunted perfusion
C. total perfusion
D. oxygen content

66d. Given: $C_cO_2 = 21.1$ vol%, $C_aO_2 = 18.8$ vol%, $C_{\bar{v}}O_2 = 14.4$ vol%. Calculate the percent shunt using the classic physiologic shunt equation. What is the interpretation?

A. 17%; mild shunt
B. 23%; moderate shunt
C. 34%; severe shunt
D. 38%; severe shunt

66e. Given: $C_cO_2 = 20.5$ vol%, $C_aO_2 = 20.1$ vol%, $C_{\bar{v}}O_2 = 13.8$ vol%. Calculate the percent shunt using the classic physiologic shunt equation. Is it normal or abnormal?

A. 6%; normal
B. 6%; abnormal
C. 12%; normal
D. 12%; abnormal

66f. A patient in the intensive care unit has the following oxygen contents: C_aO_2 = 19.7 vol%, $C_{\bar{v}}O_2$ = 13.6 vol%. If the calculated C_cO_2 is 20.8 vol%, what is the percent shunt based on the classic physiologic shunt equation? What is the interpretation?

    A. 8%; normal
    B. 10%; mild shunt
    C. 15%; mild shunt
    D. 18%; mild shunt

66g. A patient with acute respiratory distress syndrome has a P/F index of 150 mm Hg. The oxygen contents are: C_cO_2 21 vol%, C_aO_2 18.2 vol%, and $C_{\bar{v}}O_2$ 14 vol%. Use the classic physiologic shunt equation to calculate the shunt percent. Is it consistent with the diagnosis?

    A. 20%; moderate shunt, inconsistent with diagnosis
    B. 20%; severe shunt, consistent with diagnosis
    C. 40%; moderate shunt, consistent with diagnosis
    D. 40%; severe shunt, consistent with diagnosis

66h. Which of the following sets of data has the *highest* calculated physiologic shunt?

	C_cO_2	C_aO_2	$C_{\bar{v}}O_2$
A.	20	19	15
B.	19	17	14
C.	21	20	16
D.	18	17	13

66i. Which of the following sets of oxygen content measurement has the *lowest* calculated physiologic shunt?

	C_cO_2	C_aO_2	$C_{\bar{v}}O_2$
A.	20.8	18.7	14.3
B.	18.7	16.9	13.2
C.	20.1	19.0	14.6
D.	18.4	17.2	13.5

66j. Which of the following sets of oxygen content measurement represents *normal* physiologic shunt?

	C_cO_2	C_aO_2	$C_{\bar{v}}O_2$
A.	19.8	19.0	14.3
B.	20.3	18.2	13.6
C.	18.3	17.5	13.8
D.	17.1	16.8	12.9

66k. A patient has a series of four physiologic shunt measurements. Which set of data represents *severe* physiologic shunt?

	C_cO_2	C_aO_2	$C_{\bar{v}}O_2$
A.	20.3	17.8	13.6
B.	19.6	19.0	14.7
C.	19.1	17.7	13.5
D.	18.5	17.9	13.8

66l. Which of the four physiologic shunt measurements below has an interpretation of *moderate* shunt?

	C_cO_2	C_aO_2	$C_{\bar{v}}O_2$
A.	20.1	18.3	14.7
B.	19.7	18.2	14.3
C.	19.4	16.5	13.1
D.	19.3	17.6	14.2

67

Shunt Equation ($Q_{sp}/\dot{Q}_T$): Estimated

EQUATION 1

For individuals who are breathing spontaneously with or without CPAP:

$$\frac{Q_{sp}}{\dot{Q}_T} = \frac{C_cO_2 - C_aO_2}{5 + (C_cO_2 - C_aO_2)}$$

EQUATION 2

For critically ill patients who are receiving mechanical ventilation with or without *PEEP*:

$$\frac{Q_{sp}}{\dot{Q}_T} = \frac{C_cO_2 - C_aO_2}{3.5 + (C_cO_2 - C_aO_2)}$$

$Q_{sp}/\dot{Q}_T$: Physiologic shunt to total perfusion ratio in %
C_cO_2 : End-capillary oxygen content in vol%
C_aO_2 : Arterial oxygen content in vol%

NORMAL VALUE

Less than 10%

EXAMPLE 1

Given: A patient on CPAP of 5 cm H_2O

C_cO_2 = 20.4 vol%
C_aO_2 = 19.8 vol%

Use 5 vol% as the estimated $C(a-\bar{v})O_2$ and calculate $Q_{sp}/\dot{Q}_T$.

$$\frac{Q_{sp}}{\dot{Q}_T} = \frac{C_cO_2 - C_aO_2}{5 + (C_cO_2 - C_aO_2)}$$

$$= \frac{20.4 - 19.8}{5 + (20.4 - 19.8)}$$

$$= \frac{0.6}{5 + 0.6}$$

$$= \frac{0.6}{5.6}$$

$$= 0.107 \text{ or } 10.7\%$$

NOTES

The estimated shunt equation does not require a mixed venous blood sample. It is less accurate than the classic physiologic shunt equation. In normal subjects, 5 vol% is used as the estimated arterial-mixed venous oxygen content difference $[C(a-\bar{v})O_2]$.

In critically ill patients, 3.5 vol% is used because these patients typically have a lower $C(a-\bar{v})O_2$ as a result of lower oxygen extraction (consumption).

A calculated shunt of less than 10% is considered normal in clinical settings. A shunt of 10 to 20% indicates mild intrapulmonary shunting, and a shunt of 21 to 30% indicates moderate (or significant) intrapulmonary shunting. Greater than 30% of calculated shunt reflects severe (or critical) intrapulmonary shunting.

$Q_{sp}/\dot{Q}_T$ is increased in the presence of one of the following categories of shunt producing diseases: anatomic shunt (e.g., congenital heart disease, intrapulmonary fistulas, vascular lung tumors); capillary shunt (e.g., atelectasis, alveolar fluid); venous admixture (e.g., hypoventilation, uneven distribution of ventilation, diffusion defects).

EXAMPLE 2

Given: A patient on mechanical ventilation.

$C_cO_2 = 20.4$ vol%
$C_aO_2 = 19.8$ vol%

Use 3.5 vol% as the estimated $C(a-\bar{v})O_2$ and calculate $Q_{sp}/\dot{Q}_T$.

$$\frac{Q_{sp}}{\dot{Q}_T} = \frac{C_cO_2 - C_aO_2}{3.5 + (C_cO_2 - C_aO_2)}$$

$$= \frac{20.4 - 19.8}{3.5 + (20.4 - 19.8)}$$

$$= \frac{0.6}{3.5 + 0.6}$$

$$= \frac{0.6}{4.1}$$

$$= 0.146 \text{ or } 14.6\%$$

EXERCISE 1

Given: $C_cO_2 = 20.6$ vol%
$C_aO_2 = 19.8$ vol%

Use $C(a-\bar{v})O_2$ of 5 vol% and calculate the estimated $Q_{sp}/\dot{Q}_T$ of a patient. What is the interpretation?

[Answer: $Q_{sp}/\dot{Q}_T = 0.138$ or 13.8%; mild shunt.]

EXERCISE 2

Given the oxygen contents of a critically ill patient who is receiving mechanical ventilation:

$C_cO_2 = 20.6$ vol%

$C_aO_2 = 17.2$ vol%

Use $C(a-\bar{v})O_2$ of 3.5 vol% and calculate the estimated $Q_{sp}/\dot{Q}_T$ of this critically ill patient. What is the interpretation?

[Answer: $Q_{sp}/\dot{Q}_T = 0.49$ or 49%; abnormal, severe shunt.]

SELF-ASSESSMENT QUESTIONS

67a. **All of the following are true with regard to the estimated shunt equation with the *exception* of:**

A. It does not require a pulmonary artery catheter.
B. Its accuracy is same as the classic physiologic shunt equation.
C. It does not require a mixed venous sample.
D. It requires an arterial blood sample.

67b. Select the estimated physiologic shunt equation for individuals who are *breathing spontaneously*:

A. $\dfrac{C_cO_2 - C_aO_2}{C_cO_2 - C_{\bar{v}}O_2}$

B. $(C_cO_2 - C_aO_2) \times (5 + C_cO_2 - C_aO_2)$

C. $\dfrac{C_cO_2 - C_aO_2}{5 + C_cO_2 - C_aO_2}$

D. $\dfrac{C_aO_2 - C_{\bar{v}}O_2}{5 + C_cO_2 - C_aO_2}$

67c. Given the oxygen contents below for a *spontaneously breathing* person: $C_cO_2 = 20.4$ vol%, $C_aO_2 = 19.7$ vol%. Calculate the estimated $Q_{sp}/\dot{Q}_T$. What is the interpretation?

A. 12.3%; mild shunt
B. 12.3%; normal
C. 23.6%; moderate shunt
D. 23.6%; normal

67d. A *critically ill* patient has a C_aO_2 of 14.5 vol%. If the calculated end-capillary oxygen content is 16.8 vol%, what is the estimated shunt for this patient? How severe is the shunt? (Assume $C_aO_2 - C_{\bar{v}}O_2 = 3.5$ vol% for *critically ill* patients.)

A. 24.8%; mild shunt
B. 24.8%; moderate shunt
C. 39.7%; moderate shunt
D. 39.7%; severe shunt

67e. Which of the following sets of values has the *highest* estimated shunt?

	C_cO_2	C_aO_2 (vol%)
A.	20	19
B.	19	17
C.	21	20
D.	18	17

67f. Which of the following sets of values has the *lowest* estimated shunt?

	C_cO_2	C_aO_2 (vol%)
A.	20.8	18.7
B.	18.7	16.9
C.	20.1	19.0
D.	18.6	17.2

67g. Which of the following sets of values represents a *normal* estimated shunt for *non-critically ill* patients?

	C_cO_2	C_aO_2 (vol%)
A.	19.8	19.0
B.	20.3	18.2
C.	17.1	16.8
D.	18.3	17.5

67h. Mr. Tan's oxygen contents are shown below. Which of the following sets of data shows severe shunt for *critically ill* patients?

	C_cO_2	C_aO_2 (vol%)
A.	20.3	17.8
B.	19.6	19.0
C.	19.1	17.7
D.	18.5	17.9

67i. The following values are obtained from a *critically ill* patient: $C_cO_2 = 20.5$ vol%, $C_aO_2 = 18.6$ vol%, $C_{\bar{v}}O_2 = 14.8$ vol%. Calculate the percent shunt using the estimated shunt equation. What is the interpretation?

A. 35.2%; severe shunt
B. 38.5%; severe shunt
C. 41.5%; severe shunt
D. 44.8%; severe shunt

67j. The following oxygen contents are obtained from a *non-critically ill* patient: $C_cO_2 = 20.1$ vol%, $C_aO_2 = 18.6$ vol%. Calculate the percent shunt using the estimated shunt equation. What is the interpretation?

A. 9%; normal
B. 14%; mild shunt
C. 18%; mild shunt
D. 23%; moderate shunt

67k. Given the data below from a *critically ill* patient: $C_cO_2 = 18.3$ vol%, $C_aO_2 = 14.8$ vol%. What is the percent shunt using the estimated shunt equation. What is the interpretation?

A. 17%; mild shunt
B. 25%; moderate shunt
C. 32%; severe shunt
D. 50%; severe shunt

Go to **rtexam.com** for more learning resources

68

Stroke Volume (SV) and
Stroke Volume Index (SVI)

EQUATION 1

$$SV = \frac{CO}{HR}$$

EQUATION 2

$$SVI = \frac{SV}{BSA}$$

SV : Stroke volume in mL or mL/beat
SVI : Stroke volume index in mL/m² (or mL/beat/m²)
CO : Cardiac output in L/min
HR : Heart rate/min
BSA : Body surface area in m²

NORMAL VALUES

SV : 40 to 80 mL (adult)
SVI : 33 to 47 mL/m² (adult)

EXAMPLE

Given: Cardiac output = 4.0 L/min
       Heart rate   = 100/min
       Body surface area = 1.5 m²

Calculate the stroke volume and the stroke volume index.

$$SV = \frac{CO}{HR}$$

$$= \frac{4.0}{100}$$

$$= 0.04 \text{ L or } 40 \text{ mL}$$

$$SVI = \frac{SV}{BSA}$$

$$= \frac{40}{1.5}$$

$$= 26.7 \text{ mL/m}^2$$

EXERCISE

Given: Cardiac output = 5.0 L/min
       Heart rate   = 90/min
       Body surface area = 1.2 m²

Calculate the stroke volume and the stroke volume index.

[Answer: SV = 55.6 mL; SVI = 46.3 mL/m²]

NOTES

The stroke volume (SV) measures the average cardiac output per one heartbeat. Its accuracy is dependent on the method and technique used in the cardiac output measurement (e.g., Fick's method, dye-dilution, and thermodilution). The SV increases with drugs that raise cardiac contractility and during early stages of compensated septic shock. It decreases with drugs that lower cardiac contractility and during late stages of decompensated septic shock.

The stroke volume index (SVI) is used to normalize stroke volume measurement among patients of varying body size. For instance, a 50-mL stroke volume may be normal for an average-sized person but low for a large-sized person. The SVI can distinguish this difference based on the body size.

SELF-ASSESSMENT QUESTIONS

68a. **The equation for calculating the stroke volume (SV) is:**

A. Cardiac output × Heart rate

B. $\dfrac{\text{Cardiac output}}{\text{Heart rate}}$

C. $\dfrac{\text{Cardiac output} \times \text{Heart rate}}{\text{Body surface area}}$

D. $\dfrac{\text{Cardiac output} / \text{Heart rate}}{\text{Body surface area}}$

68b. **The equation for calculating the stroke volume index (SVI) is:**

A. Cardiac output × Heart rate

B. $\dfrac{\text{Cardiac output}}{\text{Heart rate}}$

C. $\dfrac{\text{Cardiac output} \times \text{Heart rate}}{\text{Body surface area}}$

D. $\dfrac{\text{Cardiac output} / \text{Heart rate}}{\text{Body surface area}}$

68c. **Given: cardiac output = 4.5 L/min, heart rate = 110/min, body surface area = 1.3 m². Calculate the stroke volume (SV) and stroke volume index (SVI).**

A. SV = 46.2 mL; SVI = 35.5 mL/m²

B. SV = 44.6 mL; SVI = 34.3 mL/m²

C. SV = 40.9 mL; SVI = 31.5 mL/m²

D. SV = 38.6 mL; SVI = 29.7 mL/m²

68d. **Given: cardiac output = 5 L/min, heart rate = 80/min, body surface area = 1.7 m². Calculate the stroke volume (SV) and stroke volume index (SVI). Are both SV and SVI normal for an adult?**

A. SV = 62.5 mL; SVI = 34.1 mL/m²; yes

B. SV = 62.5 mL; SVI = 36.8 mL/m²; yes

C. SV = 67.4 mL; SVI = 39.6 mL/m²; no

D. SV = 67.4 mL; SVI = 42.4 mL/m²; no

68e. Given: cardiac output = 5 L/min, heart rate = 80/min, body surface area = 1.1 m². Calculate the stroke volume (SV) and stroke volume index (SVI). Are both SV and SVI normal for an adult?

    A. SV = 62.5 mL; SVI = 56.8.1 mL/m²; no
    B. SV = 62.5 mL; SVI = 56.8 mL/m²; yes
    C. SV = 71.5 mL; SVI = 65 mL/m²; no
    D. SV = 71.5 mL; SVI = 65 mL/m²; yes

68f. A patient has the following data: cardiac output = 3.5 L/min, heart rate = 120/min, body surface area = 1.3 m². Calculate the stroke volume (SV) and stroke volume index (SVI).

    A. SV = 29.2 mL; SVI = 22.4 mL/m²
    B. SV = 29.2 mL; SVI = 24.7 mL/m²
    C. SV = 33.5 mL; SVI = 25.8 mL/m²
    D. SV = 33.5 mL; SVI = 27.3 mL/m²

68g. A patient whose body surface area is about 1.1 m² has the following hemodynamic measurements: cardiac output = 5.9 L/min, heart rate = 120/min. Calculate the stroke volume (SV) and stroke volume index (SVI).

    A. SV = 51.8 mL; SVI = 47.1 mL/m²
    B. SV = 51.8 mL; SVI = 50.4 mL/m²
    C. SV = 49.2 mL; SVI = 40.6 mL/m²
    D. SV = 49.2 mL; SVI = 44.7 mL/m²

68h. Given the following sets of cardiac output (CO) and heart rate (HR) data, which set has the *highest* stroke volume (SV)?

	CO (L)	HR (beats/min)
A.	4.0	80
B.	4.5	90
C.	5.5	100
D.	6.3	120

68i. Given the following sets of cardiac output (CO) and heart rate (HR) data, which set has the *lowest* stroke volume (SV)?

	CO (L)	HR (beats/min)
A.	3.2	80
B.	3.8	90
C.	4.5	100
D.	4.9	110

68j. Given the following sets of stroke volume (SV) and body surface area (BSA) data, which set has the *highest* stroke volume index (SVI)?

	SV (mL)	BSA (m^2)
A.	60	1.4
B.	55	1.2
C.	58	2.0
D.	63	1.7

68k. Given the following sets of stroke volume (SV) and body surface area (BSA) data, which set has the *lowest* stroke volume index (SVI)?

	SV (mL)	BSA (m^2)
A.	70	1.1
B.	75	1.3
C.	80	1.5
D.	85	1.7

Go to **rtexam.com** for more learning resources

69

Stroke Work: Left Ventricular (LVSW) and Index (LVSWI)

EQUATION 1 (LVSW)

$$LVSW = (MAP - PCWP) \times SV \times 0.0136$$

EQUATION 2 (LVSWI)

$$LVSWI = \frac{LVSW}{BSA}$$

LVSW	:	Left ventricular stroke work in g·m/beat
LVSWI	:	Left ventricular stroke work index in g·m/beat/m^2
MAP	:	Mean arterial pressure in mm Hg
PCWP	:	Pulmonary capillary wedge pressure in mm Hg
SV	:	Stroke volume in mL
BSA	:	Body surface area in m^2

NORMAL VALUES

LVSW = 60 to 80 g·m/beat
LVSWI = 40 to 60 g·m/beat/m^2

EXAMPLE

Given: MAP = 100 mm Hg
PCWP = 20 mm Hg
SV = 50 mL
BSA = 1.1 m^2

Calculate the left ventricular stroke work (LVSW) and index (LVSWI).

$$
\begin{aligned}
LVSW &= (MAP - PCWP) \times SV \times 0.0136 \\
&= (100 - 20) \times 50 \times 0.0136 \\
&= 80 \times 50 \times 0.0136 \\
&= 4{,}000 \times 0.0136 \\
&= 54.4 \text{ g·m/beat}
\end{aligned}
$$

$$
\begin{aligned}
LVSWI &= \frac{LVSW}{BSA} \\
&= \frac{54.4}{1.1} \\
&= 49.45 \text{ g·m/beat/m}^2
\end{aligned}
$$

NOTES

Left ventricular stroke work (LVSW) reflects the work of the left heart in providing perfusion through the systemic circulation. LVSW is directly related to the systemic vascular resistance, myocardial mass, and the volume and viscosity of the blood. In addition, tachycardia, hypoxemia, and poor contractility of the heart may further increase the stroke work of the left heart.

The pulmonary capillary wedge pressure (PCWP) is used because it approximates the mean left atrial pressure or the left ventricle end-diastolic pressure.

The constant 0.0136 in the equation is used to convert mm Hg/mL to gram·meters (g·m).

The left ventricular stroke work index (LVSWI) is used to equalize the stroke work to a person's body size. In the example shown, an apparently low left ventricular stroke work may be normal for a small person after indexing. See **Figure 69-1** Frank-Starling curve for the relationship between LVSWI and left ventricular preload (represented by PCWP). For example, when the LVSWI and PCWP readings are both low and meet in quadrant 1, hypovolemia may be present.

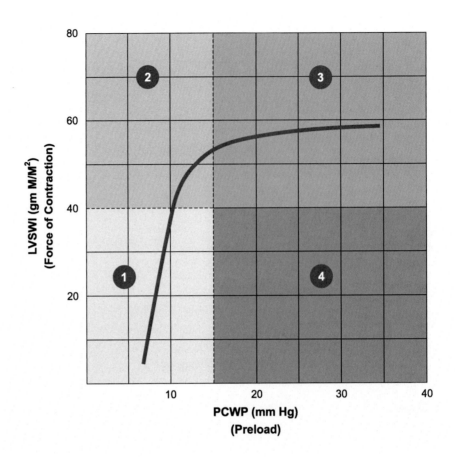

FIGURE 69-1. Frank-Starling curve. The Frank-Starling curve shows that the more the myocardial fi ber is stretched as a result of the blood pressure that develops as blood returns to the chambers of the heart during diastole, the more the heart muscle contracts during systole. In addition, it contracts with greater force. The stretch produced within the myocardium at end-diastole is called preload. Clinically, it would be best to determine the preload of the left ventricle by measuring the end-diastolic pressure of the left ventricle or left atrium. However, because it is impractical to measure that at the patient's bedside, the best preload approximation of the left heart is the pulmonary capillary wedge pressure (PCWP). As shown in this illustration, the relationship of the PCWP (preload) to the left ventricular stroke work index (LVSWI) (force of contraction) may appear in four quadrants: (1) hypovolemia, (2) optimal function, (3) hypervolemia, and (4) cardiac failure.

EXERCISE

Given: MAP   = 120 mm Hg
        PCWP = 20 mm Hg
        SV   = 45 mL
        BSA   = 1.5 m²

Calculate the LVSW and LVSWI.

[Answer: LVSW = 61.2 g·m/beat; LVSWI = 40.8 g·m/beat/m²]

SELF-ASSESSMENT QUESTIONS

69a. Calculation of the left ventricular stroke work (LVSW) and left ventricular stroke work index (LVSWI) does *not* require measurement of:

    A. mean arterial pressure
    B. mean pulmonary arterial pressure
    C. pulmonary capillary wedge pressure
    D. stroke volume

69b. The equation for calculating the left ventricular stroke work (LVSW) is:

    A. $(MAP + PCWP) \times SV$
    B. $(MAP + PCWP) \times SV \times 0.0136$
    C. $(MAP - PCWP) \times SV \times 0.0136$
    D. $(MAP - PCWP) \times SV$

69c. Given: MAP = 98 mm Hg, PCWP = 10 mm Hg, SV = 60 mL. What is the calculated left ventricular stroke work (LVSW)? Is it normal?

    A. 64.6 g·m/beat; normal
    B. 64.6 g·m/beat; abnormal
    C. 71.8 g·m/beat; normal
    D. 71.8 g·m/beat; abnormal

69d. A patient whose estimated body surface area is 1.4 m² has the following hemodynamic values: MAP = 103 mm Hg, PCWP = 15 mm Hg, SV = 48 mL. What is the patient's left ventricular stroke work index (LVSWI)? Is it normal?

    A. 41 g·m/beat/m²; normal
    B. 41 g·m/beat/m²; abnormal
    C. 57 g·m/beat/m²; normal
    D. 57 g·m/beat/m²; abnormal

69e. The hemodynamic values for a patient (body surface area = 1.3 m²) in the coronary care unit are: MAP = 94 mm Hg, CVP = 4 mm Hg, mPAP = 28 mm Hg, PCWP = 15 mm Hg, SV = 55 mL. What is the patient's left ventricular stroke work (LVSW) and index (LVSWI)?

    A. LVSW = 59.1 g·m/beat; LVSWI = 45.5 g·m/beat/m²
    B. LVSW = 59.1 g·m/beat; LVSWI = 47.7 g·m/beat/m²
    C. LVSW = 63.4 g·m/beat; LVSWI = 48.8 g·m/beat/m²
    D. LVSW = 63.4 g·m/beat; LVSWI = 52.9 g·m/beat/m²

69f. The hemodynamic values for a patient (body surface area = 1.2 m²) in the coronary care unit are: MAP = 110 mm Hg, CVP = 8 mm Hg, MPAP = 28 mm Hg, PCWP = 20 mm Hg, SV = 58 mL. Calculate the left ventricular stroke work index (LVSWI). What is the interpretation by applying the LVSWI and PCWP values to **Figure 69-1**?

A. 59.2 g·m/beat/m²; hypovolemia
B. 59.2 g·m/beat/m²; hypervolemia
C. 71 g·m/beat/m²; hypovolemia
D. 71 g·m/beat/m²; hypervolemia

69g. A patient's clinical data are provided below: BSA = 1.5 m², MAP = 70 mm Hg, CVP = 5 mm Hg, MPAP = 16 mm Hg, PCWP = 10 mm Hg, SV = 43 mL. Calculate the left ventricular stroke work index (LVSWI). What is the interpretation by applying the LVSWI and PCWP values to **Figure 69-1**?

A. 21.6 g·m/beat/m²; optimal function
B. 21.6 g·m/beat/m²; hypovolemia
C. 23.4 g·m/beat/m²; optimal function
D. 23.4 g·m/beat/m²; hypovolemia

69h. Given: BSA = 1.2 m², MAP = 82 mm Hg, CVP = 3 mm Hg, mPAP = 17 mm Hg, PCWP = 18 mm Hg, SV = 42 mL. Calculate the left ventricular stroke work index (LVSWI). What is the interpretation by applying the LVSWI and PCWP values to **Figure 69-1**?

A. 27.2 g·m/beat/m²; hypervolemia
B. 27.2 g·m/beat/m²; cardiac failure
C. 30.5 g·m/beat/m²; hypervolemia
D. 30.5 g·m/beat/m²; cardiac failure

69i. The hemodynamic values for a patient (body surface area = 1.1 m²) in the coronary care unit are: MAP = 78 mm Hg, CVP = 5 mm Hg, mPAP = 16 mm Hg, PCWP = 10 mm Hg, SV = 55 mL. Calculate the left ventricular stroke work index (LVSWI). What is the interpretation by applying the LVSWI and PCWP values to **Figure 69-1**?

A. 46.2 g·m/beat/m²; optimal function
B. 46.2 g·m/beat/m²; hypovolemia
C. 48.7 g·m/beat/m²; optimal function
D. 48.7 g·m/beat/m²; hypovolemia

69j. Four sets of hemodynamic data are shown below. Which set produces the *highest* left ventricular stroke work (LVSW)?

	MAP (mm Hg)	PCWP (mm Hg)	SV (mL)
A.	60	8	48
B.	65	10	46
C.	70	12	44
D.	75	14	42

69k. Four sets of hemodynamic data are shown below. Which set produces the *highest* left ventricular stroke work index (LVSWI)?

	MAP (mm Hg)	PCWP (mm Hg)	SV (mL)	BSA (m²)
A.	70	14	50	1.2
B.	85	12	45	1.4
C.	90	10	50	1.6
D.	95	18	45	1.8

69l. Four sets of hemodynamic data are shown below. Which set has an interpretation of *optimal function* of the heart?

	MAP (mm Hg)	PCWP (mm Hg)	SV (mL)	BSA (m²)
A.	65	8	55	1.1
B.	80	8	60	1.3
C.	75	18	55	1.1
D.	80	18	60	1.3

Go to **rtexam.com** for more learning resources

Stroke Work: Right Ventricular (RVSW) and Index (RVSWI)

70

NOTES

Right ventricular stroke work (RVSW) reflects the work of the right heart in providing perfusion through the pulmonary circulation. RVSW is directly related to the pulmonary vascular resistance, myocardial mass, and the volume and viscosity of the blood. In addition, tachycardia, hypoxemia, and poor contractility of the heart may further increase the stroke work of the right heart.

The constant 0.0136 in the equation is used to convert mm Hg/mL to gram·meters (g·m).

The right ventricular stroke work index (RVSWI) is used to equalize the stroke work to a person's body size. In the example shown, a normal RVSW (11.42 g·m/beat) may be low (6.01 g·m/beat/m²) for a large-sized person after indexing (normal RVSW, low RVSWI).

EQUATION 1
(RVSW)

$$RVSW = (\overline{PA} - \overline{RA}) \times SV \times 0.0136$$

EQUATION 2
(RVSWI)

$$RVSWI = \frac{RVSW}{BSA}$$

$RVSW$	: Right ventricular stroke work in g·m/beat
$RVSWI$	: Right ventricular stroke work index in g·m/beat/m²
$\overline{PA}$	: Mean pulmonary artery pressure in mm Hg
$\overline{RA}$	: Mean right atrial pressure (central venous pressure) in mm Hg
SV	: Stroke volume in mL
BSA	: Body surface area in m²

NORMAL VALUES

RVSW $= 10$ to 15 g·m/beat
RVSWI $= 7$ to 12 g·m/beat/m²

EXAMPLE

Given: $\overline{PA}$ = 18 mm Hg
$\overline{RA}$ = 4 mm Hg
SV = 60 mL
BSA = 1.9 m²

Calculate the right ventricular stroke work (RVSW) and its index (RVSWI).

$$
\begin{aligned}
RVSW &= (\overline{PA} - \overline{RA}) \times SV \times 0.0136 \\
&= (18 - 4) \times 60 \times 0.0136 \\
&= 14 \times 60 \times 0.0136 \\
&= 840 \times 0.0136 \\
&= 11.42 \text{ g·m/beat}
\end{aligned}
$$

$$
\begin{aligned}
RVSWI &= \frac{RVSW}{BSA} \\
&= \frac{11.42}{1.9} \\
&= 6.01 \text{ g·m/beat/m}^2
\end{aligned}
$$

EXERCISE

Given: $\overline{PA}$ = 20 mm Hg
$\overline{RA}$ = 6 mm Hg
SV = 56 mL
BSA = 1.2 m²

Calculate the RVSW and RVSWI.

[Answer: RVSW = 10.66 g·m/beat; RVSWI = 8.88 g·m/beat/m²]

SELF-ASSESSMENT QUESTIONS

70a. Which of the following is not required for calculating the right ventricular stroke work (RVSW) and right ventricular stroke work index (RVSWI)?

A. 0.0136
B. mean pulmonary artery pressure
C. mean systemic artery pressure
D. body surface area

70b. The equation for calculating the right ventricular stroke work (RVSW) is:

A. $(\overline{PA} - \overline{RA}) \times SV$
B. $(\overline{PA} + \overline{RA}) \times SV \times 0.0136$
C. $(\overline{PA} + \overline{RA}) \times SV$
D. $(\overline{PA} - \overline{RA}) \times SV \times 0.0136$

70c. Given: MPAP = 20 mm Hg, $\overline{RA}$ = 3 mm Hg, SV = 55 mL. What is the calculated right ventricular stroke work (RVSW)? Is it normal?

A. 11.4 g·m/beat; normal
B. 12.7 g·m/beat; normal
C. 13.9 g·m/beat; abnormal
D. 15.2 g·m/beat; abnormal

70d. Given: MPAP = 22 mm Hg, $\overline{RA}$ = 6 mm Hg, SV = 45 mL, BSA = 1.1 m². Calculate the right ventricular stroke work index (RVSWI). Is it normal?

A. 8.9 g·m/beat/m²; normal
B. 9.1 g·m/beat/m²; normal
C. 9.3 g·m/beat/m²; abnormal
D. 9.8 g·m/beat/m²; abnormal

70e. A patient whose estimated body surface area is 1.2 m² has the following hemodynamic values: MPAP = 18 mm Hg, $\overline{RA}$ = 3 mm Hg, SV = 60 mL. What is the patient's right ventricular stroke work (RVSW) and right ventricular stroke work index (RVSWI)?

A. RVSW = 9.8 g·m/beat; RVSWI = 8.2 g·m/beat/m²
B. RVSW = 10.3 g·m/beat; RVSWI = 8.6 g·m/beat/m²
C. RVSW = 11.6 g·m/beat; RVSWI = 9.7 g·m/beat/m²
D. RVSW = 12.2 g·m/beat; RVSWI = 10.2 g·m/beat/m²

70f. A patient in the intensive care unit whose body surface area is 2.1 m² has the following hemodynamic values: MPAP = 20 mm Hg, $\overline{RA}$ = 6 mm Hg, SV = 65 mL. What is the patient's right ventricular stroke work (RVSW) and index (RVSWI)? Is RVSWI normal?

A. RVSW = 12.4 g·m/beat; RVSWI = 9.2 g·m/beat/m²; RVSWI normal
B. RVSW = 12.4 g·m/beat; RVSWI = 5.9 g·m/beat/m²; RVSWI abnormal
C. RVSW = 16.17 g·m/beat; RVSWI = 9.2 g·m/beat/m²; RVSWI normal
D. RVSW = 16.17 g·m/beat; RVSWI = 5.9 g·m/beat/m²; RVSWI abnormal

70g. A patient's hemodynamic data are provided below: BSA = 1.1 m², MAP = 76 mm Hg, CVP ($\overline{RA}$) = 5 mm Hg, MPAP = 18 mm Hg, PCWP =10 mm Hg, SV = 50 mL. Calculate the right ventricular stroke work index (RVSWI). Is it normal?

A. 8.04 g·m/beat/m²; normal
B. 8.04 g·m/beat/m²; abnormal
C. 9.27 g·m/beat/m²; normal
D. 9.27 g·m/beat/m²; abnormal

70h. Given: BSA = 1.2 m², MAP = 86 mm Hg, CVP ($\overline{RA}$) = 3 mm Hg, MPAP = 21 mm Hg, PCWP = 16 mm Hg, SV = 55 mL. Calculate the right ventricular stroke work index (RVSWI). Is it normal?

A. 10.5 g·m/beat/m²; normal
B. 10.5 g·m/beat/m²; abnormal
C. 11.2 g·m/beat/m²; normal
D. 11.2 g·m/beat/m²; abnormal

70i. The hemodynamic data for a patient (body surface area = 1.3 m²) in the coronary care unit are: MAP = 83 mm Hg, CVP ($\overline{RA}$) = 8 mm Hg, MPAP = 18 mm Hg, PCWP = 12 mm Hg, SV = 60 mL. Calculate the right ventricular stroke work index (RVSWI). Is it normal?

A. 6.3 g·m/beat/m²; normal
B. 6.3 g·m/beat/m²; abnormal
C. 7.8 g·m/beat/m²; normal
D. 7.8 g·m/beat/m²; abnormal

70j. Four sets of hemodynamic data are shown below. Which set produces the *highest* right ventricular stroke work (RVSW)?

	$\overline{PA}$ (mm Hg)	CVP ($\overline{RA}$) (mm Hg)	SV (mL)
A.	18	6	55
B.	20	8	50
C.	22	10	45
D.	24	12	40

70k. Four sets of hemodynamic data are shown below. Which set produces the *highest* right ventricular stroke work index (RVSWI)?

	$\overline{PA}$ (mm Hg)	CVP ($\overline{RA}$) (mm Hg)	SV (mL)	BSA (m^2)
A.	16	6	50	1.3
B.	18	4	55	1.2
C.	20	6	60	1.3
D.	22	4	65	1.2

70l. Four sets of hemodynamic data are shown below. Which set produces the *lowest* right ventricular stroke work index (RVSWI)?

	$\overline{PA}$ (mm Hg)	CVP ($\overline{RA}$) (mm Hg)	SV (mL)	BSA (m^2)
A.	17	4	55	1.4
B.	18	6	60	1.5
C.	19	5	65	1.6
D.	20	8	70	1.7

71

Temperature Conversion (°C to °F)

Temperature conversion calculations are done where a conversion chart is not readily available. Since there are three main temperature conversion equations, it is essential to select the correct equation. Example shows conversion of normal body temperature (from 37°C to 98.6°F). This commonly known body temperature may be used to verify the proper equation for temperature conversion form °C to °F.

In Celsius to Fahrenheit conversion, the ratio $\frac{9}{5}$ is derived from $\frac{180}{100}$ where 180 is the Fahrenheit range (212 – 32) between the boiling point of water (212 °F) and its freezing point (32 °F); whereas 100 is the Celsius range (100 – 0) between the boiling point of water (100 °C) and its freezing point (0 °C). The fraction $\frac{9}{5}$ may be substituted with 1.8 in Celsius to Fahrenheit temperature conversions.

EQUATION

$$°F = \left(°C \times \frac{9}{5}\right) + 32$$

°F : degrees Fahrenheit (named after Daniel Fahrenheit)
°C : degrees Celsius (named after Anders Celsius)

EXAMPLE

Given: °C = 37

Calculate the degrees Fahrenheit.

$$°F = \left(°C \times \frac{9}{5}\right) + 32$$

$$= \left(37 \times \frac{9}{5}\right) + 32$$

$$= \left(\frac{333}{5}\right) + 32$$

$$= 66.6 + 32$$

$$= 98.6$$

EXERCISE 1

Given: °C = 25
Find the degrees Fahrenheit.
[Answer: °F = 77]

EXERCISE 2

Given: °C = 39
Find the degrees Fahrenheit.
[Answer: °F = 102.2]

SELF-ASSESSMENT QUESTIONS

71a. The water freezing point is 0 °C. What is it in degrees Fahrenheit?

A. 0 °F
B. 1.8 °F
C. 32 °F
D. 100 °F

71b. What is the normal body temperature (37 °C) in degrees Fahrenheit?

   A. 54.3 °F
   B. 66.6 °F
   C. 87.5 °F
   D. 98.6 °F

71c. The skin temperature of a neonate is recorded as 36 °C. What is its equivalent in degrees Fahrenheit?

   A. 96.8 °F
   B. 97.4 °F
   C. 98.3 °F
   D. 98.9 °F

71d. The core temperature of a patient being treated for hypothermia is 28 °C. What is it in degrees Fahrenheit?

   A. 79.3 °F
   B. 82.4 °F
   C. 84.7 °F
   D. 88.1 °F

Questions 71e to 71m: convert °C to °F. Write in the answers under column °F.

	°C	°F (write in)
71e.	0 °C (freezing point of water)	_____
71f.	17 °C (high temperature at Mount Everest 1st base camp)	_____
71g.	20 °C (high surface temperature on Mars)	_____
71h.	30 °C (average body temperature of reptiles)	_____
71i.	37 °C (normal body temperature of Homo sapiens)	_____
71j.	48 °C (average high temperature in August at Pikes Peak, CO)	_____
71k.	77 °C (low-temperature to roast turkey for 9 to 11 hours)	_____
71l.	100 °C (boiling point of water)	_____
71m.	177 °C (average oven temperature to bake cookies)	_____

>> Go to **rtexam.com** for more learning resources

Temperature Conversion (°C to k)

The kelvin (not capitalized being a unit of temperature just like "meter" or "gram") is primarily used in gas law calculations (i.e., Boyle's law, Charles' law, Gay-Lussac's law, and Combined Gas Law).

Kelvin temperature is also called the absolute temperature because molecular activity of gases theoretically stops at 0 K (–273 °C). In the Equation, it is essential to remember the constant number 273.

For temperature conversion from Fahrenheit (°F) to kelvin (k), change °F to °C and then change °C to k.

EQUATION

$k = °C + 273$

k : kelvin (a unit named after Lord Kelvin, not a degree)
°C : degrees Celsius (named after Anders Celsius)

EXAMPLE

Given: °C = 37. Calculate the kelvin equivalent.

$$k = °C + 273$$
$$= 37 + 273$$
$$= 310$$

EXERCISE 1

Given: °C = 25

Find the kelvin equivalent.

[Answer: k = 298]

EXERCISE 2

Given: °C = 39

Find the kelvin equivalent.

[Answer: k = 312]

SELF-ASSESSMENT QUESTIONS

72a. The equation to convert a known temperature to kelvin is:

A. 273 – °C
B. °C + 273
C. 273 – °F
D. °F + 273

72b. Given: °C = 0. Calculate the kelvin equivalent.

A. 236 k
B. 250 k
C. 273 k
D. 295 k

72c. Given: °F = 88 (31°C). Calculate the kelvin.

    A. 304 k
    B. 312 k
    C. 325 k
    D. 336 k

72d. A gas volume is measured at body temperature (37 °C). Find its equivalent in k for temperature corrections with the Combined Gas Law.

    A. 287 k
    B. 293 k
    C. 299 k
    D. 310 k

72e. Which of the following gas temperatures is the same as 310 k?

    A. 35 °C
    B. 37 °C
    C. 39 °C
    D. 94 °F

Questions 72f to 72n: convert °C to k. Write in the answers under column k.

°C	k (write in)
72f. 0 °C (freezing point of water)	_____
72g. 5.4 °C (mean annual temperature during the last ice age)	_____
72h. 8° C (average summer temperature of tundra)	_____
72i. 15 °C (summer high temperature at Glacier Bay, Alaska)	_____
72j. 29 °C (average body temperature of blue fin tuna)	_____
72k. 37 °C (normal body temperature of Homo sapiens)	_____
72l. 100 °C (boiling point of water)	_____
72m. 167 °C (surface temperature of planet Mercury)	_____
72n. 462 °C (average temperature on planet Venus)	_____

>> Go to **rtexam.com** for more learning resources

Temperature Conversion (°F to °C)

NOTES

Temperature conversion calculations are done where a conversion chart is not readily available. Since there are three main temperature conversion equations, it is essential to select the correct equation. Example shows conversion of normal body temperature (from 98.6 °F to 37 °C). This commonly known body temperature may be used to verify the correct equation for temperature conversion form °F to °C. To convert Fahrenheit to kelvins, first convert Fahrenheit to Celsius and then convert to kelvins.

The temperature constant $\frac{5}{9}$ is derived from $\frac{100}{180}$ where 100 is the Celsius range (100 – 0) between the boiling point of water (100 °C) and its freezing point (0 °C); whereas 180 is the Fahrenheit range (212 – 32) between the boiling point of water (212 °F) and its freezing point (32 °F). For precise calculations, the fraction $\frac{5}{9}$ should not be substituted with 0.56.

EQUATION

$$°C = (°F - 32) \times \frac{5}{9}$$

°C : degrees Celsius
°F : degrees Fahrenheit

EXAMPLE

Given: °F = 98.6

Calculate the degrees Celsius.

$$°C = (°F - 32) \times \frac{5}{9}$$

$$= (98.6 - 32) \times \frac{5}{9}$$

$$= (66.6) \times \frac{5}{9}$$

$$= \frac{333}{9}$$

$$= 37$$

EXERCISE

A patient is running a fever at a temperature of 103.5 °F. Calculate the degrees Celsius.

[Answer: °C = 39.72 or 39.7]

SELF-ASSESSMENT QUESTIONS

73a. **A patient has an oral temperature of 99.2°F. It is the same as:**

A. 36.8°C
B. 37.3°C
C. 37.7°C
D. 38.1°C

73b. The rectal temperature of a neonate is 101.5°F. It is equal to:

A. 37.4°C
B. 37.7°C
C. 38.6°C
D. 39.0°C

73c. A room temperature of 78°F is same as:

A. 23.3°C
B. 23.7°C
C. 24.4°C
D. 25.6°C

Questions 73d to 73o: convert °F to °C. Write in the answers under column °C.

	°F	°C (write in)
73d.	32 °F (freezing point of water)	_____
73e.	40 °F (minimum temperature to store live shellfish)	_____
73f.	52 °F (ideal temperature to serve white wine)	_____
73g.	55 °F (ideal temperature to store red or white wine)	_____
73h.	65 °F (ideal temperature to serve red wine)	_____
73i.	98.6 °F (normal body temperature of Homo sapiens)	_____
73j.	130 °F (internal temperature for medium prime rib roast)	_____
73k.	140 °F (internal temperature for well done ribeye)	_____
73l.	165 °F (internal temperature for turkey, goose, duck)	_____
73m.	212 °F (boiling point of water)	_____
73n.	400 °F (temperature to roast salmon in oven)	_____
73o.	425 °F (temperature to roast vegetables in oven)	_____

» Go to **rtexam.com** for more learning resources

Tidal Volume Based on Flow and I Time

In general, the tidal volume delivered by a constant flow is directly related to the flow rate and inspiratory time (I time). A higher flow rate or longer I time yields a larger tidal volume in the absence of severe airway obstruction or lung parenchymal disease. In addition to other ventilator settings, flow and I time should be adjusted accordingly to provide sufficient gas exchange, patient comfort, and cardiopulmonary stability.

In dual mode ventilation such as pressure-regulated volume control (PRVC), the pressure is "regulated" (lowered) by using a lower flow and a longer I time to deliver a stable tidal volume. Since $R = \dfrac{\Delta P}{\dot{V}}$ and at a constant resistance, a lower flow ($\dot{V}$) reduces the peak inspiratory pressure (ΔP). A longer I time makes up the reduced constant flow and maintains "volume control" (a stable tidal volume).

EQUATION

$V_T = \text{Flow} \times I \text{ time}$

V_T : Tidal volume in mL
Flow : Flow rate in mL/sec
I time : Inspiratory time in sec

EXAMPLE

Given: Flow $= 8$ L/min
Inspiratory time $= 0.5$ sec

Calculate the approximate tidal volume.

First change the flow rate from L/min to mL/sec. Flow rate at 8 L/min is the same as 8,000 mL/60 sec or 133 mL/sec.

$\begin{aligned} V_T &= \text{Flow} \times I \text{ time} \\ &= 133 \text{ mL/sec} \times 0.5 \text{ sec} \\ &= 66.5 \text{ mL} \end{aligned}$

EXERCISE 1

Given the following settings on a pressure-controlled ventilator: flow = 6 L/min, inspiratory time = 0.4 sec. What is the approximate tidal volume based on these settings?

[Answer: $V_T = 40$ mL]

EXERCISE 2

A patient is receiving volume-controlled ventilation with a constant (square) flow of 40 L/min and an inspiratory time of 0.8 sec. What is the approximate tidal volume based on these settings?

[Answer: $V_T = 533$ mL]

SELF-ASSESSMENT QUESTIONS

74a. Given: flow = 7 L/min, inspiratory time = 0.5 sec. Calculate the delivered tidal volume based on these settings on a constant flow time-cycled ventilator.

A. 55 mL
B. 58 mL
C. 61 mL
D. 63 mL

74b. The following settings are used on a constant flow time-cycled ventilator: flow = 8 L/min, inspiratory time = 0.4 sec. Calculate the delivered tidal volume.

A. 53 mL
B. 55 mL
C. 57 mL
D. 59 mL

74c. Given the following flow rate (Flow) and inspiratory time (*I* time). Which set of values provides the *lowest* delivered tidal volume?

	Flow (L/min)	*I* time (sec)
A.	7	0.3
B.	7	0.4
C.	6	0.4
D.	6	0.5

74d. The following sets of data are found on the flow sheet of an infant ventilator over a 3-day period. Which set of values has the *highest* calculated tidal volume?

	Flow (L/min)	*I* time (sec)
A.	7	0.5
B.	8	0.4
C.	6	0.5
D.	7	0.4

74e. Which set of data below produces the *highest* calculated tidal volume?

	Flow (L/min)	*I* time (sec)
A.	50	0.7
B.	55	0.6
C.	60	0.6
D.	65	0.5

74f. Which set of data below produces the *lowest* calculated tidal volume?

	Flow (L/min)	*I* time (sec)
A.	40	0.8
B.	45	0.7
C.	50	0.6
D.	55	0.5

» Go to **rtexam.com** for more learning resources

Unit Conversion: Length

NOTES

In Example 4: Step 4, change 63 inches to feet and inches. If a calculator is used to solve division problems, the number in front of the decimal point represents the feet. The number after the decimal point should be multiplied by 12 to obtain the remaining height in inches. In Step 4 of Example 4, (63 /12) ft = 5.25 ft. The number in front of the decimal point (5) is the height in feet. The number after the decimal point (0.25) is multiplied by 12 for the remaining height in inches. 0.25 × 12 = 3 inches. A height of 63 inches is therefore 5 feet 3 inches.

TABLE 75-1. Conversion Table (Length)

Millimeter (mm)	Centimeter (cm)	Meter (m)	Inch (in)	Foot (ft)	Yard (y)
1	0.1	0.001	0.03937	0.003281	0.001094
10	1	0.001	0.3937	0.03281	0.01094
1,000	100	1	39.37	3.281	1.0936
25.4	2.54	0.0254	1	0.0833	0.0278
304.8	30.48	0.3048	12	1	0.333
914.4	91.44	0.9144	36	3	1

Table data from unitconverters.net

EXAMPLE 1 A patient is 5'6" tall. Convert this height to meter (m).

Step 1. 5'6" = 66"

Step 2. From the conversion table, 1" = 0.0254 m

Step 3. 66" = (66 × 0.0254) m or 1.67 m

EXAMPLE 2 An athlete can run 100 meters (m) in 10 seconds. This distance is same as _____ ft.

Step 1. From the conversion table, 1 m = 3.281 ft

Step 2. 100 m = (100 × 3.281) ft or 328 ft

EXAMPLE 3 Mr. James is 5' 8" tall. This is the same as _____ centimeter (cm).

Step 1. 5' 8" = [(5 × 12) + 8] in = 68 in

Step 2. From the conversion table, 1" = 2.54 cm

Step 3. 68 in = (68 × 2.54) cm or 172.72 cm

EXAMPLE 4 Ms. Malby is 160 cm tall. How tall is she in feet and inches?

Step 1. From the conversion table, 1 cm = 0.3937 in

Step 2. 160 cm = (160 × 0.3937) in = 63 in

Step 3. From the conversion table, 1 ft = 12 in

Step 4. 63 in = (63/12) ft = 5.25 ft or 5'3"

EXERCISE 1   A patient tells you that her height is 5'5". If you need to enter her height in the pulmonary function data sheet in centimeters (cm), what should it be?

[Answer: Height in cm = 165.1 cm or 165 cm]

EXERCISE 2   Mr. Hall is 176 cm tall. Convert his height to feet and inches.

[Answer: Height in ft and in = 5'9"]

SELF-ASSESSMENT QUESTIONS

75a.   Convert 280 millimeters (mm) to inches (in).

A. 1.02 in
B. 11.02 in
C. 110.2 in
D. 7112 in

75b.   Convert 46 meters (m) to feet (ft).

A. 14 ft
B. 15.1 ft
C. 140 ft
D. 151 ft

75c.   Convert 12 inches (in) to centimeters (cm).

A. 0.30 cm
B. 3.05 cm
C. 30.48 cm
D. 304.8 cm

75d.   Convert 1.6 feet (ft) to millimeters (mm).

A. 487.7 mm
B. 4,877 mm
C. 521.4 mm
D. 5,214 mm

75e.   A patient, Ms. Smith, is 5'6" tall. What is the centimeter (cm) equivalent?

A. 154.1 cm
B. 1,541 cm
C. 167.6 cm
D. 1,676 cm

75f. Mr. Jackson is 180 cm tall. Convert this height to feet and inches.

A. 5' 8"
B. 5' 9"
C. 5'10"
D. 5'11"

75g. A patient is 163 cm tall. What is the height in feet and inches?

A. 5' 4"
B. 5' 6"
C. 5' 8"
D. 5' 10"

75h. Mr. Hall runs 1,600 meters every morning. This is the same as how many feet?

A. 524 ft
B. 4,800 ft
C. 5,250 ft
D. 48,000 ft

75i. During a 6-minute walk test, the patient walked 660 ft. This is same as:

A. 201 meters
B. 200 yards
C. 7,800 inches
D. 2,011 centimeters

75j. The predicted normal of a 6-minute walk test for a healthy adult is about 500 meters. This distance is same as:

A. 1,580 ft
B. 1,640 ft
C. 1,720 ft
D. 1,850 ft

75k. The height of a 300-lb college athlete is 6 ft 6 in. The height is same as:

A. 76 in or 186 cm
B. 76 in or 194 cm
C. 78 in or 194 cm
D. 78 in or 198 cm

Go to **rtexam.com** for more learning resources

76

Unit Conversion: Volume

TABLE 76-1. Conversion Table (Volume)

Microliter (μL)	Milliliter (mL)	Liter (L)	US Ounce (Oz)	US Pint (Pt)	US Quart (Q)
1	0.001	0.000001	0.00003381	0.000002113	0.000001057
1,000	1	0.001	0.03381	0.002113	0.00105669
1,000,000	1,000	1	33.814	2.1134	1.0567
29,573.5	29.5735	0.02957	1	0.0625	0.0315
473,176	473.176	0.4732	16.6535	1	0.4163
946,353	946.353	0.946353	32	2	1

Table data from unitconverters.net

EXAMPLE 1 Convert 12 fluid ounces (fl oz) to milliliters (mL).

Step 1. From the conversion table, 1 fl oz = 29.57 mL

Step 2. 12 fl oz = (12 × 29.57) mL or 354.84 mL

EXAMPLE 2 Convert 3.5 liters (L) to pints (pt).

Step 1. From the conversion table, 1 L = 2.11 pt

Step 2. 3.5 L = (3.5 × 2.11) pt or 7.385 pt

EXAMPLE 3 A blood gas analyzer has the capability to analyze blood samples as low as 100 microliters (μL). What is the milliliter (mL) equivalent?

Step 1. From the conversion table, 1 μL = 0.001 mL

Step 2. 100 μL = (100 × 0.001) mL = 0.1 mL

EXAMPLE 4 A large-volume aerosol unit holds 1,000 mL of sterile water. Convert this volume to fluid ounces (fl oz).

Step 1. From the conversion table, 1 mL = 0.03381 fl oz

Step 2. 1,000 mL = (1,000 × 0.03381) fl oz = 33.81 fl oz

EXERCISE 1   In order to analyze a capillary blood gas sample, a minimum sample size of 60 microliters (μL) is needed. What is the milliliter (mL) equivalent?

[Answer: Sample size in mL = 0.06 mL]

EXERCISE 2   Before using a concentrated disinfectant solution, 2 liters of water must be added. How much water in fluid ounces (fl oz) should be added to prepare this disinfectant solution before use?

[Answer: Water to be added = 67.62 fl oz]

SELF-ASSESSMENT QUESTIONS

76a.   Convert 32 fluid ounces (fl oz) to milliliters (mL).

A. 1.08 mL
B. 94.6 mL
C. 946 mL
D. 1,008 mL

76b.   Convert 6 pints (pt) to liters (L).

A. 2.12 L
B. 2.84 L
C. 21.2 L
D. 28.4 L

76c.   Convert 2 liters (L) to milliliters (mL).

A. 0.002 mL
B. 0.02 mL
C. 200 mL
D. 2,000 mL

76d.   Convert 300 microliters (μL) to milliliters (mL).

A. 0.3 mL
B. 0.03 mL
C. 3 mL
D. 30 mL

76e. A blood gas syringe contains 0.4 mL of arterial blood sample. What is the microliters (μL) equivalent?

A. 0.4 μL
B. 4 μL
C. 40 μL
D. 400 μL

76f. A heated humidifier holds 1.6 quarts of sterile water. Convert this volume to liters (L).

A. 1.51 L
B. 1.78 L
C. 15.1 L
D. 17.8 L

76g. The minimum sample size for a blood gas analyzer is 80 microliters (μL). What is the milliliter (mL) equivalent?

A. 0.008 mL
B. 0.08 mL
C. 0.8 mL
D. 8 mL

76h. A concentrated cleaning solution is being diluted with 12 quarts of water before use. How much water in fluid ounces (oz) should be added?

A. 192 oz
B. 1,920 oz
C. 384 oz
D. 3,840 oz

76i. During *RSBI* (rapid shallow breathing index) assessment, the average spontaneous tidal volume is 430 mL. Convert this volume from mL to liter for *RSBI* calculation.

A. 0.043 L
B. 0.43 L
C. 4.3 mL
D. 43 mL

76j. Use the formula below to convert mL to μL.

A. mL × 1,000
B. mL × 100
C. mL / 100
D. mL / 1,000

» Go to **rtexam.com** for more learning resources

Unit Conversion: Weight

77

NOTES

In step 2 of Example 4, the number in front of the decimal point represents the weight in lb. The number after the decimal point is multiplied by 16 to obtain the remaining weight in oz. In this example 2.76 lb, the number in front of the decimal point (2) is the weight in lb; 0.76 (the number after the decimal point) is multiplied by 16 for the remaining weight in oz: 0.76 × 16 = 12.16 oz or 12 oz. The birth weight 1,255 g = 2.76 lb = 2 lb 12 oz.

TABLE 77-1. Conversion Table (Weight)

Microgram (µg or mcg)	Milligram (mg)	Gram (g)	Kilogram (kg)	Ounce (oz)	Pound (lb)
1	0.001	0.000001	0.000000001	0.00000003527	0.000000002205
1,000	1	0.001	0.000001	0.00003527	0.000002205
1,000,000	1,000	1	0.001	0.03527	0.002205
1,000,000,000	1,000,000	1,000	1	35.27	2.205
28,349,500	28,349.5	28.35	0.02835	1	0.0625
453,592,000	453,592	453.59	0.4536	16	1

Table data from unitconverters.net

EXAMPLE 1

Convert 78 kilograms (kg) to pounds (lb).

Step 1. From the conversion table, 1 kg = 2.2 lb

Step 2. 78 kg = (78 × 2.2) lb or 171.6 lb

EXAMPLE 2

Convert 120 pounds (lb) to kilograms (kg).

Step 1. From the conversion table, 1 lb = 0.4545 kg

Step 2. 120 lb = (120 × 0.4545) or 54.54 kg

EXAMPLE 3

Convert 6 lb 7 oz to grams (g) and kilograms (kg).

Step 1. From the conversion table, 1 lb = 16 oz

Step 2. 6 lb = (6 × 16) oz = 96 oz

Step 3. 6 lb 7 oz = (96 + 7) oz = 103 oz

Step 4. From the conversion table, 1 oz = 28.35 g

Step 5. 103 oz = (103 × 28.35) g = 2,920.05 g

Step 6. From the conversion table, 1 g = 0.001 kg

Step 7. 2,920.05 g = (2,920.05 × 0.001) g = 2.92005 or 2.92 kg

6 lb 7 oz = 2,920.05 g = 2.92 kg

EXAMPLE 4   A premature infant weights 1,255 grams (g) at birth. What is this birth weight in pounds (lb) and ounces (oz)?

Step 1. From the conversion table, 1 g = 0.0022 lb

Step 2. 1,255 g = (1,255 × 0.0022) lb = 2.76 lb or 2 lb 12 oz

1,255 g = 2 lb 12 oz

EXERCISE 1   Mr. Dade, who weighs 150 lbs, is ready for the pulmonary function study. What is his weight in kilograms (kg)?

[Answer: Weight = 68.18 kg]

EXERCISE 2   The birth weight of a neonate is 3 lb 12 oz. What is this birth weight in grams (g) and kilograms (kg)?

[Answer: Birth weight = 1,701 g or 1.7 kg]

SELF-ASSESSMENT QUESTIONS

77a. **Convert 1,200 grams (g) to pounds (lb).**

A. 0.26 lb
B. 0.32 lb
C. 2.64 lb
D. 3.18 lb

77b. **Convert 150 pounds (lb) to kilograms (kg).**

A. 59.22 kg
B. 62.15 kg
C. 65.34 kg
D. 68.18 kg

77c. **Convert 77 kilograms (kg) to pounds (lb).**

A. 169.4 lb
B. 172.9 lb
C. 174.2 lb
D. 177.7 lb

77d. **Convert 8 lb 4 oz to grams (g).**

A. 3,685 g
B. 3,741 g
C. 3,790 g
D. 3,820 g

77e. Convert 8 lb 7 oz to kilograms (kg).

A. 3.66 kg
B. 3.82 kg
C. 4.17 kg
D. 4.36 kg

77f. A neonate weighs 3,500 grams (g) at birth. Record this birth weight in pounds (lb) and ounces (oz).

A. 7 lb 11 oz
B. 7 lb 15 oz
C. 8 lb 4 oz
D. 8 lb 8 oz

77g. The birth weight of a neonate is 4 lb 6 oz. What is this birth weight in grams (g) and kilograms (kg)?

A. 181.8 g; 0.1818 kg
B. 1,818 g; 1.818 kg
C. 198.5 g; 0.1985 kg
D. 1,985 g; 1.985 kg

77h. A concentration of 1 g per 100 mL is the same as ___ mg per 100 mL.

A. 10
B. 100
C. 1,000
D. 10,000

77i. An 0.5% bronchodilator solution has a concentration of 0.5 g per 100 mL. This is the same as how many milligrams per 100 mL?

A. 500 mg
B. 5,000 mg
C. 50,000 mg
D. 500,000 mg

77j. The birth weight of a neonate is 1,000 g. What is this birth weight in lb?

A. 1.6 lb
B. 1.8 lb
C. 2 lb
D. 2.2 lb

Go to **rtexam.com** for more learning resources

78

Vascular Resistance: Pulmonary

EQUATION

$$PVR = \left(\overline{PA} - PCWP\right) \times \frac{80}{CO}$$

PVR	: Pulmonary vascular resistance in dyne·sec/cm⁵
$\overline{PA}$	: Mean pulmonary artery pressure in mm Hg
$PCWP$	: Pulmonary capillary wedge pressure in mm Hg
80	: Conversion factor from mm Hg/L/min to dyne·sec/cm⁵
CO	: Cardiac output in L/min ($\dot{Q}_T$)

NORMAL VALUE

PVR = 50 to 150 dyne·sec/cm⁵

EXAMPLE

A patient with pulmonary hypertension has the following measurements. What is the calculated pulmonary vascular resistance (PVR)?

$\overline{PA}$ = 22 mm Hg
PCWP = 6 mm Hg
CO = 4.0 L/min

$$PVR = \left(\overline{PA} - PCWP\right) \times \frac{80}{CO}$$

$$= (22 - 6) \times \frac{80}{4.0}$$

$$= 16 \times \frac{80}{4.0}$$

$$= \frac{1280}{4}$$

$$= 320 \text{ dyne} \cdot \text{sec/cm}^5$$

EXERCISE

A patient has the following measurements. What is the calculated pulmonary vascular resistance (PVR)? Is it normal?

$\overline{PA}$ = 14 mm Hg
PCWP = 7 mm Hg
CO = 5.0 L/min

[Answer: PVR = 112 dyne·sec/cm⁵; normal]

NOTES

Pulmonary vascular resistance (PVR) reflects the resistance of pulmonary vessel to blood flow. A Swan-Ganz (pulmonary artery) catheter is required to measure the $\overline{PA}$ and PCWP. The cardiac output must also be known to calculate the PVR.

The factor 80 in the equation is used to convert the PVR to absolute resistance units, dyne·sec/cm⁵.

Under normal conditions, the PVR is about one-sixth of the systemic vascular resistance. An abnormally high PVR may indicate pulmonary vascular problems, such as pulmonary hypertension, reduction of capillary bed, and pulmonary embolism. An extremely low PVR may be associated with reduction in circulating blood volume, such as hypovolemic shock.

SELF-ASSESSMENT QUESTIONS

78a. In order to calculate the pulmonary vascular resistance, all of the following measurements are required with the *exception* of:

  A. mean systemic artery pressure
  B. mean pulmonary artery pressure
  C. pulmonary capillary wedge pressure
  D. cardiac output

78b. A patient has the following measurements: mean pulmonary artery pressure = 20 mm Hg, pulmonary capillary wedge pressure = 12 mm Hg, cardiac output = 5.0 L/min. What is the pulmonary vascular resistance (PVR)? Is it normal?

  A. 102 dyne · sec/cm^5; normal
  B. 128 dyne · sec/cm^5; normal
  C. 164 dyne · sec/cm^5; abnormal
  D. 223 dyne · sec/cm^5; abnormal

78c. The following hemodynamic measurements are obtained from a patient in the intensive care unit. What is the calculated pulmonary vascular resistance (PVR)? Is it normal?

Mean pulmonary artery pressure = 18 mm Hg
Pulmonary capillary wedge pressure = 8 mm Hg
Cardiac output = 4.5 L/min

  A. 112 dyne · sec/cm^5; normal
  B. 145 dyne · sec/cm^5; normal
  C. 160 dyne · sec/cm^5; abnormal
  D. 178 dyne · sec/cm^5; abnormal

78d. Calculate the patient's pulmonary vascular resistance (PVR) with the following measurements obtained during a hemodynamic study. Is it normal?

Mean pulmonary artery pressure = 15 mm Hg
Pulmonary capillary wedge pressure = 8 mm Hg
Cardiac output = 4.2 L/min

  A. 86 dyne · sec/cm^5; normal
  B. 105 dyne · sec/cm^5; normal
  C. 133 dyne · sec/cm^5; normal
  D. 163 dyne · sec/cm^5; abnormal

78e. Given the following hemodynamic data. Which set of data provides the *highest* pulmonary vascular resistance (PVR)?

	Mean PAP	PCWP	CO
A.	14	9	4
B.	15	10	4.5
C.	16	11	5
D.	17	12	5.5

78f. Given 4 sets of hemodynamic measurements. Which set of data provides the *lowest* pulmonary vascular resistance (PVR)?

	Mean PAP	PCWP	CO
A.	17	10	4.5
B.	17	11	5
C.	16	12	4.5
D.	16	13	5

78g. Hemodynamic data are obtained from 4 patients. Which patient has a *normal* pulmonary vascular resistance (PVR)?

	Mean PAP	PCWP	CO
A.	16	8	4
B.	15	10	3.5
C.	18	10	4
D.	19	10	4.5

78h. Hemodynamic data from 4 patients are shown below. Which patient has an *abnormal* pulmonary vascular resistance (PVR)?

	Mean PAP	PCWP	CO
A.	11	6	4
B.	12	7	3.5
C.	11	8	5
D.	12	9	3.5

78i. Use the hemodynamic data below to find a set of data that has the *highest* pulmonary vascular resistance (PVR).

	Mean PAP	PCWP	CO
A.	14	9	5
B.	13	7	3.5
C.	16	11	4.5
D.	17	10	4

78j. Use the hemodynamic data below to find a set of data that has the *lowest* pulmonary vascular resistance (PVR).

	Mean PAP	PCWP	CO
A.	14	9	4.7
B.	15	10	3.8
C.	16	11	4.4
D.	18	12	5.3

78k. Use the hemodynamic data below to find a set of data that has a *normal* pulmonary vascular resistance (PVR).

	Mean PAP	PCWP	CO
A.	16	7	4.5
B.	15	8	4
C.	17	8	4
D.	18	8	4.5

78l. Use the hemodynamic data below to find a set of data that has an *abnormal* pulmonary vascular resistance (PVR).

	Mean PAP	PCWP	CO
A.	15	9	5
B.	16	8	4.5
C.	17	9	4
D.	18	10	5.5

79

Vascular Resistance: Systemic

EQUATION

$$SVR = \left(MAP - \overline{RA} \right) \times \frac{80}{CO}$$

SVR : Systemic vascular resistance in dyne $\cdot$ sec/cm^5
MAP : Mean arterial pressure in mm Hg
$\overline{RA}$: Mean right atrial pressure in mm Hg, same as central venous pressure (CVP)
80 : Conversion factor from mm Hg/L/min to dyne $\cdot$ sec/cm^5
CO : Cardiac output in L/min ($\dot{Q}_T$)

NORMAL VALUE

SVR = 800 to 1,500 dyne $\cdot$ sec/cm^5

EXAMPLE

A patient has the following measurements. What is the calculated systemic vascular resistance (SVR)?

MAP = 70 mm Hg
$\overline{RA}$ = 8 mm Hg
CO = 5.0 L/min

$$SVR = \left(MAP - \overline{RA} \right) \times \frac{80}{CO}$$

$$= \left(70 - 8 \right) \times \frac{80}{5.0}$$

$$= 62 \times \frac{80}{5.0}$$

$$= \frac{4{,}960}{5}$$

$$= 992 \text{ dyne} \cdot \text{sec/cm}^5$$

EXERCISE

What is the patient's systemic vascular resistance (SVR) if the following measurements are recorded? Is it normal?

MAP = 76 mm Hg
$\overline{RA}$ = 6 mm Hg
CO = 5.0 L/min

[Answer: SVR = 1,120 dyne $\cdot$ sec/cm^5; normal]

NOTES

Systemic vascular resistance (SVR) reflects the resistance of systemic vessel to blood flow. The MAP (mean arterial pressure) in the equation is a measured value obtained from an arterial line. It may also be estimated by using the systolic and diastolic pressure readings (See *Mean Arterial Pressure*). The right atrial pressure (or central venous pressure) and the cardiac output must also be known to calculate the SVR. The constant value 80 in the equation is used to convert the SVR to absolute resistance units dyne $\cdot$ sec/cm^5.

An abnormally high SVR is indicative of systemic hypertension or fluid retention. Whereas an abnormally low SVR is indicative of hypovolemia or severe peripheral vasodilation (e.g., septic shock).

SELF-ASSESSMENT QUESTIONS

79a. To calculate a patient's systemic vascular resistance (SVR), all the following procedures or parameters are needed *except*:

A. pulmonary artery pressure
B. mean arterial pressure
C. mean right atrial pressure
D. cardiac output

79b. A patient has the following measurements: mean arterial pressure = 70 mm Hg, mean right atrial pressure = 10 mm Hg, cardiac output = 4.0 L/min. What is the systemic vascular resistance (SVR)? Is it normal?

A. 900 dyne·sec/cm^5; abnormal
B. 1,000 dyne·sec/cm^5; abnormal
C. 1,100 dyne·sec/cm^5; normal
D. 1,200 dyne·sec/cm^5; normal

79c. The following hemodynamic information is obtained from a patient's chart. What is the calculated systemic vascular resistance (SVR)? Is it normal?

Mean arterial pressure = 62 mm Hg
Mean right atrial pressure = 6 mm Hg
Cardiac output = 4.2 L/min

A. 107 dyne·sec/cm^5; abnormal
B. 667 dyne·sec/cm^5; abnormal
C. 1,067 dyne·sec/cm^5; normal
D. 1,120 dyne·sec/cm^5; normal

79d. What is the patient's systemic vascular resistance (SVR) if the following measurements are recorded? MAP = 55 mm Hg, $\overline{RA}$ = 5 mm Hg, CO = 3.8 L/min. Is it normal?

A. 226 dyne·sec/cm^5; abnormal
B. 904 dyne·sec/cm^5; normal
C. 998 dyne·sec/cm^5; normal
D. 1,053 dyne·sec/cm^5; normal

79e. The following hemodynamic measurements are obtained from a patient in the intensive care unit. Calculate the systemic vascular resistance (SVR). Is it normal?

Mean pulmonary arterial pressure = 20 mm Hg
Pulmonary capillary wedge pressure = 7 mm Hg
Mean arterial pressure = 70 mm Hg
Mean right atrial pressure = 4 mm Hg
Cardiac output = 4.2 L/min

A. 1,257 dynes·sec/cm^5; normal
B. 1,303 dynes·sec/cm^5; normal
C. 1,346 dynes·sec/cm^5; abnormal
D. 1,421 dynes·sec/cm^5; abnormal

79f. Given the following hemodynamic data. Which set of data provides the *highest* systemic vascular resistance (SVR)?

	MAP	$\overline{RA}$	CO
A.	75	9	4
B.	80	10	4.5
C.	85	11	5
D.	90	12	5.5

79g. Given 4 sets of hemodynamic measurements. Which set of data provides the *lowest* systemic vascular resistance (SVR)?

	MAP	$\overline{RA}$	CO
A.	80	10	4.5
B.	80	11	5
C.	90	12	4.5
D.	90	13	5

79h. Hemodynamic data are obtained from 4 patients. Which patient has a *normal* systemic vascular resistance (SVR)?

	MAP	$\overline{RA}$	CO
A.	95	8	4
B.	90	10	3.5
C.	100	10	4
D.	105	10	5.2

79i. Hemodynamic data from 4 patients are shown below. Which patient has an *abnormal* systemic vascular resistance (SVR)?

	MAP	$\overline{RA}$	CO
A.	105	10	5
B.	110	8	5.5
C.	70	10	5
D.	80	8	5.5

79j. Use the hemodynamic data below to find a set of data that has the *highest* systemic vascular resistance (SVR).

	MAP	$\overline{RA}$	CO
A.	80	9	5
B.	90	7	3.5
C.	105	11	4.5
D.	110	10	4

79k. Use the hemodynamic data below to find a set of data that has the *lowest* systemic vascular resistance (SVR).

	MAP	$\overline{RA}$	CO
A.	70	9	4.7
B.	75	10	3.8
C.	80	11	4.4
D.	85	12	5.3

79l. Use the hemodynamic data below to find a set of data that has a *normal* systemic vascular resistance (SVR).

	MAP	$\overline{RA}$	CO
A.	100	7	4.5
B.	90	8	4
C.	85	8	4
D.	80	8	4.5

79m. Use the hemodynamic data below to find a set of data that has an *abnormal* systemic vascular resistance (SVR).

	MAP	$\overline{RA}$	CO
A.	60	9	5
B.	70	8	4.5
C.	70	9	4
D.	60	10	5.5

Go to **rtexam.com** for more learning resources

80

Ventilator Frequency Needed for a Desired P_aCO_2

EQUATION 1

$$\text{New frequency} = \frac{\text{Frequency} \times P_aCO_2}{\text{Desired } P_aCO_2}$$

EQUATION 2

$$\text{New frequency} = \frac{(\text{Frequency} \times P_aCO_2) \times (V_T - V_D)}{\text{Desired } P_aCO_2 \times (\text{New } V_T - \text{New } V_D)}$$

Frequency	: Original ventilator frequency/min
P_aCO_2	: Original arterial carbon dioxide tension in mm Hg
Desired P_aCO_2	: Desired arterial carbon dioxide tension in mm Hg
V_T	: Original ventilator tidal volume
V_D	: Original deadspace volume
New V_T	: New ventilator tidal volume
New V_D	: New deadspace volume

NORMAL VALUE   Set frequency to provide eucapnic (patient's normal) ventilation.

EXAMPLE 1   (When ventilator tidal volume and deadspace volume remain unchanged)

The P_aCO_2 of a patient is 55 mm Hg at a ventilator frequency of 10/min. What should be the ventilator frequency if a P_aCO_2 of 40 mm Hg is desired assuming the ventilator tidal volume and spontaneous ventilation remain stable?

$$\text{New frequency} = \frac{\text{Frequency} \times P_aCO_2}{\text{Desired } P_aCO_2}$$

$$= \frac{(10 \times 55)}{40}$$

$$= \frac{550}{40}$$

$$= 13.75 \text{ or } 14/\text{min}$$

NOTES

Equation 1 assumes the following four conditions remain stable: metabolic rate (CO_2 production), ventilator tidal volume, spontaneous ventilation, and mechanical deadspace. The anatomic deadspace is not considered in this equation because it is an estimated value (based on ideal body weight) and does not change significantly in practice.

If the ventilator tidal volume or deadspace volume is changed, use Equation 2. If the ventilator tidal volume remains unchanged, new V_T = original V_T. If the deadspace volume remains unchanged, new V_D = original V_D.

EXAMPLE 2   (When ventilator tidal volume or deadspace volume is changed)

A patient has a P_aCO_2 of 25 mm Hg at a ventilator tidal volume of 800 mL, 0 mL added circuit deadspace, and a frequency of 10/min. If the ventilator tidal volume is changed to 780 mL and 50 mL of mechanical deadspace is added to the ventilator circuit, what should be the new ventilator frequency for a desired P_aCO_2 of 40 mm Hg?

$$\text{New frequency} = \frac{\left(\text{Frequency} \times P_aCO_2\right) \times \left(V_T - V_D\right)}{\text{Desired } P_aCO_2 \times \left(\text{New } V_T - \text{New } V_D\right)}$$

$$= \frac{\left(10 \times 25\right) \times \left(800 - 0\right)}{40 \times \left(780 - 50\right)}$$

$$= \frac{\left(250\right) \times \left(800\right)}{40 \times \left(730\right)}$$

$$= \frac{200,000}{29,200}$$

$$= 6.85 \text{ or } 7/\text{min}$$

EXERCISE 1   At a ventilator frequency of 8/min a patient's P_aCO_2 is 55 mm Hg. Calculate the new ventilator frequency if a P_aCO_2 of 40 mm Hg is desired (assuming the ventilator tidal volume and spontaneous ventilation remain unchanged).

[Answer: New frequency = 11/min]

EXERCISE 2   A patient has a P_aCO_2 of 30 mm Hg at a ventilator tidal volume of 700 mL and a frequency of 8/min. If 50 mL of mechanical deadspace is added to the ventilator circuit, what should be the new ventilator frequency for a desired P_aCO_2 of 40 mm Hg? What should be the calculated new frequency if no mechanical deadspace is used?

[Answer: New frequency = 6.46 or 7/min; new frequency without deadspace = 6/min]

SELF-ASSESSMENT QUESTIONS

80a. Given: P_aCO_2 = 60 mm Hg, ventilator frequency = 12/min. Calculate the estimated ventilator frequency for a P_aCO_2 of 45 mm Hg (assuming the ventilator tidal volume and spontaneous ventilation remain unchanged).

   A. 14/min
   B. 15/min
   C. 16/min
   D. 17/min

80b. Given: P_aCO_2 = 30 mm Hg, ventilator frequency = 16/min. Calculate the estimated ventilator frequency for a P_aCO_2 of 40 mm Hg (assuming the ventilator tidal volume and spontaneous ventilation remain unchanged).

   A. 11/min
   B. 12/min
   C. 13/min
   D. 14/min

80c. The P_aCO_2 of a patient is 48 mm Hg at a ventilator frequency of 12/min. What should be the ventilator frequency if a P_aCO_2 of 36 mm Hg is desired (assuming the ventilator tidal volume and spontaneous ventilation remain unchanged)?

   A. 13/min
   B. 14/min
   C. 15/min
   D. 16/min

80d. Given: P_aCO_2 52 mm Hg and ventilator frequency 10/min. What should be the ventilator frequency if a P_aCO_2 of 40 mm Hg is desired?

   A. 12/min
   B. 13/min
   C. 14/min
   D. 15/min

80e. Given: P_aCO_2 34 mm Hg and ventilator frequency 12/min. What should be the ventilator frequency if a P_aCO_2 of 40 mm Hg is desired?

   A. 10/min
   B. 11/min
   C. 12/min
   D. 13/min

80f. A patient's arterial blood gas results show pH 7.30, P_aCO_2 48 mm Hg, P_aO_2 84 mm Hg. The ventilator frequency is 14/min. Calculate the ventilator frequency for a desired P_aCO_2 of 40 mm Hg.

A. 15/min

B. 16/min

C. 17/min

D. 18/min

80g. A patient has a P_aCO_2 of 22 mm Hg at a ventilator tidal volume of 650 mL and a frequency of 12/min. If 50 mL of mechanical deadspace is added to the ventilator circuit, what should be the new ventilator frequency for a desired P_aCO_2 of 35 mm Hg?

A. 7/min

B. 8/min

C. 9/min

D. 10/min

80h. A patient has a P_aCO_2 of 45 mm Hg at a ventilator tidal volume of 540 mL and a frequency of 12/min. If the ventilator tidal volume is changed to 600 mL, what should be the new ventilator frequency for a desired P_aCO_2 of 40 mm Hg?

A. 12/min

B. 13/min

C. 14/min

D. 15/min

80i. The P_aCO_2 of a patient is 35 mm Hg at a ventilator tidal volume of 650 mL and a frequency of 14/min. If the ventilator tidal volume is decreased to 600 mL, what should be the new ventilator frequency for a desired P_aCO_2 of 40 mm Hg?

A. 10/min

B. 11/min

C. 12/min

D. 13/min

80j. A patient's arterial blood gas results show pH 7.46, P_aCO_2 34 mm Hg, P_aO_2 76 mm Hg. The ventilator settings are tidal volume 600 mL, frequency 12/min. If a deadspace volume of 100 mL is added, calculate the ventilator frequency for a desired P_aCO_2 of 40 mm Hg.

A. 10/min

B. 11/min

C. 12/min

D. 13/min

80k. A patient's ABG results show pH 7.35, P_aCO_2 46 mm Hg, P_aO_2 68 mm Hg. The ventilator settings are tidal volume 600 mL, frequency 14/min. If the tidal volume is changed to 650 mL, calculate the ventilator frequency for a desired P_aCO_2 of 40 mm Hg.

A. 15/min
B. 16/min
C. 17/min
D. 18/min

80l. A patient recently admitted to the Neuro ICU with head injury has these ABG results: pH 7.38, P_aCO_2 42 mm Hg, P_aO_2 98 mm Hg. The ventilator settings are tidal volume 550 mL, frequency 12/min. The physician wants to hyperventilate the patient to reduce the intracranial pressure. What should be the new ventilator frequency for a desired P_aCO_2 of 30 mm Hg if the tidal volume is changed to 580 mL?

A. 14/min
B. 15/min
C. 16/min
D. 17/min

Go to **rtexam.com** for more learning resources

81

Weaning Index: Rapid Shallow Breathing (RSBI)

NOTES

Failure of weaning from mechanical ventilation may be related to a spontaneous breathing pattern that is rapid (high frequency) and shallow (low tidal volume). The relationship between spontaneous frequency and spontaneous tidal volume (in liters) has been used to evaluate the presence and severity of this breathing pattern.

Rapid shallow breathing index is expressed as f (frequency or breaths per minute) divided by the V_T in liters. A rapid shallow breathing pattern leads to an increased deadspace ventilation. A f/V_T index >100 breaths/min/L (rounded from 103 breaths/min/L) correlates with weaning or extubation failure. On the other hand, absence of rapid shallow breathing, as defined by an f/V_T index of ≤100 breaths/min/L, correlates with weaning or extubation success.

To measure the f/V_T ratio, the patient is put on the spontaneous mode and allowed to breathe spontaneously for 1 to 3 minutes. Invalid breathing status may occur if measurements are done before the patient reaches a stable spontaneous breathing pattern. Ventilator modes that provide assisted breaths (e.g., SIMV) or excessive pressure support ventilation (PSV >5 cm H_2O) will underestimate the RSBI measurements.

EQUATION

$RSBI = f/V_T$

$RSBI$: Rapid Shallow Breathing Index, in breaths/min/L or cycles/L

f : Spontaneous frequency in breaths/min (cycles)

V_T : Spontaneous tidal volume, in liters

NORMAL VALUE

≤100 breaths/min/L or cycles/L
(rounded from <103 breaths/min/L)

EXAMPLE

A mechanically ventilated patient is being evaluated for weaning trial.

While breathing spontaneously, the minute ventilation is 4.5 L/min at a frequency of 18/min. What is the average spontaneous tidal volume, in liters? What is the calculated Rapid Shallow Breathing Index (f/V_T)? Does this index suggest a successful weaning outcome?

$$\text{Average spontaneous } V_T = \text{minute ventilation/frequency}$$
$$= 4.5\,L/18$$
$$= 0.25\,L$$

$$\text{Rapid Shallow Breathing Index} = f/V_T$$
$$= 18/0.25$$
$$= 72 \text{ breaths/min/L}$$

Because the Rapid Shallow Breathing Index is less than 100, the calculated RSBI suggests a successful weaning outcome.

EXERCISE

A mechanically ventilated patient is being evaluated for weaning trial. The spontaneous minute ventilation and spontaneous frequency are 7.6 L/min and 36/min, respectively. What is the average spontaneous tidal volume, in liters? What is the calculated Rapid Shallow Breathing Index (f/V_T)? Does this index indicate a successful weaning outcome?

[Answer: Average spontaneous V_T = 0.21 L; Rapid Shallow Breathing Index = 171 breaths/min/L; the RSBI is >100 breaths/min/L and it suggests a poor weaning outcome.]

SELF-ASSESSMENT QUESTIONS

81a. **Successful weaning from mechanical ventilation is likely when the RSBI is:**

A. greater than 100 breaths/min/L
B. less than 100 breaths/min/L
C. greater than 100 L
D. less than 100 L

81b. **RSBI requires measurements of the patient's _____ minute ventilation and spontaneous _____.**

A. mechanical; frequency
B. mechanical; tidal volume
C. spontaneous; frequency
D. spontaneous; tidal volume

81c. **RSBI is calculated by:**

A. dividing a patient's spontaneous tidal volume by frequency
B. multiplying a patient's spontaneous tidal volume and frequency
C. dividing a patient's spontaneous frequency by tidal volume
D. multiplying a patient's spontaneous minute ventilation and frequency

81d. **Given the following measurements: spontaneous minute ventilation = 6 L/min, spontaneous frequency = 20/min. What is the average spontaneous tidal volume, in liters?**

A. 0.15 L
B. 0.2 L
C. 0.25 L
D. 0.3 L

81e. **Given the following measurements: spontaneous minute ventilation = 5.6 L/min, spontaneous frequency = 16/min. What is the calculated RSBI? Does the RSBI indicate a successful weaning outcome?**

A. 46 breaths/min/L; yes
B. 46 breaths/min/L; no
C. 90 breaths/min/L; yes
D. 90 breaths/min/L; no

NOTES *(continued)*

The minute expired volume (V_E) measured by the ventilator or a respirometer is divided by the frequency to obtain the average spontaneous tidal volume (V_T). The RSBI is calculated by dividing the f by average spontaneous V_T (L). Note that the V_T in the equation is in liters.

An alternate equation for RSBI is f^2/V_E.

81f. Given the following measurements: spontaneous minute ventilation = 9.9 L/min, spontaneous frequency = 22/min. What is the average spontaneous tidal volume, in liters?

A. 0.36 L
B. 0.38 L
C. 0.41 L
D. 0.45 L

81g. Given the following measurements: spontaneous minute ventilation = 5.5 L/min, spontaneous frequency = 25/min. What is the calculated RSBI? Does the RSBI indicate a successful weaning outcome?

A. 114 breaths/min/L; yes
B. 114 breaths/min/L; no
C. 138 breaths/min/L; yes
D. 138 breaths/min/L; no

81h. Mr. Johns, a mechanically ventilated patient, is being evaluated for weaning attempt. His spontaneous minute ventilation and frequency are 7.7 L/min and 22/min, respectively. What is the average spontaneous tidal volume, in liters? What is the calculated Rapid Shallow Breathing Weaning Index (f/V_T)? Does the calculated RSBI suggest a successful weaning outcome?

A. average spontaneous V_T = 0.35 L; *RSBI* = 63 breaths/min/L; yes
B. average spontaneous V_T = 0.35 L; *RSBI* = 112 breaths/min/L; no
C. average spontaneous V_T = 0.45 L; *RSBI* = 49 breaths/min/L; yes
D. average spontaneous V_T = 0.45 L; *RSBI* = 125 breaths/min/L; no

81i. The spontaneous minute ventilation and frequency of a mechanically ventilated patient are 6.2 L/min and 20/min respectively. Calculate the average spontaneous tidal volume, in liters, and the Rapid Shallow Breathing Index (f/V_T). Does the calculated RSBI indicate a successful weaning outcome?

A. average spontaneous V_T = 0.27 L; RSBI = 74 breaths/min/L; yes
B. average spontaneous V_T = 0.27 L; RSBI = 114 breaths/min/L; no
C. average spontaneous V_T = 0.31 L; RSBI = 65 breaths/min/L; yes
D. average spontaneous V_T = 0.31 L; RSBI = 108 breaths/min/L; no

81j. Which of the following sets of data provides the *highest* average spontaneous tidal volume?

	V_E (L/min)	f (/min)
A.	4.6	14
B.	5.2	16
C.	5.8	18
D.	6.4	20

81k. Which of the following sets of data provides the *lowest* average spontaneous tidal volume?

	V_E (L/min)	f (/min)
A.	6.7	22
B.	6.9	24
C.	7.2	26
D.	7.5	28

81l. Four sets of weaning parameters are shown below. Which set of data indicates a *successful* weaning outcome?

	V_E (L/min)	f (/min)
A.	6.3	26
B.	6.8	24
C.	7.2	28
D.	7.8	30

81m. Four sets of weaning parameters are listed below. Which set of data indicates an *unsuccessful* weaning outcome?

	V_E (L/min)	f (/min)
A.	6.8	22
B.	6.9	24
C.	7.6	26
D.	7.8	29

81n. An alternate equation for RSBI calculation is:

A. f / V_E
B. f^2 / V_E
C. $f \times V_E$
D. $f^2 \times V_E$

Ventilator Waveform

The ventilator waveforms presented in this section are for illustration purposes.
Actual changes in the waveforms are influenced by other factors such as dual-mode settings and other co-existing patient conditions affecting the airflow resistance and lung compliance.

Contents

Volume-Time Waveforms

Constant Flow

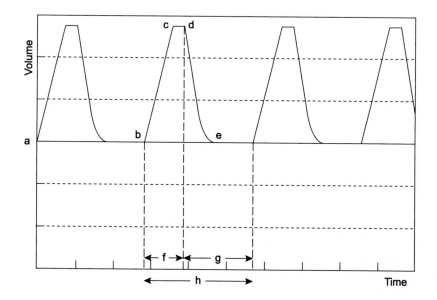

FIGURE 3-1. Normal

x-axis (time)
y-axis (volume)

a.   baseline volume
b.   beginning inspiration
c.   end inspiration
b to c. inspiratory tidal volume
d.   beginning expiration
c to d. inspiratory pause
e.   end expiration
d to e. expiratory tidal volume
f.   inspiratory time
g.   expiratory time
h.   respiratory cycle time

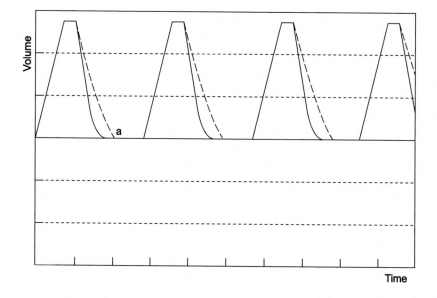

FIGURE 3-2. Increased Resistance

Solid line (normal)
Dotted line (increased resistance)

a. *slower* exponential decay to baseline volume (dotted line)

[*unchanged* inspiratory volume, pause time, expiratory volume, inspiratory time, expiratory time, and respiratory cycle time]

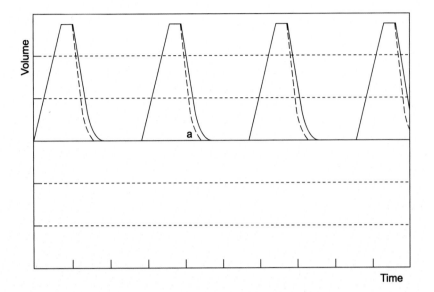

FIGURE 3-3. Decreased Compliance

Solid line (normal)
Dotted line (decreased compliance)
a. *faster* exponential decay to baseline volume (dotted line)
[unchanged inspiratory volume, pause time, expiratory volume, inspiratory time, expiratory time, and respiratory cycle time]

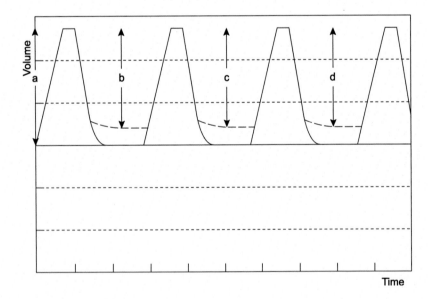

FIGURE 3-4. Air Leak

Solid line (normal)
Dotted line (air leak)
a. inspiratory tidal volume
b. expiratory tidal volume
   (expired volume < inspired volume)
c. expiratory tidal volume
   (expired volume < inspired volume)
d. expiratory tidal volume
   (expired volume < inspired volume)
[in air leaks, every expiratory tidal volume is less than the inspiratory tidal volume]

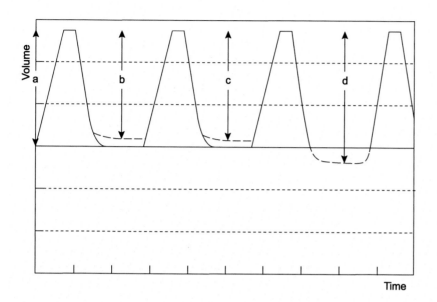

FIGURE 3–5. Air Trapping

Solid line (normal)
Dotted line (air trapping)
a. inspiratory tidal volume
b. expiratory tidal volume
   (expired volume < inspired volume)
c. expiratory tidal volume
   (expired volume < inspired volume)
d. expiratory tidal volume
   (expired volume > inspired volume)
[in air trapping, tidal volume and previously trapped air are exhaled every 2 to 3 breaths, resulting in an expired volume that is *larger* than the inspired volume]

Volume–Time Waveforms

Pressure-Controlled

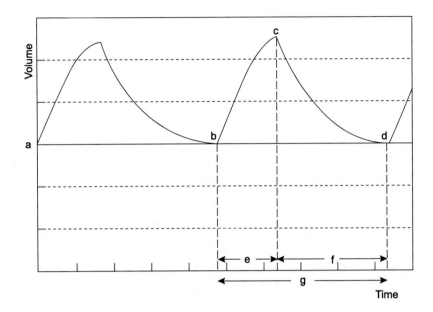

FIGURE 3-6. Normal

x-axis (time)
y-axis (volume)

a.   baseline volume
b.   beginning inspiration
c.   end inspiration/beginning expiration
b to c. inspiratory tidal volume
d.   end expiration
c to d. expiratory tidal volume
e.   inspiratory time
f.   expiratory time
g.   respiratory cycle time

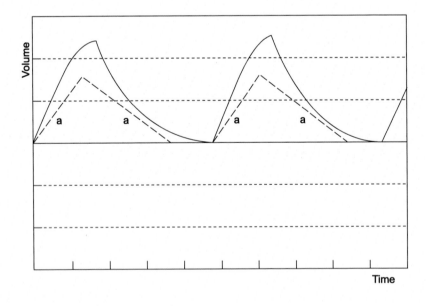

FIGURE 3-7. Increased Resistance

Solid line (normal)
Dotted line (increased resistance)

a. *smaller* inspiratory and expiratory tidal volumes
   (dotted line)

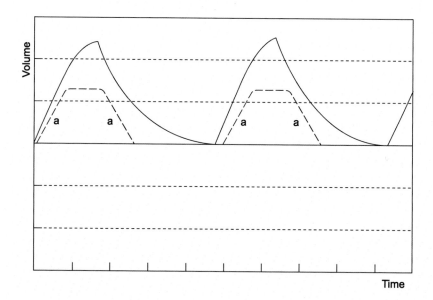

FIGURE 3-8. Decreased Compliance

Solid line (normal)
Dotted line (decreased compliance)
a. *smaller* inspiratory and expiratory tidal volumes
   (dotted line)

Pressure–Time Waveforms

Constant Flow

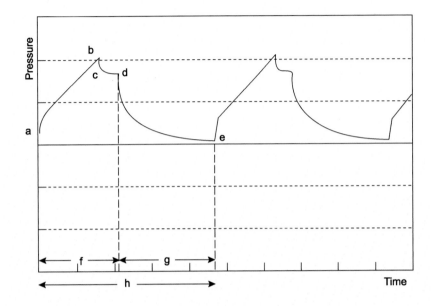

FIGURE 3-9. Normal

x-axis (time)
y-axis (pressure)
a.   beginning inspiration
b.   peak inspiratory pressure
c.   beginning inspiratory pause
b to c. air flow resistance
d.   end inspiratory pause/beginning expiration
c to d. plateau pressure (i.e., P_{PLAT}, static pressure)
e.   end expiration
f.   inspiratory time
g.   expiratory time
h.   respiratory cycle time

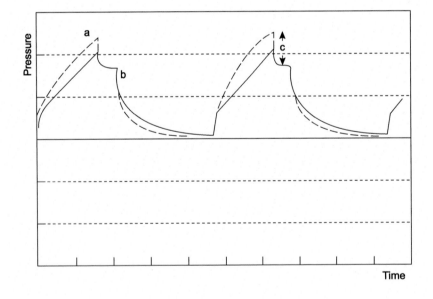

FIGURE 3-10. Increased Resistance

Solid line (normal)
Dotted line (increased resistance)
a. *higher* PIP
b. *unchanged* P_{PLAT}
c. larger difference between PIP and P_{PLAT}

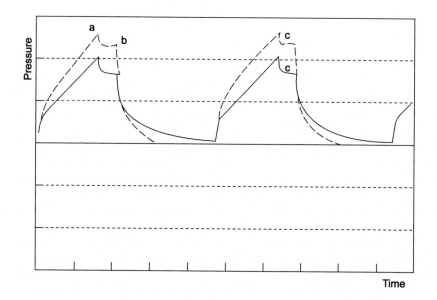

FIGURE 3-11. Decreased Compliance

Solid line (normal)
Dotted line (decreased compliance)
a. *higher* PIP
b. *higher* P_{PLAT}
c. unchanged difference between PIP and P_{PLAT}
(a-b)

Pressure-Time Waveforms

Pressure-Controlled

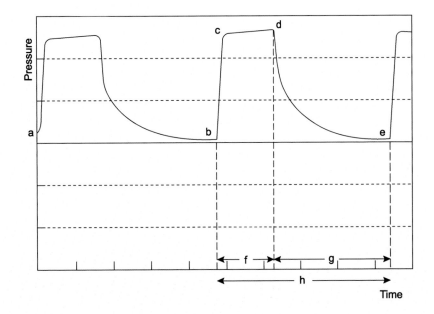

FIGURE 3-12. Normal

x-axis (time)
y-axis (pressure)
a. beginning inspiration
b. beginning inspiration/baseline pressure
c. peak inspiratory pressure
d. end inspiratory/beginning expiration
e. end expiration
f. inspiratory time
g. expiratory time
h. respiratory cycle time

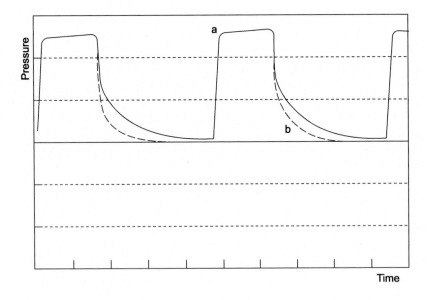

FIGURE 3-13. Increased Resistance

Solid line (normal)
Dotted line (increased resistance)
a. unchanged inspiratory phase
b. rapid decay to the second portion of pressure tracing

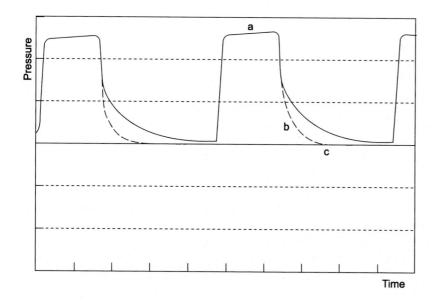

FIGURE 3-14. Decreased Compliance

Solid line (normal)
Dotted line (decreased compliance)
a. unchanged inspiratory phase
b. rapid decay of pressure tracing
c. expiratory pressure reaches baseline sooner

Flow–Time Waveforms

Constant Flow

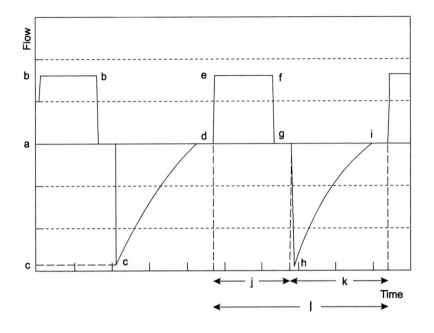

FIGURE 3-15. Normal

x-axis (time)
y-axis (flow)
a.　baseline (separates inspiratory and expiratory flow patterns)
b.　peak inspiratory flow
c.　peak expiratory flow
d.　beginning inspiration
e.　peak inspiratory flow at beginning inspiration
f.　peak inspiratory flow at end inspiration/ beginning expiration
e to f. constant flow pattern
g.　inspiratory pause
h.　peak expiratory flow
i.　end expiration (expiratory flow returns to baseline)
j.　inspiratory time (includes pause time)
k.　expiratory time (does not include pause time)
l.　respiratory cycle time

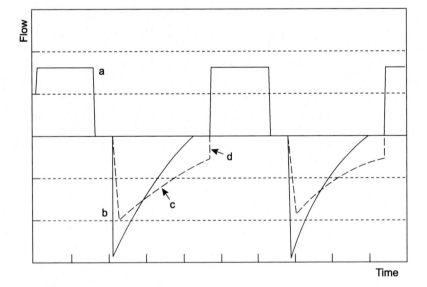

FIGURE 3-16. Increased Resistance

Solid line (normal)
Dotted line (increased resistance)
a. inspiratory phase does not change
b. *lower* expiratory flow as a result of increased airflow resistance during expiration
c. *slower* expiratory flow decay to baseline
d. air-trapping as expiratory flow does not reach baseline at end expiration (auto-**PEEP** may be observed in pressure-time waveform)

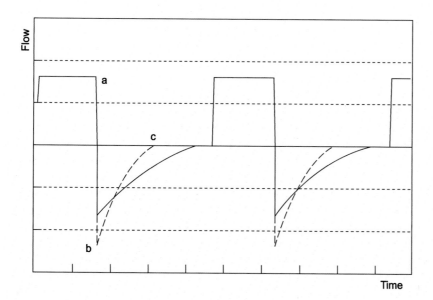

FIGURE 3–17. Decreased Compliance

Solid line (normal)
Dotted line (decreased compliance)
a. inspiratory phase does not change
b. *higher* peak expiratory flow as a result of increased lung recoil (↑ elastance/↓ compliance)
c. *faster* expiratory flow decay to baseline as a result of increased lung recoil (↑ elastance/↓ compliance)

Flow-Time Waveforms

Pressure-Controlled

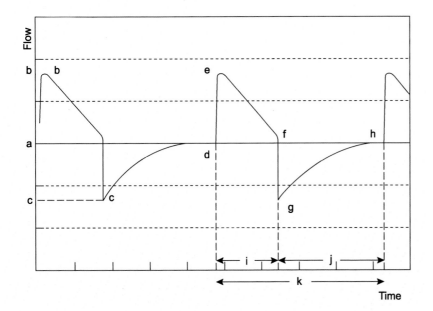

FIGURE 3-18. Normal

x-axis (time)
y-axis (flow)
a. baseline (separates inspiratory and expiratory flow patterns)
b. peak inspiratory flow
c. peak expiratory flow
d. beginning inspiration
e. peak inspiratory flow at beginning inspiration
f. inspiratory flow at end inspiration/beginning expiration
e to f. descending flow pattern
g. peak expiratory flow
h. end expiration (expiratory flow returns to baseline)
i. inspiratory time
j. expiratory time
k. respiratory cycle time

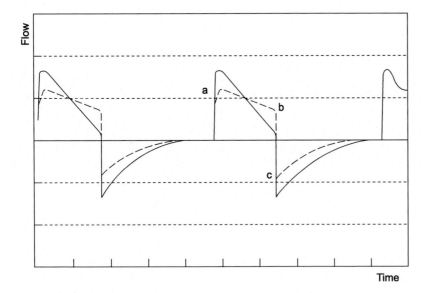

FIGURE 3-19. Increased Resistance

Solid line (normal)
Dotted line (increased resistance)
a. *lower* peak inspiratory flow
b. inspiratory flow stops before reaching baseline
c. *lower* peak expiratory flow

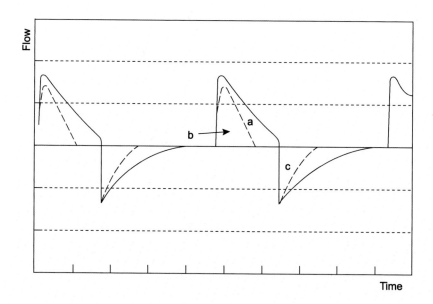

FIGURE 3-20. Decreased Compliance

Solid line (normal)
Dotted line (decreased compliance)
a. *faster* inspiratory flow decay to baseline before end of set inspiratory time
b. *lower* delivered tidal volume as a result of smaller flow-time area
c. *faster* expiratory flow decay to baseline as a result of increased lung recoil (↑ elastance/↓ compliance)

Volume–Pressure Waveforms

Constant Flow

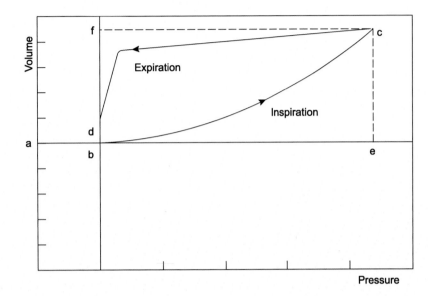

FIGURE 3-21. Normal

x-axis (pressure)
y-axis (volume)
a. baseline pressure/volume
b. beginning inspiration
c. end inspiration/beginning expiration
d. end expiration
e. peak inspiratory pressure
f. inspired volume (expired volume may differ in air leak or air trapping)

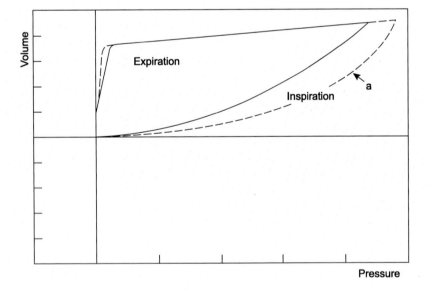

FIGURE 3-22. Increased Resistance

a. increase of pressure throughout the volume-pressure loop (inspiratory and expiratory phases)

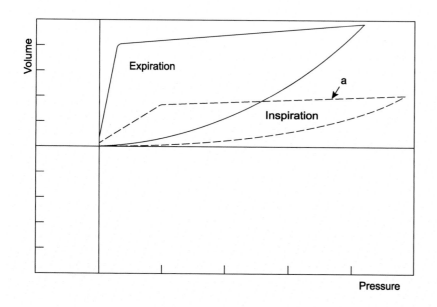

FIGURE 3-23. Decreased Compliance

a. shift of the volume-pressure loop toward the pressure-axis (usually x-axis)

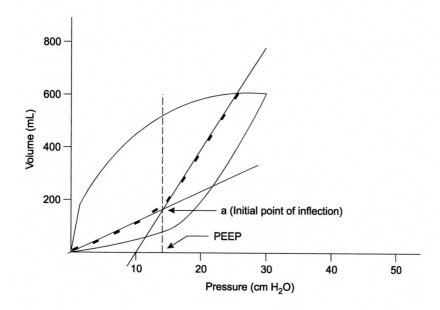

FIGURE 3-24. Initial Point of Inflection (Ipi)

a. change of slope from low compliance to improved compliance
[Because lung recruitment is likely to occur over the entire inspiratory inflation volume-pressure curve, the Ipi is only an approximation of the pressure at which the low compliance shows improvement. A **PEEP** level slightly higher than the Ipi (e.g., 2 cm H_2O) may be used initially to reduce the alveolar opening pressure.]

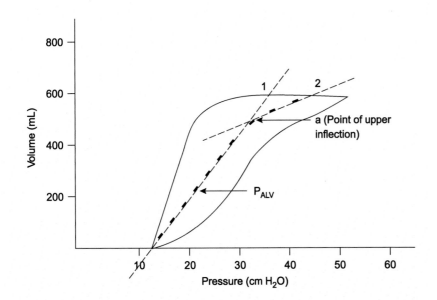

FIGURE 3-25. Point of Upper Inflection (Ipu)

a. change of slope from normal to reduced compliance as a result of overdistention of alveoli
[The Ipu is an approximation of the inspiratory pressure at which the compliance shows deterioration. The tidal volume may be reduced initially until the Ipu (duckbill) disappears, pending further evaluation of presence of overdistention.]

Flow–Volume Waveform

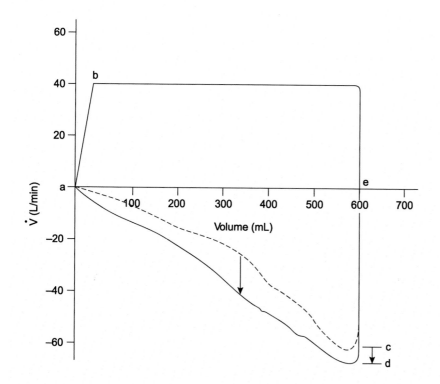

FIGURE 3-26. Decreased Airflow Resistance

x-axis (volume)
y-axis (inspiratory flow; expiratory flow)
a.   baseline flow/volume
b.   peak inspiratory flow
c.   abnormal peak expiratory flow
     (before bronchodilator)
d.   normal peak expiratory flow
     (after bronchodilator)
c to d. improvement of peak expiratory flow
     (i.e., decreased airflow resistance)
e.   tidal volume

Basic Statistics and Educational Calculations

Statistics Terminology

Coefficient of Variation (CV)

Expresses the standard deviation as a percent of the mean:

$$CV = \left(\frac{s}{\overline{X}}\right) \times 100\%$$

The coefficient of variation (CV) is useful in comparing the dispersion of two or more sets of data measured by different instruments or methods. For example, if set A of measurements has a CV of 25% and set B of measurements has a CV of 14%, we can infer that the measuring instrument or method for set A has more random errors than that for set B. (See sample calculation in this section.)

Confidence Level

Probability level. The confidence level is usually set at 95% (0.05 level), which means that there is a 95% probability that the sample population is distributed in the same way as the whole population. For example, if statistical analysis provides a conclusion that is accepted at the 0.05 level, the researcher can be 95% confident that the conclusion can be applied to the whole population.

Control Group

A group of subjects whose selection and experiences are identical in every way possible to those of the treatment (experimental) group except that they do not receive the treatment.

Control Variable

A variable in the experimental design that is neutralized or canceled out by the researcher. This is the factor controlled by the researcher to neutralize any undesirable effect that might otherwise distort the observed outcome.

Correlation Coefficient (r)

Describes the relationship between two interval variables. It ranges from –1 (most negative relationship) to +1 (most positive relationship). For example, the coefficient may be positively related ($r = 0.86$) as in P_IO_2 and P_aO_2, or it may be negatively related ($r = -0.77$) as in alveolar ventilation and P_aCO_2.

If a regression line is constructed from the data points, it can "predict" one interval variable given the other interval variable.

Cut Score	The minimal passing score of an objective test or questionnaire. It is determined by a formula using the consensus of a group of subject-matter experts. (See sample calculation in this section.)
Dependent Variable	A response or output caused by the use of treatment or placebo. This is the factor observed and measured by the researcher to determine the effect of the independent variable.
Hypothesis	A suggested solution to a problem. It has the following characteristics: (1) It should have a statement based on logical derivation of a conclusion from facts; (2) it should be stated clearly and concisely in the form of a declarative sentence; and (3) it should be testable.
Independent Variable	A variable or input that operates within a person or an object that affects behavior or outcome. This is the factor selected and manipulated by the researcher to determine the relationship to an observed outcome.
Interval Variable	Lists the order of data and sets the distance between measurements. Heart rate, oxygen saturation, and drug dosages are interval variables because their measurements are equally spaced.
Kuder-Richardson Reliability Coefficient (K-R21)	A test reliability formula that is equivalent to the average of all possible split-half reliability coefficients. (See sample calculation in this section.) $$\text{K-R21} = 1 - \frac{\bar{X}\left(n - \bar{X}\right)}{ns^2}$$ K-R21 = Kuder-Richardson reliability coefficient, Formula 21 $\bar{X}$ = Mean score on the test n = Number of items in the test s^2 = Test variance
Likert Scale	A three-point or five-point scale is often used in surveys because it can easily record the extent of agreement or disagreement with a statement. The scale does not provide interval data and should not be used in statistical calculations.

Mean	The average measurement. It is computed by adding all measurements and then dividing by the number of measurements. (See sample calculation in this section.)
Median	The measurement in the middle of a ranked distribution; 50% of the measurements fall above it, and the other 50% fall below it. (See sample calculation in this section.)
Mode	The most frequently occurring measurement in a ranked distribution. If two measurements share the highest frequency count, the ranked distribution is called bimodal. (See example in this section.)
Nominal Variable	Also called categorical variable. The term "nominal" means "to name." A nominal variable classifies data into categories with no relation existing between the categories. For example, three categories of disease: chronic obstructive pulmonary disease, congestive heart failure, cystic fibrosis.
Null Hypothesis	A negative or "no differences" version of a hypothesis. When a null hypothesis is rejected, a significant difference between the two means is said to have occurred in a research study. (See *t*-test in this section.)
Ordinal Variable	The term "ordinal" means "to rank in order." An ordinal scale ranks data in terms of more than or less than. For example, no cyanosis, mild cyanosis, moderate cyanosis, severe cyanosis.
Placebo	An inert substance given to the control group in the same manner as to the treatment group. Placebos are often used in medical research to make it impossible for the subjects to determine whether they are receiving the active substance under study.
Range	The distance or measurement between the lowest and highest measurements. (See example in this section.)

Rating Scale	A device that can be used to summarize the observed activity. This scale may have three, five, seven, or an infinite number of points on a line with descriptive statements on both ends.
Ratio Scale	Data of physical science measurements including a true zero value such as blood pressure, arterial PO_2, height, and weight.
Reliability	Consistency. A *reliable* research study yields *consistent* results when the study is repeated. Reliability ranges from 0% (least reliable) to 100% (most reliable).
Revised Nedelsky Procedure	A three-step procedure to calculate the Cut Score of an evaluation instrument such as a multiple-choice exam. (See sample calculations in this section.)
Spearman-Brown Formula	A formula to calculate the whole test reliability (r_2). (See sample calculation in this section.) $$r_2 = \frac{n(r_1)}{1+(n-1)r_1}$$ r_2 = whole test reliability n = number of parts (for halves, $n = 2$) r_1 = correlation coefficient
Split-Half Reliability	A reliability index of the internal consistency of a test that enables a researcher to determine whether the halves of a test are measuring the same quality or characteristic. The test is divided into halves, usually the odd-numbered items and the even-numbered items. The correlation coefficient (r_1) is calculated by using the scores obtained by all students on one half of the exam and those obtained on the other half of the same exam. For a group of 30 students, 30 pairs of scores (30 scores for odd-numbered items and 30 scores for even-numbered items) would be used to calculate the correlation coefficient (r_1). From the correlation coefficient (r_1), the whole test reliability (r_2) can be calculated by the Spearman-Brown formula.

Standard Deviation (s)	A measure of the spread or dispersion of a distribution of measurements. $N - 1$ in the equation is the degree of freedom. (See sample calculation in this section.) In text, the abbreviation for standard deviation is SD.
	In the blood gas laboratory, standard deviation is used along with the mean to create a Levey-Jennings chart for graphic illustration of quality control results. Results falling within two standard deviations (± 2 SD) from the mean are considered "in control." Results falling outside two standard deviations from the mean are considered "out of control," and corrective actions must be taken to bring the results within two standard deviations.
Standard (z) Scores	A standard (z) score reflects the distance (in terms of standard deviations) of a measurement away from the mean. A z score of $+ 1.5$ means that the measurement is 1.5 standard deviations *above* the mean. A z score of $- 1.5$ means that the measurement is 1.5 standard deviations *below* the mean. (See sample calculation in this section.)
t-test	The *t*-test allows a researcher to compare two means to determine the probability that the difference between the means is a real difference rather than a chance difference.
	If the calculated *t* value is greater than the table *t* value at a specific confidence (p) level, then null hypothesis (i.e., that the means are equal) can be rejected at the p level. In other words, there is a statistical difference between the two means.
	If the calculated *t* value is smaller than the table *t* value, there is no statistical difference between the means.
Treatment Group	A group of subjects whose selection and experiences are identical in every way possible to those of the control group. This is the group that receives the treatment.
Validity	The precision with which a research study measures what it purports to measure.
Variance (s^2)	The square of the standard deviation. (See example calculation in this section.)
REFERENCES	Chatburn; Gross; Nedelsky; Tuckman; White

Measures of Central Tendency

EXAMPLES 1–8 Ten scores from a 100-item final exam are ranked and listed as follows: 66, 66, 66, 73, 75, 79, 82, 84, 87, and 87. For examples 1 through 8, write or calculate the (1) range, (2) mode, (3) mean, (4) median, (5) standard deviation, (6) variance, (7) coefficient of variation, and (8) standard scores for 73 points and 82 points on the exam.

SOLUTION 1 *Range*: The range for the 10 exam scores is 66 to 87 points (21 points).

SOLUTION 2 *Mode*: The most frequently occurring measurement of these 10 exam scores is 66 points.

SOLUTION 3 *Mean ($\bar{X}$):*

$$\bar{X} = \frac{\text{Sum of exam scores}}{\text{Number of scores}}$$

$$= \frac{66 + 66 + 66 + 73 + 75 + 79 + 82 + 84 + 87 + 87}{10}$$

$$= \frac{765}{10}$$

$$= 76.5 \text{ points}$$

SOLUTION 4 *Median*: Because the median is the measurement in the middle of this ranked 10-number distribution, it falls between 75 (the fifth number) and 79 (the sixth number). The median is therefore

$$\frac{75 + 79}{2} = \frac{154}{2} = 77 \text{ points}$$

SOLUTION 5 *Standard deviation (s):*

Value of X	Mean ($\bar{X}$)	$(X - \bar{X})$	$(X - \bar{X})^2$
66	76.5	−10.5	110.25
66	76.5	−10.5	110.25
66	76.5	−10.5	110.25
73	76.5	−3.5	12.25
75	76.5	−1.5	2.25
79	76.5	2.5	6.25
82	76.5	5.5	30.25
84	76.5	7.5	56.25
87	76.5	10.5	110.25
87	76.5	10.5	110.25
		0	658.50

$$s = \sqrt{\dfrac{\text{Sum of } (X - \bar{X})^2}{\text{Degree of freedom}}}$$

$$= \sqrt{\dfrac{\text{Sum of } (X - \bar{X})^2}{(\text{Number of scores} - 1)}}$$

$$= \sqrt{\dfrac{\text{Sum of } (X - \bar{X})^2}{(N - 1)}}$$

$$= \sqrt{\dfrac{658.5}{(10 - 1)}}$$

$$= \sqrt{\dfrac{658.5}{9}}$$

$$= \sqrt{73.17}$$

$$= 8.554 \text{ points}$$

SOLUTION 6   *Variance (s^2)*: Because variance is the square of the standard deviation, it is 73.17 (8.554^2).

SOLUTION 7   *Coefficient of Variation (CV)*:

$$CV = \left(\dfrac{\text{standard deviation}}{\text{mean}}\right) \times 100\%$$

$$= \left(\dfrac{s}{\bar{X}}\right) \times 100\%$$

$$= \left(\dfrac{8.554}{76.5}\right) \times 100\%$$

$$= 0.1118 \times 100\%$$

$$= 11.18\%$$

SOLUTION 8   *Standard (z) Scores*: For a score of 73 points on the exam, the standard score (z) is calculated as follows:

$$z = \dfrac{X - \bar{X}}{s}$$

$$= \dfrac{73 - 76.5}{8.554}$$

$$= \dfrac{-3.5}{8.554}$$

$$= -0.41$$

The *z* score for 73 is 0.41 standard deviation *below* the mean.

For a score of 82 points on the exam, the standard score (z) is calculated as follows:

$$z = \frac{X - \bar{X}}{s}$$

$$= \frac{82 - 76.5}{8.554}$$

$$= \frac{5.5}{8.554}$$

$$= 0.64$$

The z score for 82 is 0.64 standard deviation *above* the mean.

EXAMPLE 9

The mean and one standard deviation for a series of PO_2 calibration measurements are 157 mm Hg and ±3 mm Hg, respectively. If two standard deviations from the mean are used to set the limit of acceptance, which of the following six PO_2 calibration points is out of range? 155, 160, 153, 157, 164, 163 mm Hg.

SOLUTION 9

164 mm Hg is out of range.

A mean PO_2 of 157 mm Hg with one standard deviation (SD) of ±3 mm Hg would have two SD of ±6 mm Hg. Therefore, the acceptable range for PO_2 calibration is 151 (157 – 6) mm Hg to 163 (157 + 6) mm Hg. Of the six calibration points, 164 mm Hg is the only one outside this acceptable range.

EXAMPLE 10

The mean and one standard deviation for a series of normal pH calibration measurements are 7.375 and ±0.002, respectively. If measurements falling within two standard deviations from the mean are considered acceptable, which of the following seven pH calibration points is out of range? 7.379, 7.376, 7.374, 7.377, 7.370, 7375, and 7.376.

SOLUTION 10

7.370 is out of range.

A mean pH of 7.375 with one standard deviation (SD) of ±0.002 would have two SD of ±0.004. The acceptable range for pH calibration is therefore 7.371 (7.375 – 0.004) to 7.379 (7.375 + 0.004). Of the seven calibration points, 7.370 is the only one outside this acceptable range.

Exercises

EXERCISE 1–8   Nine mixed-venous oxygen content measurements in volume percent (vol%) are ranked and listed as follows: 12, 14, 14, 15, 15, 16, 16, 16, and 17. Write or calculate the (1) range, (2) mode, (3) mean, (4) median, (5) standard deviation, (6) variance, (7) coefficient of variation, and (8) standard scores for 12 vol% and 16 vol%.

SOLUTION 1   *Range*: The range for the nine measurements is 12 to 17 vol% (5 vol%).

SOLUTION 2   *Mode*: The most frequently occurring measurement of these nine values is 16 vol%.

SOLUTION 3   *Mean ($\bar{X}$):*

$$\bar{X} = \frac{\text{Sum of } C_{\bar{v}}O_2 \text{ measurements}}{\text{Number of measurements}}$$

$$= \frac{12+14+14+15+15+16+16+16+17}{9}$$

$$= \frac{135}{9}$$

$$= 15 \text{ vol\%}$$

SOLUTION 4   *Median*: Rank the nine numbers as follows:

12, 14, 14, 15, 15, 16, 16, 16, 17.

As the median is the measurement in the middle of this ranked nine-number distribution, it falls between the fourth number and the sixth number. The median is therefore 15 vol% — the second 15 having four numbers before it and four numbers behind it.

SOLUTION 5   *Standard deviation (s):*

Value of X	Mean ($\bar{X}$)	($X - \bar{X}$)	($X - \bar{X}$)²
12	1.5	−3	9
14	1.5	−1	1
14	1.5	−1	1
15	1.5	0	0
15	1.5	0	0
16	1.5	1	1
16	1.5	1	1
16	1.5	1	1
17	1.5	2	4
		0	18

$$s = \sqrt{\frac{\text{Sum of } (X - \bar{X})^2}{\text{Degree of freedom}}}$$

$$= \sqrt{\frac{\text{Sum of } (X - \bar{X})^2}{(\text{Number of } C_{\bar{v}}O_2 \text{ measurements} - 1)}}$$

$$= \sqrt{\frac{\text{Sum of } (X - \bar{X})^2}{(N - 1)}}$$

$$= \sqrt{\frac{18}{(9 - 1)}}$$

$$= \sqrt{\frac{18}{8}}$$

$$= \sqrt{2.25}$$

$$= 1.5 \text{ vol\%}$$

SOLUTION 6 *Variance (s^2)*: As the variance is the square of the standard deviation, it is therefore 2.25 (1.5^2).

SOLUTION 7 *Coefficient of Variation (CV)*:

$$CV = \left(\frac{\text{standard deviation}}{\text{mean}} \right) \times 100\%$$

$$= \left(\frac{s}{\bar{X}} \right) \times 100\%$$

$$= \left(\frac{1.5}{15} \right) \times 100\%$$

$$= 0.1 \times 100\%$$

$$= 10\%$$

SOLUTION 8 *Standard (z) Scores*: For 12 vol%, the standard score (z) is calculated as follows:

$$z = \frac{X - \bar{X}}{s}$$

$$= \frac{12 - 15}{1.5}$$

$$= \frac{-3}{1.5}$$

$$= -2$$

The z score for 12 vol% is 2 standard deviations *below* the mean.

For a score of 16, the standard score (z) is calculated as follows:

$$z = \frac{X - \bar{X}}{s}$$

$$= \frac{16 - 15}{1.5}$$

$$= \frac{1}{1.5}$$

$$= 0.67$$

The z score for 16 vol% is 0.67 standard deviations *above* the mean.

EXAMPLE 9   The mean and one standard deviation for a series of PO_2 calibration measurements are 102 mm Hg and ±1 mm Hg, respectively. If two standard deviations from the mean are used to set the limit of acceptance, which of the following five PO_2 calibration points is out of range? 102, 103, 99, 104, and 100 mm Hg.

SOLUTION 9   99 mm Hg is out of range.

A mean PO_2 of 102 mm Hg with one standard deviation (SD) of ±1 mm Hg would have two SD of ±2 mm Hg. Therefore, the acceptable range for PO_2 calibration is 100 (102 − 2) mm Hg to 104 (102 + 2) mm Hg. Of the five calibration points, 99 mm Hg is the only one outside this acceptable range.

EXAMPLE 10   The mean and one standard deviation for a series of acidotic pH calibration measurements are 7.135 and ±0.015, respectively. If measurements falling within two standard deviations from the mean are considered acceptable, which of the following six pH calibration points is out of range? 7.137, 7.165, 7.175, 7.125, 7,106, and 7.135.

SOLUTION 10   7.175 is out of range.

A mean pH of 7.135 with one standard deviation (SD) of ±0.015 would have two SD of ±0.030. The acceptable range for pH calibration is therefore 7.105 (7.135 − 0.030) to 7.165 (7.135 + 0.030). Of the six calibration points, 7.175 is the only one outside this acceptable range.

EXERCISE 11   The mean and one standard deviation for a series of PCO_2 calibration measurements are 44.9 mm Hg and ±0.5 mm Hg, respectively. Which of the following five PCO_2 calibration points (44.0, 45.6, 43.5, 45.0, and 46.5 mm Hg) is out of range if (A) *two* standard deviations from the mean are used to set the limit of acceptance; (B) *three* standard deviations from the mean are used to set the limit of acceptance.

SOLUTION 11   (A) 43.5 and 46.5 mm Hg are out of range; (B) 46.5 mm Hg is out of range.

(A) A mean PCO_2 of 44.9 mm Hg with one standard deviation (SD) of ±0.5 mm Hg would have two SD of ±1.0 mm Hg. Therefore, the acceptable range for PCO_2 calibration is 43.9 (44.9 – 1.0) mm Hg to 45.9 (44.9 + 1.0) mm Hg. Of the five calibration points, 43.5 mm Hg and 46.5 mm Hg are the PCO_2 measurements outside this acceptable range.

(B) If three standard deviations (±1.5 mm 1 Hg) were used, the acceptable range for PCO_2 calibration would become 43.4 (44.9 – 1.5) mm Hg to 46.4 (44.9 + 1.5) mm Hg. Of the five calibration points, 46.5 mm Hg is the PCO_2 outside this acceptable range.

Test Reliability

Kuder-Richardson Reliability Coefficient (K-R21)

The Kuder-Richardson reliability coefficient calculates test reliability when the following are known: (1) mean score of the test, (2) variance of the test, and (3) number of items in the test. The reliability coefficient ranges from 0 (least reliable) to 1 (most reliable).

EXAMPLE

Ten scores from a 100-item final exam are ranked and listed as follows: 66, 66, 66, 73, 75, 79, 72, 84, 87, and 87. Calculate the reliability index of this exam using the Kuder-Richardson reliability coefficient (K-R21) formula. From previous examples, the mean (Example 3) and variance (Example 6) have been calculated and obtained. The reliability index may be calculated as follows:

$\bar{X}$ (mean score) $\qquad\qquad$ = 76.5
n (number of items in the test) = 100
s^2 (variance) $\qquad\qquad\quad$ = 73.17

$$
\begin{aligned}
\text{K-R21} &= 1 - \frac{\bar{X}(n - \bar{X})}{ns^2} \\[2mm]
&= 1 - \frac{76.5(100 - 76.5)}{100(73.17)} \\[2mm]
&= 1 - \frac{76.5(23.5)}{7317} \\[2mm]
&= 1 - \frac{1797.75}{7317} \\[2mm]
&= 1 - 0.2457 \\[2mm]
&= 0.7543 \text{ or } 75.43\%
\end{aligned}
$$

The test reliability based on the K-R21 formula is 75.43%.

EXERCISE 1

The mean score and variance of a 90-item exam are 72.8 and 66.2, respectively. Calculate the reliability of this exam using the Kuder-Richardson reliability coefficient (K-R21) formula.

SOLUTION 1

$\bar{X}$ (mean score) $\quad = 72.8$
n (number of items in the test) $= 90$
s^2 (variance) $\quad = 66.2$

$$\text{K-R21} = 1 - \frac{\bar{X}(n - \bar{X})}{ns^2}$$

$$= 1 - \frac{72.8(90 - 72.8)}{90(66.2)}$$

$$= 1 - \frac{72.8(17.2)}{5958}$$

$$= 1 - \frac{1252.16}{5958}$$

$$= 1 - 0.2102$$

$$= 0.7898 \text{ or } 78.98\%$$

The test reliability based on the K-R21 formula is 78.98%.

EXERCISE 2

On a standardized 160-item comprehensive exam, the mean score and variance are 129.3 and 110.8, respectively. Use the Kuder-Richardson reliability coefficient (K-R21) formula to calculate the reliability of this exam.

SOLUTION 2

$\bar{X}$ (mean score) $\quad = 129.3$
n (number of items in the test) $= 160$
s^2 (variance) $\quad = 110.8$

$$\text{K-R21} = 1 - \frac{\bar{X}(n - \bar{X})}{ns^2}$$

$$= 1 - \frac{129.3(160 - 129.3)}{160(110.8)}$$

$$= 1 - \frac{129.3(30.7)}{17728}$$

$$= 1 - \frac{3969.51}{17728}$$

$$= 1 - 0.2239$$

$$= 0.7761 \text{ or } 77.61\%$$

The test reliability based on the K-R21 formula is 77.61%.

Spearman – Brown Formula

The Spearman-Brown Formula calculates the whole test reliability when the correlation coefficient of the split-half scores is known. The split-half technique separates the exam into two halves, usually the odd-numbered and even-numbered exam items. Pairs of scores from the exam are then used to calculate the correlation coefficient. The whole test reliability index ranges from 0 (least reliable) to 1 (most reliable).

EXAMPLE

On a 60-item exam, the scores obtained by each student on the odd-numbered items and the even-numbered items are compared. The correlation coefficient (r_1) of the split-half technique is 0.67 for the entire class of 28 students (28 pairs of scores). Based on the information given, calculate the whole test reliability (r_2) with the Spearman-Brown formula.

r_2: whole test reliability
n (number of parts; for halves, $n = 2$) = 2
r_1 (correlation coefficient) = 0.67

$$r_2 = 1 - \frac{\bar{X}(n - \bar{X})}{ns^2}$$

$$= \frac{2(0.67)}{1 + (2-1)0.67}$$

$$= \frac{1.34}{1 + (1)0.67}$$

$$= \frac{1.34}{1 + 0.67}$$

$$= \frac{1.34}{1.67}$$

$$= 0.8024 \text{ or } 80.24\%$$

The whole test reliability based on the Spearman-Brown formula is 80.24%.

EXERCISE 1

A 90-item exam was given to a class of 34 students. The 34 pairs of scores were obtained by splitting and scoring the exam by odd-numbered and even-numbered items. The correlation coefficient (r_1) for the 34 pairs of scores by this split-half technique is 0.58.

Based on the information given, calculate the whole test reliability (r_2) with the Spearman-Brown formula.

SOLUTION 1

r_2: whole test reliability
n (number of parts; for halves, $n = 2$) $= 2$
r_1 (correlation coefficient) $= 0.58$

$$r_2 = 1 - \frac{\bar{X}(n-\bar{X})}{ns^2}$$

$$= \frac{2(0.58)}{1+(2-1)0.58}$$

$$= \frac{1.16}{1+(1)0.58}$$

$$= \frac{1.16}{1+0.58}$$

$$= \frac{1.16}{1.58}$$

$$= 0.7342 \text{ or } 73.42\%$$

The whole test reliability based on the Spearman-Brown formula is 73.42%.

EXERCISE 2

Twenty pairs of scores are recorded from a 60-item exam administered to a class of 20 students. Each pair of scores represents the number of correct answers obtained by each student from the odd-numbered and even-numbered exam items. The correlation coefficient (r_1) for the 20 pairs of scores is 0.75. Based on the information given, what is the calculated whole test reliability (r_2) with the Spearman-Brown formula?

SOLUTION 2

r_2: whole test reliability
n (number of parts; for halves, $n = 2$) $= 2$
r_1 (correlation coefficient) $= 0.75$

$$r_2 = 1 - \frac{\bar{X}(n-\bar{X})}{ns^2}$$

$$= \frac{2(0.75)}{1+(2-1)0.75}$$

$$= \frac{1.5}{1+(1)0.75}$$

$$= \frac{1.5}{1+0.75}$$

$$= \frac{1.5}{1.75}$$

$$= 0.8571 \text{ or } 85.71\%$$

The whole test reliability based on the Spearman-Brown formula is 85.71%.

Cut Score: Revised Nedelsky Procedure

In 1954, Leo Nedelsky published a procedure to compute the cut score (minimum passing score) of a multiple-choice exam. Among other factors that make an exam item "difficult" or "easy," the Nedelsky procedure accounts for the degree of difficulty of the distractors in a multiple-choice exam item.

The original procedure was revised by Leon J. Gross in 1985. In this revised procedure, a three-point distribution (0 to 2) is used. The revised procedure by Gross is summarized as follows.

STEP 1	All responses to a multiple-choice exam item are evaluated by a group of subject-matter experts. Consensus is then obtained from these experts, and points ranging from 0 to 2 are assigned to each response.
	The one *correct response* is scored *2 points* (weight of correct response).
	Each *plausible but incorrect response* is scored *1 point* (weight of plausible, incorrect response). This represents an "acceptable" error for the minimally competent examinee.
	Each *implausible and incorrect response* is scored *0 points* (weight of implausible, incorrect response). This represents an unacceptable error that should have been avoided even by the minimally competent examinee.
STEP 2	The minimal pass index (MPI) for each exam item is calculated by:

$$MPI = \frac{\text{Weight of correct response}}{\text{Sum of all weights for each item}}$$

STEP 3	Cut score = MPI of all exam items × 95%.
	A value of 95% is used to avoid extreme cut scores in the original Nedelsky procedure. This value may be adjusted up or down depending on the degree of chance and perfection (number of responses) in each exam item.
EXAMPLE 1	Find the minimal pass index (MPI) of the multiple-choice exam item below.
	Under normal tidal volume and respiratory rate, the F_1O_2 provided by a nasal cannula at 2 L/min of oxygen is about

A. 21%
B. 24%
C. 28%
D. 32%

STEP 1

The four responses are evaluated by a group of experts. Their consensus and point assignments to each response are as follows.

A. 21%: 0 points
B. 24%: 1 point
C. 28%: 2 points
D. 32%: 1 point

Response (A) is scored 0 points because even the minimally competent examinee should be able to eliminate this option since the F_IO_2 provided by a nasal cannula at 2 L/min of oxygen must be greater than 21% (F_IO_2 of room air).

Responses (B) and (D) are scored 1 point each because they are incorrect but plausible responses.

Response (C) is scored 2 points because it is the correct response.

STEP 2

The minimal pass index (MPI) of this exam item is therefore:

$$\text{MPI} = \frac{\text{Weight of correct response}}{\text{Sum of all weights for each item}}$$

$$= \frac{2 \text{ points}}{(0+1+2+1) \text{ points}}$$

$$= \frac{2}{4}$$

$$= 0.5$$

EXAMPLE 2

Calculate the cut score of a 10-item multiple-choice exam with the following minimal pass indices (MPI) for the 10 exam items: 0.67, 0.5, 1.0, 0.67, 0.4, 0.5, 0.4, 0.67, 0.5, and 1.0.

$$\begin{aligned}
\text{Cut score} &= \text{MPI of all exam items} \times 95\% \\
&= (0.67 + 0.5 + 1.0 + 0.67 + 0.4 + 0.5 \\
&\quad + 0.4 + 0.67 + 0.5 + 1.0) \times 95\% \\
&= 6.31 \times 95\% \\
&= 5.99 \text{ or } 6 \text{ points}
\end{aligned}$$

The cut score (minimal passing score) of this 10-item multiple-choice exam is 6 points.

EXERCISE 1   As shown below, the point assignments for each response to an exam item are provided by a group of experts. What is the minimal pass index (MPI) of this exam item?

The preferred puncture site for arterial blood gas sampling in an adult is the:

A.   radial artery: 2 points
B.   umbilical artery: 0 points
C.   brachial artery: 1 point
D.   coronary artery: 0 points

SOLUTION 1

$$MPI = \frac{\text{Weight of correct response}}{\text{Sum of all weights for each item}}$$

$$= \frac{2 \text{ points}}{3 \text{ points}}$$

$$= 0.67$$

EXERCISE 2   Use the revised Nedelsky procedure to calculate the cut score of a nine-item multiple-choice exam with the following minimal pass indices for the nine exam items: 0.5, 1.0, 0.67, 0.4, 0.4, 0.67, 0.5, 0.67, and 0.4.

SOLUTION 2

$$
\begin{aligned}
\text{Cut score} &= \text{MPI of all exam items} \times 95\% \\
&= (0.5 + 1.0 + 0.67 + 0.4 + 0.4 + 0.67 + 0.5 \\
&\quad + 0.67 + 0.4) \times 95\% \\
&= 5.21 \times 95\% \\
&= 4.95 \text{ or } 5 \text{ points}
\end{aligned}
$$

EXERCISE 3   If the sum of all minimal pass indices (MPI) in a 98-item multiple-choice exam is 81, what is the cut score using the revised Nedelsky procedure?

SOLUTION 3

$$
\begin{aligned}
\text{Cut score} &= \text{MPI of all exam items} \times 95\% \\
&= 81 \times 95\% \\
&= 76.95 \text{ or } 77 \text{ points}
\end{aligned}
$$

REFERENCES   Gross; Nedelsky

Answer Key to
Self-Assessment Questions

1a.	A	8a.	B	13e.	C
1b.	B	8b.	A	13f.	B
1c.	B	8c.	D	13g.	A
1d.	C	8d.	C	13h.	D
1e.	D	8e.	B	13i.	B
2a.	D	9a.	B	14a.	D
2b.	D	9b.	D	14b.	A
2c.	C	9c.	D	14c.	D
2d.	A	9d.	C	14d.	B
2e.	C	9e.	A	14e.	B
				14f.	A
3a.	A	10a.	A	14g.	C
3b.	B	10b.	B	14h.	C
3c.	D	10c.	A		
3d.	C	10d.	D	15a.	A
3e.	D	10e.	C	15b.	B
				15c.	D
4a.	C	11a.	B	15d.	D
4b.	D	11b.	D	15e.	C
4c.	B	11c.	D		
4d.	D	11d.	A	16a.	D
4e.	A	11e.	C	16b.	C
		11f.	B	16c.	B
5a.	B	11g.	D	16d.	A
5b.	A	11h.	C	16e.	C
5c.	B	11i.	A		
5d.	C			17a.	D
5e	D	12a.	B	17b.	C
		12b.	A	17c.	A
6a.	B	12c.	B	17d.	B
6b.	B	12d.	C	17e.	C
6c.	C	12e.	D	17f.	A
6d.	D	12f.	D	17g.	B
6e.	C	12g.	C	17h.	D
		12h.	A		
7a.	C	12i.	D	18a.	A
7b.	A			18b.	B
7c.	B	13a.	A	18c.	D
7d.	D	13b.	D	18d.	A
7e.	A	13c.	B	18e.	C
		13d.	C		

19a.	C	24d.	A	28g.	C
19b.	B	24e.	A		
19c.	D	24f.	D	29a.	A
19d.	A	24g.	B	29b.	C
19e.	A			29c.	B
		25a.	D	29d.	A
20a.	C	25b.	C	29e.	D
20b.	A	25c.	A	29f.	D
20c.	D	25d.	D	29g.	B
20d.	A	25e.	A		
20e.	D	25f.	B	30a.	B
20f.	B	25g.	B	30b.	C
20g.	C			30c.	A
20h.	B	26a.	B	30d.	D
		26b.	A	30e.	A
21a.	B	26c.	C	30f.	B
21b.	A	26d.	D	30g.	D
21c.	C	26e.	A		
21d.	D	26f.	C	31a.	B
21e.	A	26g.	D	31b.	C
21f.	D	26h.	B	31c.	D
21g.	B			31d.	B
		27a.	C	31e.	A
22a.	D	27b.	D	31f.	C
22b.	A	27c.	B	31g.	D
22c.	C	27d.	C		
22d.	B	27e.	A	32a.	D
22e.	A	27f.	D	32b.	C
22f.	C	27g.	A	32c.	A
22g.	B	27h.	B	32d.	B
		27i.	D	32e.	D
23a.	D	27j.	B		
23b.	B	27k.	A	33a.	D
23c.	C	27l.	B	33b.	C
23d.	A	27m.	C	33c.	B
23e.	D			33d.	D
23f.	C	28a.	D	33e.	A
23g.	A	28b.	C	33f.	B
		28c.	D	33g.	A
24a.	C	28d.	A		
24b.	B	28e.	B	34a.	D
24c.	D	28f.	A	34b.	A

34c.	A	40g.	C	45e.	C
34d.	B	40h.	B	45f.	A
34e.	B	40i.	D	45g.	A
		40j.	B	45h.	B
35a.	D	40k.	A	45i.	B
35b.	C	40l.	D	45j.	A
35c.	B			45k.	B
35d.	A	41a.	D	45l.	C
35e.	B	41b.	A	45m.	B
		41c.	C	45n.	D
36a.	C	41d.	B	45o.	C
36b.	D	41e.	A	45p.	A
36c.	A	41f.	C	45q.	D
36d.	A	41g.	B	45r.	A
36e.	B			45s.	D
		42a.	C	45t.	D
37a.	$FEV_1 = 0.75$ L	42b.	A	45u.	B
	$FVC = 3.5$ L	42c.	D		
	$FEV_1\% = 21.4\%$	42d.	B	46a.	C
	Abnormal	42e.	B	46b.	D
37b.	$FEV_2 = 2.15$ L	42f.	C	46c.	A
	$FVC = 4.5$ L			46d.	A
	$FEV_2\% = 47.8\%$	43a.	D	46e.	D
	Abnormal	43b.	C	46f.	B
37c.	$FEV_3 = 4.0$ L	43c.	D	46g.	C
	$FVC = 5.5$ L	43d.	A	46h.	B
	$FEV_3\% = 72.7\%$	43e.	B	46i.	D
	Abnormal	43f.	A	46j.	C
		43g.	C	46k.	A
38a.	$FEF_{200-1200} = 0.6$ L/sec			46l.	D
38b.	$FEF_{200-1200} = 1.1$ L/sec			46m.	D
38c.	$FEF_{200-1200} = 1.8$ L/sec	44a.	B	46n.	D
		44b.	A	46o.	B
39a.	$FEF_{25-75\%} = 0.5$ L/sec	44c.	D	46p.	B
39b.	$FEF_{25-75\%} = 0.75$ L/sec	44d.	C	46q.	A
39c.	$FEF_{25-75\%} = 1.15$ L/sec	44e.	A	46r.	A
		44f.	B	46s.	B
40a.	D	44g.	D	46t.	A
40b.	C				
40c.	A	45a.	C	47a.	A
40d.	A	45b.	C	47b.	C
40e.	C	45c.	C	47c.	B
40f.	B	45d.	D		

47d.	D	51h.	B	55a.	B
47e.	B			55b.	D
47f.	C	52a.	C	55c.	C
47g.	D	52b.	C	55d.	A
		52c.	D	55e.	A
48a.	B	52d.	A	55f.	C
48b.	D	52e.	B	55g.	B
48c.	C	52f.	B	55h.	D
48d.	D	52g.	D	55i.	B
48e.	A	52h.	A	55j.	C
48f.	A	52i.	C	55k.	A
		52j.	D	55l.	D
49a.	B	52k.	B		
49b.	D	52l.	B	56a.	C
49c.	C	52m.	C	56b.	D
49d.	B	52n.	D	56c.	A
49e.	D	52o.	C	56d.	B
49f.	A	52p.	B	56e.	D
49g.	B	52q.	A	56f.	A
49h.	D			56g.	B
49i.	C	53a.	C	56h.	C
49j.	B	53b.	B	56i.	B
49k.	A	53c.	D	56j.	A
49l.	C	53d.	A		
49m.	A	53e.	D	57a.	B
		53f.	D	57b.	D
50a.	B	53g.	B	57c.	C
50b.	A	53h.	A	57d.	B
50c.	D	53i.	C	57e.	C
50d.	C	53j.	A	57f.	B
50e.	D			57g.	A
50f.	A	54a.	A	57h.	D
50g.	A	54b.	B	57i.	A
50h.	D	54c.	A	57j.	D
		54d.	B		
51a.	A	54e.	D	58a.	B
51b.	C	54f.	C	58b.	A
51c.	D	54g.	D	58c.	C
51d.	D	54h.	D	58d.	C
51e.	B	54i.	C	58e.	C
51f.	A	54j.	A	58f.	D
51g.	C			58g.	D

58h.	A	62f.	A	67a.	B		
58i.	D			67b.	C		
		63a.	B	67c.	A		
59a.	C	63b.	A	67d.	D		
59b.	B	63c.	B	67e.	B		
59c.	D	63d.	C	67f.	C		
59d.	A	63e.	D	67g.	C		
59e.	B	63f.	C	67h.	A		
59f.	B	63g.	A	67i.	A		
59g.	A	63h.	D	67j.	D		
59h.	C	63i.	C	67k.	D		
59i.	C	63j.	A				
		63k.	D	68a.	B		
60a.	C	63l.	B	68b.	D		
60b.	D			68c.	C		
60c.	A	64a.	C	68d.	B		
60d.	C	64b.	B	68e.	A		
60e.	A	64c.	D	68f.	A		
60f.	B	64d.	A	68g.	D		
60g.	B	64e.	B	68h.	C		
60h.	D	64f.	D	68i.	A		
60i.	B	64g.	A	68j.	B		
60j.	C			68k.	D		
		65a.	A				
61a.	C	65b.	D	69a.	B		
61b.	D	65c.	C	69b.	C		
61c.	C	65d.	C	69c.	C		
61d.	C	65e.	B	69d.	A		
61e.	A	65f.	A	69e.	A		
61f.	B			69f.	B		
61g.	A	66a.	A	69g.	D		
61h.	B	66b.	D	69h.	D		
61i.	B	66c.	B	69i.	A		
61j.	D	66d.	C	69j.	D		
61k.	A	66e.	A	69k.	C		
61l.	D	66f.	C	69l.	B		
		66g.	D				
62a.	D	66h.	B	70a.	C		
62b.	D	66i.	C	70b.	D		
62c.	C	66j.	D	70c.	B		
62d.	B	66k.	A	70d.	A		
62e.	C	66l.	B	70e.	D		

70f.	B	**73f.**	11.1 °C	**77b.**	D		
70g.	A	**73g.**	12.8 °C	**77c.**	A		
70h.	C	**73h.**	18.3 °C	**77d.**	B		
70i.	B	**73i.**	37 °C	**77e.**	B		
70j.	A	**73j.**	54.4 °C	**77f.**	A		
70k.	D	**73k.**	60 °C	**77g.**	D		
70l.	B	**73l.**	73.9 °C	**77h.**	C		
		73m.	100 °C	**77i.**	A		
71a.	C	**73n.**	204.4 °C	**77j.**	D		
71b.	D	**73o.**	218.3 °C				
71c.	A			**78a.**	A		
71d.	B	**74a.**	B	**78b.**	B		
71e.	32 °F	**74b.**	A	**78c.**	D		
71f.	62.6 °F	**74c.**	B	**78d.**	C		
71g.	68 °F	**74d.**	A	**78e.**	A		
71h.	86 °F	**74e.**	C	**78f.**	D		
71i.	98.6 °F	**74f.**	D	**78g.**	B		
71j.	118.4 °F			**78h.**	C		
71k.	170.6 °F	**75a.**	B	**78i.**	D		
71l.	212 °F	**75b.**	D	**78j.**	A		
71m.	350.6 °F	**75c.**	C	**78k.**	B		
		75d.	A	**78l.**	C		
72a.	B	**75e.**	C				
72b.	C	**75f.**	D	**79a.**	A		
72c.	A	**75g.**	A	**79b.**	D		
72d.	D	**75h.**	C	**79c.**	C		
72e.	B	**75i.**	A	**79d.**	D		
72f.	273 k	**75j.**	B	**79e.**	A		
72g.	278.4 k	**75k.**	D	**79f.**	A		
72h.	281 k			**79g.**	B		
72i.	288 k	**76a.**	C	**79h.**	D		
72j.	302 k	**76b.**	B	**79i.**	A		
72k.	310 k	**76c.**	D	**79j.**	D		
72l.	373 k	**76d.**	A	**79k.**	A		
72m.	440 k	**76e.**	D	**79l.**	D		
72n.	735 k	**76f.**	A	**79m.**	D		
		76g.	B				
73a.	B	**76h.**	C	**80a.**	C		
73b.	C	**76i.**	B	**80b.**	B		
73c.	D	**76j.**	A	**80c.**	D		
73d.	0 °C			**80d.**	B		
73e.	4.4 °C	**77a.**	C	**80e.**	A		

80f.	C	81a.	B	81h.	A
80g.	B	81b.	C	81i.	C
80h.	A	81c.	C	81j.	A
80i.	D	81d.	D	81k.	D
80j.	C	81e.	A	81l.	B
80k.	A	81f.	D	81m.	D
80l.	C	81g.	B	81n.	B

Symbols and Abbreviations

Symbols and Abbreviations Commonly Used in Respiratory Physiology

Primary symbols

GAS SYMBOLS		BLOOD SYMBOLS	
P	Pressure	Q	Blood volume
V	Gas volume	$\dot{Q}$	Blood flow
$\dot{V}$	Gas volume per unit of time, or flow	C	Content in blood
F	Fractional concentration of gas	S	Saturation

Secondary symbols

GAS SYMBOLS		BLOOD SYMBOLS	
I	Inspired	a	Arterial
E	Expired	c	Capillary
A	Alveolar	v	Venous
T	Tidal	$\bar{v}$	Mixed venous
D	Deadspace		

Abbreviations

%	Percent
%g	Percent of gas in the mixture
a/A ratio	Arterial/alveolar oxygen tension ratio in %
BD	Base deficit in mEq/L, negative base excess (−BE)
$BP_{systolic}$	Systolic blood pressure in mm Hg
$BP_{diastolic}$	Diastolic blood pressure in mm Hg
BSA	Body surface area in m²
C	Compliance in mL/cm H_2O or L/cm H_2O
°C	degree Celsius
C_{dyn}	Dynamic compliance in mL/cm H_2O
C_{st}	Static compliance in mL/cm H_2O
C_aO_2	Arterial oxygen content in vol%
Capacity	Maximum amount of water that air can hold at a given temperature in mg/L or mm Hg
$C(a-\bar{v})O_2$	Arterial-mixed venous oxygen content difference in vol%
C_cO_2	End-capillary oxygen content in vol%
CI	Cardiac index in L/min/m²
Cl⁻	Serum chloride concentration in mEq/L
cm H_2O	Centimeters of water, a unit of pressure measurement
CO	Cardiac output in L/min ($\dot{Q}_T$)
$C_{\bar{v}}O_2$	Mixed venous oxygen content in vol%
CVP	Central venous pressure in mm Hg
D	Density of gas in g/L
dyne·sec/cm⁵	dyne·second/centimeter⁵, a vascular resistance unit
E	Elastance in cm H_2O/L
ERV	Expiratory reserve volume in mL or L
Expired V_T	Expired tidal volume in mL or L
°F	degree Fahrenheit
f	Frequency per minute; respiratory rate (RR)
f_{MECH}	Mechanical ventilator frequency per minute
f_{SPON}	Patient's spontaneous frequency per minute
$FEF_{25-75\%}$	Forced Expiratory Flow of the middle 50% of vital capacity in L/sec
$FEF_{200-1,200}$	Forced Expiratory Flow of 200 to 1,200 mL of vital capacity in L/sec
FEV_t	Forced Expiratory Volume (timed) in L
$FEV_t\%$	Forced Expiratory Volume (timed percent) in %
F_IO_2	Inspired oxygen concentration in %
Flow	Flow rate in L/sec or L/min
FRC	Functional residual capacity in mL or L
g	gram
g·m/beat	gram·meter/beat, a ventricular stroke work unit
g·m/beat/m²	gram·meter/beat/meter², a ventricular stroke work index unit
gmw	Gram molecular weight in g
HCO_3^-	(1) Serum bicarbonate concentration in mEq/L
	(2) Sodium bicarbonate needed to correct base deficit, in mEq/L

H_2CO_3	Carbonate acid in mEq/L
Hb	Hemoglobin content in g%
HD	Humidity deficit in mg/L
HR	Heart rate per minute
IC	Inspiratory capacity in mL or L
ID	Internal diameter of endotracheal tube in mm
I time	Inspiratory time in sec
IRV	Inspiratory reserve volume in mL or L
°K	Kelvin
K	Serum potassium concentration in mEq/L
kg	Body weight in kilograms
kPa	International System (SI) unit for pressure (kilopascal); 1 kPa equals 7.5 torr or mm Hg
L	Liter
L/min	Liters per minute
log	logarithm
LVSW	Left ventricular stroke work in g·m/beat
LVSWI	Left ventricular stroke work index in g·m/beat/m²
MAP	Mean arterial pressure in mm Hg
min	Minute
mL	Milliliter
mm Hg	Millimeters of mercury, a unit of pressure measurement (torr); equal to 0.1333 kPa
Na^+	Serum sodium concentration in mEq/L
O_2 : air	Oxygen : air ratio
O_2 consumption	Estimated to be $130 \times BSA$ in mL/min ($\dot{V}O_2$)
P	Pressure in cm H_2O or mm Hg
P/F index	P_aO_2/F_IO_2 index
ΔP	Pressure change in cm H_2O
$\overline{PA}$	Mean pulmonary artery pressure in mm Hg
PAP	Pulmonary artery pressure in mm Hg
$PA_{systolic}$	Systolic pulmonary artery pressure in mm Hg
$P(A-a)O_2$	Alveolar-arterial oxygen tension gradient in mm Hg
P_aCO_2	Arterial carbon dioxide tension in mm Hg
P_AO_2	Alveolar oxygen tension in mm Hg
P_aO_2	Arterial oxygen tension in mm Hg
$\overline{P}aw$	Mean airway pressure in cm H_2O
P_B	Barometric pressure in mm Hg
PCWP	Pulmonary capillary wedge pressure in mm Hg
P_ECO_2	Mixed expired carbon dioxide tension in mm Hg
PEEP	Positive end-expiratory pressure in cm H_2O
P_g	Partial pressure of a dry gas
pH	Puissance hydrogen, negative logarithm of H ion concentration
P_{H_2O}	Water vapor pressure, 47 mm Hg saturated at 37°C
PIP	Peak inspiratory pressure in cm H_2O
P_{max}	Maximum airway pressure in cm H_2O (peak inspiratory pressure)
P_{PLAT}	Plateau pressure in cm H_2O

psig	Pounds per square inch, a gauge pressure
P_{st}	Static pressure in cm H_2O (P_{PLAT})
$P_{\bar{v}}O_2$	Mixed venous oxygen tension in mm Hg
PVR	Pulmonary vascular resistance in dyne·sec/cm^5
$Q_{sp}/\dot{Q}_T$	Physiologic shunt to total perfusion ratio in %
Q_T	Total perfusion in L/min; cardiac output (CO)
R	Resistance in cm H_2O/L/sec
RAP	Right atrial pressure in mm Hg
$\overline{RA}$	Mean right atrial pressure in mm Hg
R_{aw}	Airway resistance in cm H_2O/L/sec
RH	Relative humidity in %
RR	Respiratory rate per minute; frequency (f)
RSBI	Rapid Shallow Breathing Index
RV	Residual volume in mL or L
RVSW	Right ventricular stroke work in g·m/beat
RVSWI	Right ventricular stroke work index in g·m/beat/m^2
S_aO_2	Arterial oxygen saturation in %
sec	Second
SV	Stroke volume in mL or L
SVI	Stroke volume index in mL/m^2
$S_{\bar{v}}O_2$	Mixed venous oxygen saturation in vol%
SVR	Systemic vascular resistance in dyne·sec/cm^5
t	Time constant in seconds
TLC	Total lung capacity in mL or L
torr	Unit of pressure measurement (mm Hg); 1 torr equals 0.1333 kPa
V	(1) Volume in mL or L
	(2) Corrected tidal volume in mL or L
ΔV	Volume change in mL or L
$\dot{V}$	Minute volume or flow in L/min
$\dot{V}_A$	Alveolar minute ventilation in L
VC	Vital capacity in mL or L
V_D	Deadspace volume in mL or L
V_D/V_T	Deadspace to tidal volume ratio in %
$\dot{V}_E$	Expired minute ventilation in L
$\dot{V}O_2$	O_2 consumption in mL/min
V_T	Tidal volume in mL or L
V_T mech	Mechanical ventilator tidal volume in mL
V_T spon	Patient's spontaneous tidal volume in mL
Vol%	Volume percent
Volume$_{ATPS}$	Gas volume saturated with water at ambient (room) temperature and pressure
Volume$_{BTPS}$	Gas volume saturated with water at body temperature (37°C) and ambient pressure

SECTION

7

Appendices

Listing of Appendices

A   Barometric Pressures at Selected Altitudes

B   Conversion Factors for Duration of Gas Cylinders

C   Electrolyte Concentrations in Plasma

D   Endotracheal Tubes and Suction Catheters

E   Energy Expenditure, Resting and Total

F   French and Millimeter Conversion

G   Harris Benedict Formula

H   Hemodynamic Normal Ranges

I   Humidity Capacity of Saturated Gas at Selected Temperatures

J   Logarithm Table

K   Lung Volumes, Capacity and Ventilation

L   Oxygen Transport

M $P_A O_2$ at Selected $F_I O_2$

N   Partial Pressure (in mm Hg) of Gases in the Air, Alveoli, and Blood

O   Pressure Conversions

Barometric Pressures at Selected Altitudes

	Feet	Meters	P_B (mm Hg)
Below sea level	−66	−20	2,280
	−33	−10	1,520
Sea level	0	0	760
Above sea level	2,000	610	707
	4,000	1,219	656
	6,000(a)	1,829	609
	8,000	2,438	564
	10,000	3,048	523
	12,000	3,658	483
	14,000(b)	4,267	446
	16,000	4,877	412
	18,000	5,486	379
	20,000	6,096	349
	22,000	6,706	321
	24,000	7,315	294
	26,000	7,925	270
	28,000	8,534	247
	30,000(c)	9,144	226
	32,000	9,754	206
	34,000	10,363	187
	36,000	10,973	170
	40,000	12,192	141
	50,000	15,240	87
	63,000	19,202	47

(a) Denver, Colorado, 5,280 ft
(b) Mount Elbert, Colorado, 14,433 ft
(c) Mount Everest, 29,028 ft

B

Conversion Factors for Duration of Gas Cylinders

Cylinder size	B/BB	D/DD	E	M	G	H/K
Carbon Dioxide (CO_2)	0.17	0.43	0.72	3.44	5.59	7.18
Carbon Dioxide/Oxygen (CO_2/O_2)		0.18	0.3	1.36	2.42	2.73
Cyclopropane (C_3H_6)	0.17	0.40				
Helium (He)		0.14	0.23	1.03	1.82	2.73
Helium/Oxygen (He/O_2)			0.23	1.03	1.82	2.05
Nitrous Oxide (N_2O)		0.43	0.72	3.44	6.27	7.18
Oxygen (O_2)	0.09	0.18	0.28	1.57	2.41	3.14
Air (N_2/O_2)		0.17	0.28	1.49	2.30	2.98
Nitrogen (N_2)			0.28			2.91

(Conversion factors are based on full cylinder at pressure of 2,200 psig.)

To calculate duration of gas cylinder at a constant liter flow: (1) multiply the conversion factor by the pressure reading on the gas gauge; (2) divide the product from (1) by the liter flow in use; (3) answer equals the duration, in minutes, of gas cylinder at the same liter flow.

$$\text{Duration} = \frac{\text{Conversion factor} \times \text{Psig}}{\text{Liter flow}}$$

For example, see Oxygen Duration of E Cylinder and Oxygen Duration of H or K Cylinder.

C

Electrolyte Concentrations in Plasma

Cations	Concentration (Range) mEq/L	Anions	Concentration (Range) mEq/L
Na^+	140 (138 to 142)	Cl^-	103 (101 to 105)
K^+	4 (3 to 5)	HCO_3^-	25 (23 to 27)
Ca^{++}	5 (4.5 to 5.5)	Protein	16 (14 to 18)
Mg^{++}	2 (1.5 to 2.5)	$HPO_4^{--}, H_2PO_4^-$	2 (1.5 to 2.5)
		SO_4^{--}	1 (0.8 to 1.2)
Total	151	Organic acids	4 (3.5 to 4.5)
		Total	151

Endotracheal Tubes and Suction Catheters

Age	Weight (g/kg)	Internal Diameter (ID) (mm)	Oral Length* (cm)	Suction Catheter (French)
Newborn (<28 weeks)	<1,000 g	2.5	7	5 or 6
Newborn (28–34 weeks)	1,000–2,000 g	3.0	8	6 or 8
Newborn (34–38 weeks)	2,000–3,000 g	3.5	9	8
Newborn (>38 weeks)	>3,000 g	3.5–4.0	10	8 for 3.5 mm 10 for 4.0 mm
Infant under 6 months		3.5–4.0	10	8
Infant under 1 year		4.0–4.5	11	8
Child under 2 years		4.5–5.0	12	8
Child over 2 years		(Age/4) + 4	(Age/2) + 12	10
Adult female		7.0–8.0	20–22	12
Adult male		8.0–8.5	20–22	14

Notes: Use uncuffed ET tube for children under age 8 years (normal narrowing at cricoids serves as natural cuff).
*ET tube with one marking at bottom of tube: the marking should be at vocal cord level.
ET tube with two markings at bottom of tube: the vocal cords should be between these two markings.

REFERENCE

fpnotebook.com/lung/Procedure/EndtrchlTb.htm

Energy Expenditure, Resting and Total

CALCULATION OF RESTING ENERGY EXPENDITURE (REE)

REE for men in kcal/day = 66 + (13.7 × kg) + (5.0 × cm) − (6.8 × years)
REE for women in kcal/day = 655 + (9.6 × kg) + (1.85 × cm) − (4.7 × years)

CALCULATION OF TOTAL ENERGY EXPENDITURE (TEE)

TEE for men in kcal/day = REE × Activity Factor × Stress Factor
TEE for women in kcal/day = REE × Activity Factor × Stress Factor

Activity Factor
    Confined to bed × 1.2
    Out of bed × 1.3

Stress Factor
    Minor operation × 1.20
    Skeletal trauma × 1.35
    Major sepsis × 1.60
    Severe thermal burn × 2.10

French and Millimeter Conversion

Millimeter (mm)	French (Fr)
1	3
0.33	1

G

Harris Benedict Formula

To determine the total daily calorie needs, multiply the Harris Benedict Formula (BMR) by the appropriate activity factor:

Sedentary (little or no exercise): Calories = BMR × 1.2

Lightly active (light exercise/sports 1–3 days/week): Calories = BMR × 1.375

Moderately active (moderate exercise/sports 3–5 days/week): Calories = BMR × 1.55

Very active (hard exercise/sports 6–7 days a week): Calories = BMR × 1.725

Extra active (very hard exercise/sports and physical job or 2× training): Calories = BMR × 1.9

REFERENCES

bmi-calculator.net/bmr-calculator/harris-benedict-equation/

bmi-calculator.net/bmi-chart.php (Body Mass Index or BMI)

Hemodynamic Normal Ranges

Hemodynamic Values Directly Obtained by Pulmonary Artery Catheter

Hemodynamic Value	Abbreviation	Normal Range
Central venous pressure	CVP	1 to 7 mm Hg
Right atrial pressure	RAP	1 to 7 mm Hg
Mean pulmonary artery pressure	$\overline{PA}$	15 mm Hg
Pulmonary capillary wedge pressure	PCWP	8 to 12 mm Hg
(also called pulmonary artery wedge pressure;	PAWP	
pulmonary artery occlusion pressure)	PAOP	
Cardiac output	CO	4 to 8 L/min

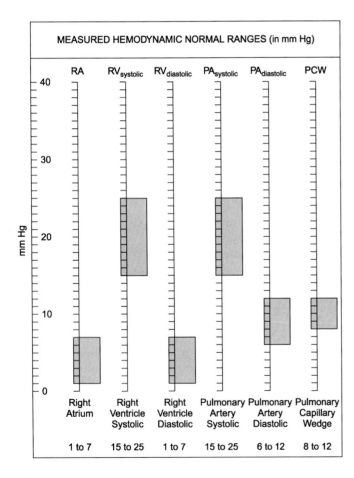

Adapted from Des Jardins, T.R. *Cardiopulmonary Anatomy and Physiology: Essentials for Respiratory Care,* 5th ed. Clifton Park, NY: Delmar Cengage Learning, 2008.

Computed Hemodynamic Values

Hemodynamic Value	Abbreviation	Normal Range
Stroke volume	SV	40 to 80 mL
Stroke volume index	SVI	33 to 47 L/beat/m^2
Cardiac index	CI	2.5 to 3.5 L/min/m^2
Right ventricular stroke work index	RVSWI	7 to 12 g·m/beat/m^2
Left ventricular stroke work index	LVSWI	40 to 60 g·m/beat/m^2
Pulmonary vascular resistance	PVR	50 to 150 dyne·sec/cm^5
Systemic vascular resistance	SVR	800 to 1500 dyne·sec/cm^5

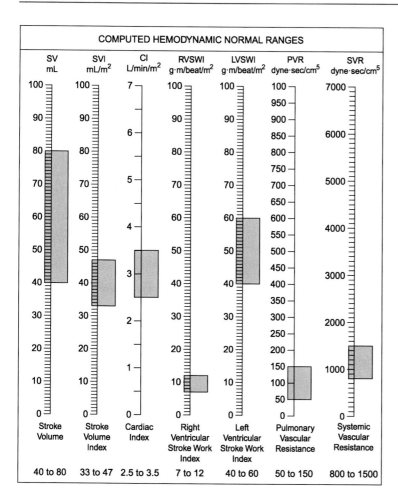

Modified from Des Jardins, T.R. *Cardiopulmonary Anatomy and Physiology: Essentials for Respiratory Care*, 5th ed. Clifton Park, NY: Delmar Cengage Learning, 2008.

Humidity Capacity of Saturated Gas at Selected Temperatures

Gas Temperature (°C)	Water Content (mg/L)	Water Vapor Pressure (mm Hg)
0	4.9	4.6
5	6.8	6.6
10	9.4	9.3
17	14.5	14.6
18	15.4	15.6
19	16.3	16.5
20	17.3	17.5
21	18.4	18.7
22	19.4	19.8
23	20.6	21.1
24	21.8	22.4
25	23.1	23.8
26	24.4	25.2
27	25.8	26.7
28	27.2	28.3
29	28.8	30.0
30	30.4	31.8
31	32.0	33.7
32	33.8	35.7
33	35.6	37.7
34	37.6	39.9
35	39.6	42.2
36	41.7	44.6
37	43.9	47.0
38	46.2	49.8
39	48.6	52.5
40	51.1	55.4
41	53.7	58.4
42	56.5	61.6
43	59.5	64.9

J

Logarithm Table

TERMINOLOGY

$$\log 20 = 1.301$$
$$\downarrow \downarrow \quad \downarrow \downarrow$$
$$a \ b \quad c \ d$$

a: logarithm, b: number, c: characteristic, d: mantissa.

EXAMPLE 1

Find the logarithm for 30.4.

Step 1. From the log table find the number 30 along the vertical column (N).
Step 2. Find the number 4 along the horizontal row (N).
Step 3. The mantissa intersected by the column and row should read 4829.
Step 4. Since the number 30.4 has two digits in front of the decimal point, use 1. in front of the mantissa.

Log 30.4 becomes 1.4829.

NOTE

The characteristic is determined by the number of digits in front of the decimal point. The characteristic is 0. for one digit in front of the decimal point; 1. for two digits; 2. for three digits; and so on.

For example, the answer for log 304 is 2.4829. You may notice that the mantissa for 304 is same as that for 30.4 and that the only change is in the characteristic. The following examples should clarify this point:

$$\log 0.0304 = \overline{2}.4829$$
$$\log 0.304 = \overline{1}.4829$$
$$\log 3.04 = 0.4829$$
$$\log 30.4 = 1.4829$$
$$\log 304 = 2.4829$$
$$\log 3040 = 3.4829$$

EXAMPLE 2

Find the logarithms for 18.7 and 187.

Step 1. From the log table find the number 18 along the vertical column (N).
Step 2. Find the number 7 along the horizontal row (N).
Step 3. The mantissa intersected by the column and row should read 2718.
Step 4. Because the number 18.7 has two digits in front of the decimal point, use 1. in front of the mantissa. Log 18.7 becomes 1.2718. Because the number 187 has three digits in front of the decimal point, use 2. in front of the mantissa.

Log 187 becomes 2.2718.

EXERCISE 1   Find the logarithm for 22.2.

[Answer: log 22.2 = 1.3464]

EXERCISE 2   Find the logarithm for 30.15.

[Answer: log 30.15 = 1.4793. Look for the mantissas under 1 and 2 and find the average.]

Common Logarithms of Numbers[a]

N	0	1	2	3	4	5	6	7	8	9
10	0000	0043	0086	0128	0170	0212	0253	0294	0334	0374
11	0414	0453	0492	0531	0569	0607	0645	0682	0719	0755
12	0792	0828	0864	0899	0934	0969	1004	1038	1072	1106
13	1139	1173	1206	1239	1271	1303	1335	1367	1399	1430
14	1461	1492	1523	1553	1584	1614	1644	1673	1703	1732
15	1761	1790	1818	1847	1875	1903	1931	1959	1987	2014
16	2041	2068	2095	2122	2148	2175	2201	2227	2253	2279
17	2304	2330	2335	2380	2405	2430	2455	2480	2504	2529
18	2553	2577	2601	2625	2648	2672	2695	2718	2742	2765
19	2788	2810	2833	2856	2878	2900	2923	2945	2967	2989
20	3010	3032	3054	3075	3096	3118	3139	3160	3181	3201
21	3222	3243	3263	3284	3304	3324	3345	3365	3385	3404
22	3424	3444	3464	3483	3502	3522	3541	3560	3579	3598
23	3617	3636	3655	3674	3692	3711	3729	3747	3766	3784
24	3802	3820	3838	3856	3874	3892	3909	3927	3945	3962
25	3979	3997	4014	4031	4048	4065	4082	4099	4116	4133
26	4150	4166	4183	4200	4216	4232	4249	4265	4281	4298
27	4314	4330	4346	4362	4378	4393	4409	4425	4440	4456
28	4472	4487	4502	4518	4533	4548	4564	4579	4594	4609
29	4624	4639	4654	4669	4683	4698	4713	4728	4742	4757
30	4771	4786	4800	4814	4829	4843	4857	4871	4886	4900
31	4914	4928	4942	4955	4969	4983	4997	5011	5024	5038
32	5051	5065	5079	5092	5105	5119	5132	5145	5159	5172
33	5185	5198	5211	5224	5237	5250	5263	5276	5289	5302
34	5315	5328	5340	5353	5366	5378	5391	5403	5416	5428
35	5441	5453	5465	5478	5490	5502	5514	5527	5539	5551
36	5563	5575	5587	5599	5611	5623	5635	5647	5658	5670
37	5682	5694	5705	5717	5729	5740	5752	5763	5775	5786
38	5798	5809	5821	5832	5843	5855	5866	5877	5888	5899
39	5911	5922	5933	5944	5955	5966	5977	5988	5999	6010
40	6021	6031	6042	6053	6064	6075	6085	6096	6107	6117
41	6128	6138	6149	6160	6170	6180	6191	6201	6212	6222
42	6232	6243	6253	6263	6274	6284	6294	6304	6314	6325
43	6335	6345	6355	6365	6375	6385	6395	6405	6415	6425
44	6435	6444	6454	6464	6474	6484	6493	6503	6513	6522
45	6532	6542	6551	6561	6571	6580	6590	6599	6609	6618
46	6628	6637	6646	6656	6665	6675	6684	6693	6702	6712
47	6721	6730	6739	6749	6758	6767	6776	6785	6794	6803
48	6812	6821	6830	6839	6848	6857	6866	6875	6884	6893
49	6902	6911	6920	6928	6937	6946	6955	6964	6972	6981
50	6990	6998	7007	7016	7024	7033	7042	7050	7059	7067
51	7076	7084	7093	7101	7110	7118	7126	7135	7143	7152
52	7160	7168	7177	7185	7193	7202	7210	7218	7226	7235
53	7243	7251	7259	7267	7275	7284	7292	7300	7308	7316
54	7324	7332	7340	7348	7356	7364	7372	7380	7388	7396

N	0	1	2	3	4	5	6	7	8	9
55	7404	7412	7419	7427	7435	7443	7451	7459	7466	7474
56	7482	7490	7497	7505	7513	7520	7528	7536	7543	7551
57	7559	7566	7574	7582	7589	7597	7604	7612	7619	7627
58	7634	7642	7649	7657	7664	7672	7679	7686	7694	7701
59	7709	7716	7723	7731	7738	7745	7752	7760	7767	7774
60	7782	7789	7796	7803	7810	7818	7825	7832	7839	7846
61	7853	7860	7868	7875	7892	7889	7896	7903	7910	7917
62	7924	7931	7938	7945	7952	7959	7966	7973	7980	7987
63	7993	8000	8007	8014	8021	8028	8035	8041	8048	8055
64	8062	8069	8075	8082	8089	8096	8102	8109	8116	8122
65	8129	8136	8142	8149	8156	8162	8169	8176	8182	8189
66	8195	8202	8209	8215	8222	8228	8235	8241	8248	8254
67	8261	8267	8274	8280	8287	8293	8299	8306	8312	8319
68	8325	8331	8338	8344	8351	8357	8363	8370	8376	8382
69	8388	8395	8401	8407	8414	8420	8426	8432	8439	8445
70	8451	8457	8463	8470	8476	8482	8488	8494	8500	8506
71	8513	8519	8525	8531	8537	8543	8549	8555	8561	8567
72	8573	8579	8585	8591	8597	8603	8609	8615	8621	8627
73	8633	8639	8645	8651	8657	8663	8669	8675	8681	8686
74	8692	8698	8704	8710	8716	8722	8727	8733	8739	8745
75	8751	8756	8762	8768	8774	8779	8785	8791	8797	8802
76	8808	8814	8820	8825	8831	8837	8842	8848	8854	8859
77	8865	8871	8876	8882	8887	8893	8899	8904	8910	8915
78	8921	8927	8932	8938	8943	8949	8954	8960	8965	8971
79	8976	8982	8987	8993	8998	9004	9009	9015	9020	9025
80	9031	9036	9042	9047	9053	9058	9063	9069	9074	9079
81	9085	9090	9096	9101	9106	9112	9117	9122	9128	9133
82	9138	9143	9149	9154	9159	9165	9170	9175	9180	9186
83	9191	9196	9201	9206	9212	9217	9222	9227	9232	9238
84	9243	9248	9253	9258	9263	9269	9274	9279	9284	9289
85	9294	9299	9304	9309	9315	9320	9325	9330	9335	9340
86	9345	9350	9355	9360	9365	9370	9375	9380	9385	9390
87	9395	9400	9405	9410	9415	9420	9425	9430	9435	9440
88	9445	9450	9455	9460	9465	9469	9474	9479	9484	9489
89	9494	9499	9504	9509	9513	9518	9523	9528	9533	9538
90	9542	9547	9552	9557	9562	9566	9571	9576	9581	9586
91	9590	9595	9600	9605	9609	9614	9619	9624	9628	9633
92	9638	9643	9647	9652	9657	9661	9666	9671	9675	9680
93	9685	9689	9694	9699	9703	9708	9713	9714	9722	9727
94	9731	9736	9741	9745	9750	9754	9759	9763	9768	9773
95	9777	9782	9786	9791	9795	9800	9805	9809	9814	9818
96	9823	9827	9832	9836	9841	9845	9850	9854	9859	9863
97	9868	9872	9877	9881	9886	9890	9894	9899	9903	9908
98	9912	9917	9921	9926	9930	9934	9939	9943	9948	9952
99	9956	9961	9965	9969	9974	9978	9983	9987	9991	9996

a This table gives the mantissas of numbers with the decimal point omitted in each case. Characteristics are determined by inspection from the numbers.
From Wojciechowski, W.V. Respiratory Care Sciences: An Integrated Approach, 4th ed. Clifton Park, NY: Delmar Cengage Learning 2006.

Lung Volumes, Capacity and Ventilation

Volume	Newborn infant	Yound Adult Male	Approx % of TLC (Young Adult Male)
V_T (mL)	15	500	8 to 10
IRV (mL)	60	3100	50
ERV (mL)	40	1200	20
RV (mL)	40	1200	20
IC (mL)	75	3600	60
FRC (mL)	80	2400	40
VC (mL)	115	4800	80
TLC (mL)	155	6000	100
f (bpm)	35 to 50	12 to 20	
$\dot{V}_E$	525 to 750 mL/min	6 to 10 L/min	

Modified from Madama, V.C. *Pulmonary Function Testing and Cardiopulmonary Stress Testing*, 2nd ed. Clifton Park, NY: Delmar Cengage Learning 1998.

L

Oxygen Transport

SHADED AREAS REPRESENT NORMAL RANGES

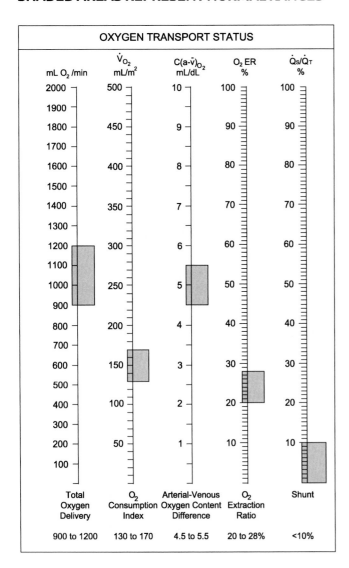

		OXYGEN TRANSPORT STATUS			
mL O_2 /min	$\dot{V}_{O_2}$ mL/m²	$C(a-\bar{v})_{O_2}$ mL/dL	O_2 ER %	$\dot{Q}s/\dot{Q}_T$ %

Total Oxygen Delivery	O_2 Consumption Index	Arterial-Venous Oxygen Content Difference	O_2 Extraction Ratio	Shunt
900 to 1200	130 to 170	4.5 to 5.5	20 to 28%	<10%

From Des Jardins, T.R. *Cardiopulmonary Anatomy and Physiology: Essentials for Respiratory Care,* 5th ed. Clifton Park, NY: Delmar Cengage Learning, 2008.

P_AO_2 at Selected F_IO_2

F_IO_2*	Calculated P_AO_2**
21%	100
25%	128
30%	164
35%	200
40%	235
45%	271
50%	307
55%	342
60%	388
65%	423
70%	459
75%	495
80%	530
85%	566
90%	602
95%	637
100%	673

* At F_IO_2 of 60% or higher, the factor 1.25 in the equation is omitted.
** The calculated P_AO_2 is based on a PCO_2 of 40 mm Hg, saturated at 37°C, PB of 760 mm Hg.
$P_AO_2 = (P_B - 47) \times F_IO_2 - (PCO_2 \times 1.25)$.

Partial Pressure (in mm Hg) of Gases in the Air, Alveoli, and Blood

Gases	Dry Air	Alveolar Gas	Arterial Blood	Venous Blood
PO_2	159.0	100.0	95.0	40.0
PCO_2	0.2	40.0	40.0	46.0
PH_2O (water vapor)	0.0	47.0	47.0	47.0
PN_2 (and other gases in minute quantities)	600.8	573.0	573.0	573.0
Total	760.0	760.0	755.0	706.0

* The values shown are based upon standard pressure and temperature.
From Des Jardins, T.R. *Cardiopulmonary Anatomy and Physiology: Essentials for Respiratory Care*, 5th ed. Clifton Park, NY: Delmar Cengage Learning, 2008.

O

Pressure Conversions

Atmosphere	cm H$_2$O	mm Hg	psig	kPa
1	1033	760	14.7	101.325
0.000968	1	0.735	0.0142	0.09806
0.001316	1.36	1	0.0193	0.1333
0.068	70.31	51.7	1	6.895
0.00987	10.197	7.501	0.145	1

REFERENCE

http://www.onlineconversion.com/pressure.htm

Bibliography

BMI Calculator – Harris Benedict Equation. (2018). Available at: http://www.bmi-calculator.net/bmr-calculator/harris-benedict-equation/ [Accessed February 14, 2018]

Burton, G. G., et al. (1997). *Respiratory Care: A Guide to Clinical Practice*. 4th ed. Philadelphia, PA: Lippincott Williams & Wilkins.

Chang, D. W. (2013). *Clinical Application of Mechanical Ventilation*. 4th ed. Clifton Park, NY: Delmar Cengage Learning.

Chatburn, R. L., et al. (2009). *Handbook for Health Care Research*. 2nd ed. Sudbury, MA: Jones & Bartlett Publishers.

Des Jardins, T. R. (2012). *Cardiopulmonary Anatomy and Physiology: Essentials for Respiratory Care*. 6th ed. Clifton Park, NY: Delmar Cengage Learning.

Dosage Help. (2018). Available at: http://www.dosagehelp.com/ [Accessed February 14, 2018]

Dubois, E. F. (1924). *Basal Metabolism in Health and Disease*. Philadelphia, PA: Lea and Febiger.

Gardenhire, D. S. (2015). *Rau's Respiratory Care Pharmacology*. 9th ed. St. Louis, MO: Elsevier.

Gross, L. J. (1985). Setting cutoff scores on credentialing examinations: a refinement in the Nedetsky Procedure. *Evaluation and the Health Professions,* 8(4), pp. 469-493.

Hegstad, L. N., et al. (2000). *Essential Drug Dosage Calculations*. 4th ed. Upper Saddle River, NJ: Prentice Hall.

Hess, D. R. (2015). *Respiratory Care: Principles and Practice*. 3rd ed. Burlington, MA: Jones & Bartlett Learning.

Heuer, A., et al. (2013). *Wilkin's Clinical Assessment in Respiratory Care*. 7th ed. St. Louis, MO: Elsevier.

Kacmarek, R. M., et al. (2016). *Egan's Fundamentals of Respiratory Care*. 11th ed. St. Louis, MO: Elsevier.

Koff, P. B., et al. (2005). *Neonatal and Pediatric Respiratory Care*. 2nd ed. St. Louis, MO: Mosby-Year Book.

Mottram, C. D. (2017). *Ruppel's Manual of Pulmonary Function Testing*. 11th ed. St. Louis, MO: Elsevier.

Nedelsky, L. (1954). Absolute grading standards for objective tests. *Educational and Psychologic Measurement*, 4, pp. 3-19.

Shapiro, B. A., et al. (1994). *Clinical Application of Blood Gases*. 5th ed. St. Louis, MO: Mosby Year Book.

Tobin, M . J., et al. (1986). The pattern of breathing during successful and unsuccessful trials of weaning from mechanical ventilation. *Am Rev Respir Dis*, 134(6), pp. 1111-1118.

Tuckman , R. W. (1993). *Conducting Educational Research*. 4th ed. Boston, MA: Houghton Mifflin Harcourt.

Unit Converters. (2018). Available at: https://www.unitconverters.net/ [Accessed February 14, 2018]

White, G.C. (2014). *Equipment Theory for Respiratory Care*. 5th ed. Clifton Park, NY: Delmar Cengage Learning.

Wojciechowski, W. V. (2014). *Respiratory Care Sciences: An integrated Approach*. 5th ed. Clifton Park, NY: Delmar Cengage Learning.

Yang, K. L., et al. (1991). A prospective study of indexes predicting the outcome of trials of weaning from mechanical ventilation. *N Engl J Med*, 324, pp. 1445-1450.

Index by Alphabetical Listing